INTRAUTERINE GROWTH RETARDATION

Intrauterine Growth Retardation

Editor

Jacques Senterre, M.D., Ph.D.

Professor of Neonatology
State University of Liège
Liège, Belgium

Nestlé Nutrition
Workshop Series
Volume 18

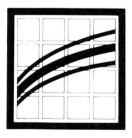

NESTLÉ NUTRITION

RAVEN PRESS ■ NEW YORK

Nestec Ltd., Avenue Nestlé, 1800 Vevey, Switzerland
Raven Press, Ltd., 1185 Avenue of the Americas, New York,
New York 10036

© 1989 by Nestec Ltd. and Raven Press, Ltd. All rights reserved. This book is
protected by copyright. No part of it may be reproduced, stored in a retrieval
system, or transmitted, in any form or by any means, electronical, mechanical,
photocopying, or recording, or otherwise, without the prior written permission
of Nestec and Raven Press.

Made in the United States of America

Library of Congress Cataloging-in-Publication Data

Intrauterine growth retardation.

    (Nestlé Nutrition workshop series ; v. 18)
    Includes bibliographical references.
    1. Fetus—Growth retardation.   I. Senterre, Jacques.   II. Series.
RG629.G76I55   1989   618.3'2   89-10735
ISBN 0-88167-557-1

   The material contained in this volume was submitted as previously
unpublished material, except in the instances in which credit has been given to
the source from which some of the illustrative material was derived.
   Great care has been taken to maintain the accuracy of the information
contained in the volume. However, neither Nestec nor Raven Press can be held
responsible for errors or for any consequences arising from the use of the
information contained herein.

9 8 7 6 5 4 3 2 1

Preface

Intrauterine growth retardation is a worldwide problem. In the more affluent societies, one-third of the low birthweight babies are small-for-dates, yet in communities with poor socioeconomic conditions the incidence of growth retardation due to intrauterine malnutrition can increase to 80% of low birthweight infants.

Perinatal mortality and morbidity are substantially increased in the intrauterine growth-retarded fetus. Short-term sequelae include perinatal asphyxia, meconium aspiration, hypoglycemia, and polycythemia. Long-term sequelae include continued growth retardation as well as learning and behavior problems, which depend on the type of growth inhibition and its duration and severity.

Despite numerous studies in this field, key aspects of intrauterine growth retardation remain undefined. There are still variations in definitions, classifications, and applicable birthweight standards. The factors responsible for fetal growth retardation are numerous but their hierarchic responsibility is not well understood. The question of how chronic reduction of uterine blood flow may affect the supply of oxygen and nutrients to the fetus is far from being answered. Most of the studies on placental circulation, hormonal regulation of fetal growth, and fetal metabolism have been carried out on animals of different species.

In the countries where the proportion of low birthweight infants is the highest, the relative influence of genetic and environmental factors is still poorly elucidated. There is a tendency to relate the high incidence of low birthweight infants to maternal undernutrition, but the benefit of food supplements during pregnancy is still a matter for discussion. Other environmental characteristics of poor socioeconomic conditions, such as maternal height, birth interval, parity, malaria, anemia, lack of perinatal care, and smoking habits, can result in lower birthweights.

The aim of the workshop on which this volume is based was to shed some light on all these factors affecting fetal growth retardation by bringing together international investigators of various disciplines interested in this area. Although much remains to be learned, considerable progress in the approach to intrauterine growth retardation has been made in recent years. In the late 1960s endocrine assessment of fetal placental growth and ultrasound measurement of fetal heart rate and biparietal diameter were revolutionary. In the late 1980s, the advent of Doppler techniques makes possible the verification of basic research done on animals and the evaluation of the dynamic aspects of the materno-fetal circulation.

The emphasis is placed more and more on anticipating perinatal complications, and the obstetrician is under pressure to predict the weight and the degree of maturity of the fetus and to decide when, where, and how the baby should be delivered. Although the mother remains the best incubator, intrauterine growth-retarded fetuses should be delivered at any time when intrauterine conditions for fetal survival seem less favorable than those offered in extrauterine life. It is quite clear that the decision will depend on medical facilities and on socioeconomic factors. In cases of newborn babies with intrauterine growth retardation, one of the therapeutical problems challenging the neonatologist is the decision as to when, what, and how to feed the baby in order to obtain a catch-up of growth.

All these aspects, including the pathogenesis, the epidemiology, the endocrine and ultrasound assessment, the clinical management, and the prevention of intrauterine growth retardation, are covered in this volume, which will be of interest not only to obstetricians, pediatricians, neonatologists, and epidemiologists but also to everyone who is interested in improving the health of mothers and children throughout the world. The interest of this book lies just as much in the discussions as in the core of the chapters.

I believe that this workshop and this volume may have contributed to a better definition of the problems they address and hence, may stimulate further research and promote measures aimed at reducing the incidence of intrauterine growth retardation.

JACQUES SENTERRE

Foreword

In the eyes of a non-specialist, all low birthweight infants are premature. In actual fact, low birthweight infants should be categorized into real prematures and infants suffering from intrauterine growth retardation (IUGR) who may either have been born at term or prematurely. Despite the fact that in many countries it is somewhat difficult to evaluate the date of conception, this distinction is not purely academic because pathology and mortality of the infant differ in relation to organ and function maturation, frequency and epidemiology vary, and, depending on etiology, prevention would be different.

In developing countries, IUGR is the most frequent disease of the newborn. The rate can be as high as 17% if we take 2.5 kg as the limit, whereas in advanced industrialized countries the rate is less than 3%.

This also raises the question of the definition of low birthweight. Should we adopt the same weight in all countries, for all races, and for all socioeconomic groups? We probably should, because in developing countries, term newborns from high socioeconomic groups weigh the same as their counterparts from industrialized countries, and when people move from developing to industrialized countries, the birthweight rapidly increases.

This volume reviews the various causes of IUGR—vascular, endocrine, nutritional—as well as the diagnosis of such problems during pregnancy through the use of traditional methods available everywhere or the more sophisticated methods which so far are only available in industrialized countries. The consequences of IUGR immediately after birth and during the following weeks are exposed, and the management of the baby suffering from IUGR reviewed. Finally, the importance of prevention is restated and the possible methods of treatment debated, thus ensuring that this volume should become a very useful tool for obstetricians as well as neonatologists and pediatricians in varying environments.

PIERRE R. GUESRY, M.D.
Vice-President
Nestlé Products Technical Assistance Co. Ltd.

Acknowledgments

I would like to express my gratitude to Professor Navantino Alves Filho, President of the Brazilian Pediatric Society, and to the Brazilian colleagues, doctors, and nurses who were our hosts; as well as to Nestlé Nutrition which initiated and made possible this fruitful workshop and this timely and comprehensive volume.

JACQUES SENTERRE

Contents

xi

Contributors

*Navantino Alves Filho

c/o Department of Pediatrics
Faculdade de Ninas Gerais
Avenue Boindeirantes
30000 Belo Horizonte, Brazil

*Fábio Ancona Lopez

Department of Pediatrics
Escola Paulista de Medicina
Rua Traipu 1251
01235 Perdizes, Sao Paulo, Brazil

*José M. Belizan

Centro Rosarino de Estudios Perinatales
Orono 500
2000 Rosario, Argentina

*Hans Bossart

Département de gynécologie-obstétrique
Centre Hospitalier Universitaire Vaudois
1011 Lausanne, Switzerland

*Cipriano A. Canosa

Department of Pediatrics
Children's Hospital "La Fe"
Avda. Campanar 21
46009 Valencia, Spain

*Louise Cédard

Unité 166 INSERM et Laboratoire de
    Chimie Hormonale
Maternité Baudelocque
123 Blvd. de Port Royal
75014 Paris, France

*Philippe Chessex

Centre de recherche et service de
    néonatologie
Hôpital Sainte-Justine
3175 Côte Ste-Catherine
Montréal H3T 1C5 PQ, Canada

*Joseph M. Ernest

Department of Obstetrics and Gynecology
Bowman Gray School of Medicine
Wake Forest University
300 South Hawthorne Road
Winston-Salem, North Carolina 27103

*Jean Girard

Centre de Recherche sur la Nutrition
    (CNRS)
9 Rue Jules Hetzel
92190 Meudon-Bellevue, France

*William W. Hay, Jr.

Associate Professor of Pediatrics
Head, Division of Perinatal Medicine
Department of Pediatrics
University of Colorado School of
    Medicine
4200 E. 9th Ave.
Denver, Colorado 80262

M.S. Keita

Human Reproduction Unit
Université Libre de Bruxelles
Hôpital Saint-Pierre
322 Rue Haute
1000 Brussels, Belgium

J. Leblond

Unité 166 INSERM et Laboratoire de
    Chimie Hormonale
Maternité Baudelocque
123 Blvd. de Port Royal
75014 Paris, France

*Antonio Marini

Neonatal Division
Institute of Obstetrics and Gynecology
    "L. Mangiagalli"
University of Milan
20120 Milan, Italy

*Workshop participants.

S. Meuris
Human Reproduction Unit
Université Libre de Bruxelles
Hôpital Saint Pierre
322 Rue Haute
1000 Brussels, Belgium

José O. Mora
Senior Medical Nutritionist
LTS International Nutritinut Junit
Bogotá, Colombia

Fernando José de Nóbrega
Department of Pediatrics
Escola Paulista de Medicina
Rua Traipu 1251
01235 Perdizes, Sao Paulo, Brazil

*Richard G. Pearse
Neonatal Intensive Care Unit
The Jessop Hospital for Women
Leavygreave Road
Sheffield S3 7RE, England

*Claude Robyn
Human Reproduction Unit
Université Libre de Bruxelles
Hôpital Saint Pierre
322 Rue Haute
1000 Brussels, Belgium

*Pedro Rosso
Department of Pediatrics
School of Medicine
Pontifical Catholic University of Chile
Casilla 114-D
Santiago, Chile

*John W. Seeds
Department of Obstetrics and Gynecology
University of North Carolina at Chapel Hill
214 MacNider Building 202H
Chapel Hill, North Carolina 27514

Conceição A.M. Segre
Department of Pediatrics
Escola Paulista de Medicina
Rua Traipu 1251
01235 Perdizes, Sao Paulo, Brazil

Jacques Senterre
Department of Pediatrics
University Hospital
4000 Liège, Belgium

Vincent Smeriglio
Department of Maternal and Child Health
School of Hygiene and Public Health
The Johns Hopkins University
Baltimore, Maryland 21218

Jorge Suescun
Department of Pediatrics
Medical School of Colombia
Bogotá, Colombia

G. Tanguy
Unité 166 INSERM et Laboratoire de Chimie Hormonale
Maternité Baudelocque
123 Blvd. de Port Royal
75014 Paris, France

*Paul L. Toubas
University of Oklahoma Health Sciences Center
Department of Pediatrics
Neonatology Section
P.O. Box 26901
Oklahoma City, Oklahoma 73190

Chiara Vegni
Neonatal Division
Institute of Obstetrics & Gynecology "L. Mangiagalli"
University of Milan
Milan, Italy

José Villar
Prevention Research Program
National Institute of Child Health and Human Development
National Institutes of Health
Executive Plaza North
Bethesda, Maryland 20892

*Brian Wharton
University of Glasgow
Department of Human Nutrition
Yorkhill Hospitals
Glasgow G3 8SJ, Scotland

Invited Attendees

N. Adeeb/*Kuala Lumpur, Malaysia*
N. Albano/*Rio de Janeiro, Brazil*
M.A. Barbieri/*Ribeirao Preto, Brazil*
G. Bogg/*Brest, France*
R. Bracci/*Siena, Italy*
A. Desai/*Ahmedabad, India*
A.Di Comite/*Taranto, Italy*
R.M. Fiori/*Porto Alegre, Brazil*
A. Jacob/*Agadir, Morocco*
H. Jeng-Hsiu/*People's Republic of China*
B. Kopelman/*Sao Paulo, Brazil*
A. Kuletharn/*Kuala Lumpur, Malaysia*
M. Lahrech/*Rabat, Morocco*

A. Latronico/*Milan, Italy*
L. Magni/*Milan, Italy*
C. Panero/*Florence, Italy*
A. Priolisi/*Palermo, Italy*
S. Rachagan/*Kuala Lumpur, Malaysia*
J. Ritter/*Strasbourg, France*
G. Rondini/*Pavia, Italy*
A.M. Segre/*Sao Paulo, Brazil*
G. Serra/*Genoa, Italy*
R. Tahiri/*Rabat, Morocco*
S. Tonete/*Sao Paulo, Brazil*
D. Tudehope/*Brisbane, Australia*
L.E. Vaz/*Miranda, Rio de Janeiro, Brazil*
L. Ziino/*Palermo, Italy*

Nestlé Participants

Pierre R. Guesry
Nestec Ltd.
Vevey, Switzerland
Philippe Goyens
Nestec Ltd.
Vevey, Switzerland
José Roberto Abreu de Souza
Nestlé Industrial e Comercial
Sao Paulo, Brazil
Feliz Romeo Braun
Nestlé Industrial e Comercial
Sao Paulo, Brazil

Adriano de Castro
Nestlé Industrial e Comercial
Sao Paulo, Brazil
Zulmiro Favoretto
Nestlé Industrial e Comercial
Sao Paulo, Brazil
Wilber Marquez Antunes
Nestlé Industrial e Comercial
Sao Paulo, Brazil

Nestlé Nutrition Workshop Series

INTRAUTERINE GROWTH RETARDATION

Intrauterine Growth Retardation, edited by
Jacques Senterre. Nestlé Nutrition Workshop
Series, Vol. 18. Nestec Ltd., Vevey/Raven Press,
Ltd., New York © 1989.

Placental Circulation and Fetal Growth

Paul L. Toubas

*Associate Professor of Pediatrics, University of Oklahoma Health Sciences Center,
Department of Pediatrics, Neonatology Section,
Oklahoma City, Oklahoma 73190*

Fetal growth retardation is a universal problem. The growth-retarded fetus carries a substantially increased perinatal mortality (1,2) and morbidity in the neonatal period and during infancy (2,3). Short-term sequelae include perinatal asphyxia (4), hypoglycemia, hypocalcemia, hypothermia, and polycythemia (2). Long-term neurological sequelae depend on the type of growth inhibition, its duration within a specific maternal environment, as well as concomitant hypoxic and/or asphyxic events. Sudden Infant Death Syndrome (SIDS) is not uncommonly associated with intrauterine growth retardation (5). The factors responsible for fetal growth retardation are numerous but their hierarchic responsibility is not well understood. However, once chromosomal abnormalities and genetic factors have been excluded, it is likely that nutrient and oxygen delivery to the fetus are essential determinants of harmonious intrauterine growth. The undisturbed perfusion of the intervillous chambers of the placenta is a prerequisite to fetal growth.

Today the accent is increasingly placed on anticipating neonatal complications, and there is pressure on the obstetrician to predict the weight and degree of maturity of the infant. Technical advances have permitted the survival of smaller and smaller infants, but quality of survival is the subject of intense investigation and is not always cost effective. The best incubator still remains the mother, but a fetus with a severely compromised uteroplacental circulation will not benefit from prolonged gestation.

The placental circulation has been extremely difficult to study and most of the research performed to establish its function has been done in a great variety of mammals. There are very few chronic studies of this ephemeral circulation and most of them are extraordinarily invasive. More recently, the advent of ultrasound techniques has allowed us to begin to verify the basic research done in animals and has provided a means of evaluating the materno-fetal circulation. In the late sixties, the continuous measurement of the heart rate and biparietal diameter was a revolution. In the late eighties, a multiplicity of Doppler techniques provides an intrauterine examination of the fetus and allows for the detection of feto-placental abnormalities. These techniques are in continuous progress and promise to tell more about the dy-

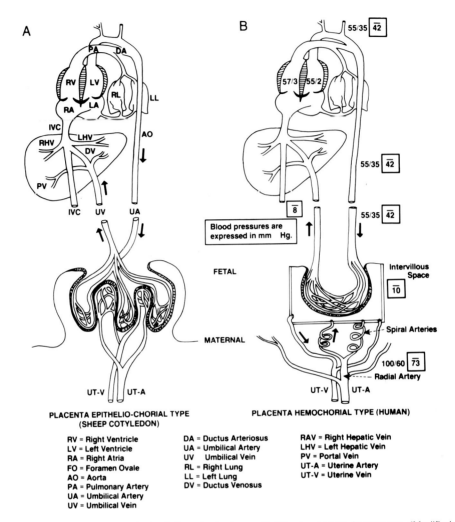

FIG. 1. The human fetal circulation. **A:** Anatomy. **B:** Blood pressure in squares. (Modified from ref. 69.)

namic aspects of the materno-fetal circulation. They also give the fetus the status of an infant, with legal and ethical implications.

Implantation, placentation, and development of the utero-placental vascular bed are important aspects of any consideration of fetal growth. The maternal cardiovascular system undergoes significant changes during pregnancy in order to comply with the blood flow of the new utero-placental vascular bed.

This chapter will provide an overview of the physiological hemodynamic transformations of the utero-placental and feto-placental circulations and identify some of the factors which may affect materno-fetal circulation in the delivery and transport of oxygen and nutrients.

ANATOMY OF UTERO-PLACENTAL CIRCULATION

In the human species the uterine arteries branch on the sides of the uterus and then travel through approximately one-third of the myometrium before they divide further into the arcuate arteries. The arcuate arteries then encircle the uterus parallel to the surface and form multiple anastomoses with the contralateral arcuate arteries near the midline. Arising from the arcuate arteries and running approximately at right angles to them are the radial arteries which travel through the middle third of the myometrium before dividing into the basal arteries, which supply the basal endometrium; and into the spiral arteries which supply the decidua and the intervillous space (Fig. 1A).

During normal pregnancy, the trophoblast invades the superficial portions of the myometrium and migrates through the entire length of the spiral arteries by about the twentieth postmenstrual week (6). This has two effects. First, the spiral artery is stripped of its musculoelastic coat, which reduces the peripheral resistance and hence the blood pressure. The systemic blood pressure falls to its lowest level at about 20 weeks (7), the time at which trophoblastic invasion is complete. Second, there is little or no resistance to blood flow from the radial artery into the intervillous space. Typically, the blood pressure at the level of the radial arteries is 70–80 mm Hg, while the pressure at the intervillous space is 10 mm Hg (8). This pressure gradient has an obvious advantage to the fetus in that it gives optimum time for materno-fetal exchange (Fig. 1B).

Early in pregnancy, 50% of the increase in cardiac output is distributed to the uterus. This is the period when the fetal membranes develop, together with the uterine endometrium and caruncles and the initation of placentation (9). Thereafter, the uterine blood flow (UBF) is redistributed as placental blood flow increases, such that near term in the sheep, blood flow to the placental cotyledons accounts for nearly all of the total UBF (10) (Fig. 2).

The pattern of change in placental blood flow during the course of normal ovine pregnancy is illustrated in Fig. 3. There are two obvious stages in the development of the utero-placental circulation. The first stage covers the first two-thirds of gestation and terminates with the completion of placentation. During this time the placenta reaches its maximal weight and placental blood flow reaches 400–500 ml/min. The second stage covers the last third of the gestation. During this period there is no further placental growth. It is during this stage that placental blood flow reaches a maximum of around 1000 ml/min (10).

In morphometric studies performed in the ovine placenta, Teasdale (11) has shown that the number of maternal placental vessels is at its maximum at the end of the first stage and does not change thereafter. The human placenta displays a similar pattern. Absolute growth of the placenta as determined by deoxyribonucleic acid (DNA), ribonuleic acid (RNA), and protein content continues to the 36th week of gestation. Thereafter, proliferation of cells does not normally occur, and the placenta undergoes only further maturational changes (12). Previous studies have suggested that the villous surface continues to expand to between 11 and 13 m^2 at term,

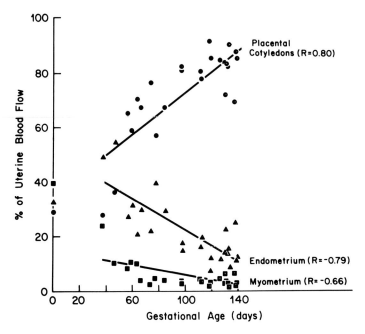

FIG. 2. The distribution of uterine blood flow during ovine pregnancy (Term = 144 ± 5 days). Flows were determined by the microsphere technique. Correlation coefficients for linear regressions are noted, p <0.01. ● = placental cotyledon; ▲ = endometrium; ■ = myometrium. (From ref. 14.)

whereas Teasdale's measurements suggest that a maximum of 10.6 m^2 is reached at 36 weeks, decreasing to 9.4 m^2 at term.

MATERNAL CARDIOVASCULAR CHANGES DURING PREGNANCY

The study of the growth and development of the utero-placental vascular bed in women is difficult. The chronic fetal sheep preparation has provided an unstressed animal model allowing simultaneous study of the mother and the fetus. Despite arguments about species differences, the cardiovascular changes observed during pregnancy in the ewe are close to those observed in women. In the early seventies, the use of radioactively labeled microspheres (13) allowed the measurement of the cardiac output and its distribution in the sheep model. Total UBF has been assessed by a variety of techniques ranging from implanted electromagnetic flow probes to diffusion-equilibration and microsphere methods. Heart rate, blood pressure, blood flow, blood gases, and nutrient transfer can thus be studied simultaneously in both mother and fetus.

In ovine pregnancy, as in the human, there are significant increases in the cardiac output and heart rate resulting in an increase in stroke volume (14). A general decrease in vascular resistance leads to a slight fall in mean arterial pressure. A 30 to

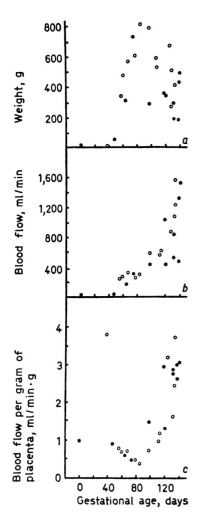

FIG. 3. Placental cotyledons: **(a)** weight, **(b)** blood flow, **(c)** blood flow per gram of placenta, plotted against gestational age. The observations on the pregnant animals represent weight and flow to the sites of implantation (caruncles) in oophorectomized ewes. The placental weight of twin gestation is the sum of the weights of the two placentas. Likewise, placental blood flow of twin gestation is the sum of the placental flows of each twin. ■ = non-pregnant; ● = singleton gestation; ○ = twin gestation. (From ref. 10.)

40% expansion in blood volume occurs in normal pregnancy. In the non-pregnant animal, 0.5% of the cardiac output is directed to the uterus (14). In the pregnant animal the percent of cardiac output redistributed to the uterus increases dramatically to reach 8% at midpregnancy and 16% or greater near term. This increase in uterine blood flow (Fig. 4) represents flows of approximately 25 ml/min, 500 ml/min, and more than 1,300 ml/min, respectively. The progressive rise in UBF is also associated with a marked increase in the weight of the utero-placental-fetal unit. If the blood flow is expressed in milliliters per gram of metabolically active tissue, it is found to be at its highest during implantation and placentation. The UBF (ml/min-g) subsequently decreases during the last third of pregnancy when the pattern of fetal growth is logarithmic (10). Despite a decrease in the percent of distribution of

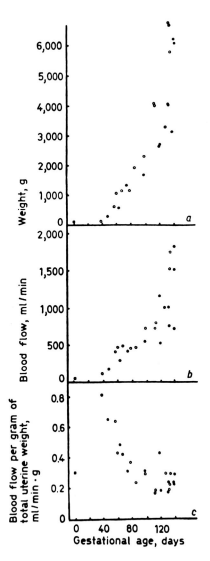

FIG. 4. The uterus: **(a)** total weight, **(b)** blood flow, **(c)** blood flow per gram of total weight, plotted against gestational age. Total uterine weight is the sum of myometrial, endometrial, placental, fetal membranes and fetal body weights. Uterine blood flow is the flow to all uterine tissues (cervix excluded) as determined by the microsphere technique. ■ = non-pregnant; ● = singleton gestation; ○ = twin gestation. (From ref. 10.)

cardiac output to other organs, the actual blood flows remain unchanged, stressing the importance of an expanded maternal blood volume.

UTERO-PLACENTAL BLOOD FLOW AND PLACENTAL TRANSPORT

The fetus depends on the placental blood flow to receive the substrate necessary for fetal growth. A reduction in utero-placental perfusion, as induced by ritodrine in the pregnant ewe, does not produce a parallel decrease in fetal-placental blood flow

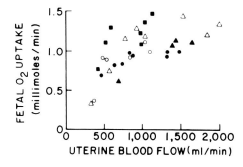

FIG. 5. Relationship of fetal O_2 uptake to uterine blood flow. Five pregnant ewes were studied. Animal no./symbol: ● = 1; ○ = 2; ▲ = 3; △ = 4; ■ = 5. (From ref. 16.)

(15). For example, over a wide range of placental blood flow the placental clearance of ethanol is not affected by a decrease of uteroplacental flow in the fetal lamb so long as it does not decrease below 500 ml/min. Fetal oxygen uptake has been found to be positively correlated with changes of uterine blood flow (Fig. 5). An even better relationship is illustrated in Fig. 6 between fetal oxygen uptake and uterine oxygen delivery (the product of uterine blood flow and arterial oxygen content) (16). Under normal circumstances, when umbilical flow is maintained, uterine oxygen delivery far exceeds the fetal needs for oxidative metabolism. The fetus thrives within a wide safety margin. However, oxygen deprivation may be the cause of fetal growth retardation. Pregnancies complicated by cyanotic maternal heart disease usually result in intrauterine growth retardation (IUGR), but it is unclear whether abnormal maternal hemodynamics or the reduction in oxygen saturation is responsible for poor fetal growth. The question of how chronic reduction of uterine blood flow may affect the delivery of nutrients to the fetus is far from being answered.

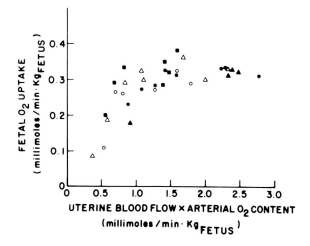

FIG. 6. Relationship of fetal O_2 uptake to rate of O_2 delivery to pregnant uterus. Five pregnant ewes were studied. Animal no./symbol: ● = 1; ○ = 2; ▲ = 3; △ = 4; ■ = 5. (From ref. 16.)

REGULATION OF UTERO-PLACENTAL BLOOD FLOW

In a quiet animal, blood flow to the gravid uterus remains virtually constant for hours (17), though some diurnal fluctuations may be observed (18). The highest values for amniotic fluid and blood pressure are recorded during daytime, whereas the highest uterine artery blood flow tends to occur at night.

There is now evidence that the partial pressures of oxygen and carbon dioxide do not exert any appreciable direct control on the placental circulation (17). Failure to demonstrate any short-term direct regulation of placental blood flow by respiratory gases does not preclude the possibility of chronic effects on the growth of the placental vasculature. The high incidence of placental hypertrophy in patients with severe anemia provides evidence for placental adaptation to anemic hypoxia (19).

Umbilical blood flow is unaffected by acute moderate hypoxia (20). However, significant increases of utero-placental vascular resistance have been observed in severe hypoxia (21,22), hypercapnia (23), hypocapnia (24), and metabolic alkalosis (25,26). These results are consistent with the concept that anesthesia and/or pronounced disturbances of oxygenation cause the release of vasoactive substances in the circulation and the activation of vasomotor nerves. During asphyxia in diving mammals, the blood flow to the gravid uterus remains relatively constant in comparison to the dramatic reduction in renal blood flow (27).

Rosenfeld et al. (28) found that the injection of estradiol 17β in pregnant ewes increases the blood flow to the myometrium, endometrium, and placental cotyledons, though blood flow to the latter increased only during the early phase of pregnancy. The mechanism by which the placental vasculature becomes refractory to vasodilation by exogenous estrogens is unknown.

The infusion of catecholamines into pregnant ewes produces a dose-dependent decrease of UBF. The vasoconstrictive effect within the uterus was more pronounced in the endometrium and myometrium than in the placental cotyledons (29,30). The reduction of utero-placental blood flow by epinephrine and norepinephrine can be blocked by phenoxybenzamine. The vascular bed of the ovine placenta is unresponsive to β-adrenergic agonists. In contrast, the administration of a β-adrenergic agent (metaproterenol) improved utero-placental blood flow in anesthetized rhesus monkeys. It is not known if this effect is direct or indirect, through relaxation of the uterine musculature (31).

The physiological role of prostaglandins in regulating the utero-placental blood flow is still obscure. The administration of prostaglandin inhibitors has led to contradictory results (32–35). The injection of PGE_2 and PGF_2 into the maternal circulation caused uterine contractions and a decrease of placental blood flow in the sheep (33,35). Indomethacin, an inhibitor of prostaglandin synthesis, produces an increased uterine blood flow late in pregnancy in the dog and sheep (34,35).

Catecholamine-induced vasoconstriction is smaller in the placental vascular beds than in the myoendometrial vasculature (30). The opposite has been reported to occur with systemic infusions of angiotensin II. Chesley, Gant, and others (36,37) have shown that a characteristic of human pregnancy is the development of a blunted response to the pressor effects of infused angiotensin II, and these results have been confirmed by other authors (38). The systemic infusion of hypertonic saline increases the systemic response to infused angiotensin II, but has no effect on the uterine vascular resistance. More recently, Leffler (39) showed in the pregnant sheep that the reduction of utero-placental perfusion pressure causes hypertension only in NaCl-supplemented animals.

Adrenergic innervation of the uterus is present in every species examined, whereas cholinergic innervation is either scarce or absent (40,41). In the non-pregnant guinea pig the whole uterus has fibers that can be stained by the catecholamine fluorescent technique. When the animal becomes pregnant, the fluorescence gradually disappears. In non-pregnant animals the norepinephrine content of the uterus increases under estrogen stimulation and decreases under the influence of progesterone (42,43). Thus, the response of the uterine adrenergic nerves to pregnancy is part of a regulatory mechanism mediated by steroid hormones. Data from experiments on dogs (44) indicate that the uterine circulation becomes insensitive to catecholamines as pregnancy progresses. Fluorescence histochemical examination of uteri from dogs in early or late gestation has revealed a total disappearance of adrenergic innervation to the myometrium and only sparsé fibers associated with uterine vessels. Data obtained in sheep have failed to demonstrate any substantial difference between non-pregnant and pregnant animals.

Can one apply this knowledge to the human? Ramsey et al. (45), using cineangiography, have suggested from data obtained in the primate that similar factors may affect placental blood flow in the human. They have proposed in addition that some other factors may alter placental blood flow, such as intrauterine pressure, changes in the pattern of uterine contractility, and contour of the individual uterine contraction wave. They also called attention to the non-homogeneity of the blood in the intervillous space and to the fact that the endometrial spiral arterioles act independently of one another.

ALTERATIONS IN UTERO-PLACENTAL PERFUSION AND FETAL GROWTH

Experimental animal studies suggest that alterations in utero-placental perfusion affect the growth of the feto-placental unit. In the pregnant rat, ligation of the uterine artery of one horn results in IUGR of the fetuses closest to the arterial constriction (46). In guinea pigs, mice, and rabbits, arterial perfusion is lowest in the middle of each uterine horn. The weight of the fetus and placenta is the lowest at this location (47). Creasy et al. (48) produced repetitive embolization of the uterine vascular blood flow (using 15 μm microspheres) during the last quarter of gestation in the pregnant ewe. This resulted in a 40% reduction in placental weight and alterations in organ growth patterns similar to those observed in growth-retarded fetuses from pregnancies complicated with hypertension. Examination of the placenta showed localized hyalinization and fibrinoid changes. Umbilical blood flow was reduced and fetal oxidative metabolism was decreased (48). In humans, the utero-placental blood flow decreases in pregnancies complicated by maternal hypertension. The clearance of radioactive sodium from the intervillous space is reduced in preeclamptic hypertensive pregnancies or in prolonged gestation (49).

The mechanism of the decreased uterine blood flow in IUGR is complex. Some workers have shown evidence of narrowing of the iliac and uterine vessels in pregnant women with hypertension (50). Others have reported that the site of implantation of the placenta in pregnancy complicated by preeclampsia and IUGR is subject to obstructive arterionecrosis which in turn produces ischemia of the villi (51). Normally, trophoblastic cells intermingle extensively with decidua basalis at the site of implantation. Cytotrophoblastic cells enter the open mouths of maternal arterioles and penetrate along their endothelial lining. Some other cells invade the spiral arteries from the outside. Incomplete invasion of the decidual part of the spiral arteries may result in the retention of the musculo-elastic coat. This may have various effects. First, the spiral arteries may remain sensitive to local or systemic pressor agents (which may be an etiological factor in pregnancy-induced hypertension). Second, the reduction of local uterine blood flow leads to the reduction of perfusion of the intervillous space with its corollary: inadequate exchange of nutrients and fetal growth retardation. There are also reports that abnormal sympathetic innervation of internal iliac arteries predisposes to IUGR (52). Other reports mention abnormal vascularization of an unicornuate uterus (53). Recurrent antepartum hemorrhage from either premature separation of the placenta or placenta previa is associated with an increased incidence of IUGR (54).

Clinically evident maternal vascular disease and the presumed decrease in utero-placental perfusion can account for 25% to 30% of cases of IUGR. Recent techniques using Doppler velocity measurements of uterine blood flow allow more precise and non-invasive documentation of utero-placental circulatory dysfunction (55). Such an evaluation may allow detection of IUGR far in advance of other biochemical and ultrasonic methods. The description of this technique and the practical assessment of fetal growth using ultrasound are described elsewhere in this volume. The use of a pulsatility index allows quantification and comparison of measurements during pregnancy. The pulsatility index is an indication of vascular resistance. Griffin et al. (56) have assessed uterine arcuate flow in normal and IUGR pregnancies and have reported raised pulsatility indices and lower diastolic frequencies in IUGR pregnancies. Fleisher et al. (57), using Doppler velocimetry of the uterine arteries, showed that when the systolic/diastolic ratio is >2.6 there is a notch in the waveform and the pregnancy is complicated by stillbirth, premature birth, IUGR, and maternal pre-eclampsia. According to Fleisher et al., the predictive value of the examination is around 90% (57).

Other techniques allow calculation of the intervillous blood flow (IVBF). The method is based on the use of ^{133}Xe. Kaar et al. (58) injected ^{133}Xe intravenously in normal and pathologic pregnancies. The mean IVBF in normal pregnancies was 140 ml per 100 ml of intervillous space/min. The lowest flow values were observed in pregnancies complicated by hypertension, severe pre-eclampsia and diabetes (class B-E). In this study, growth retardation, although associated with decreased IVBF, was not as low as found in the groups listed above. Other authors (59), using the accumulation methods, found that placental uptake of tracer in pregnancies in growth-retarded babies was significantly reduced. In the human species, ritodrine, a potent β-adrenergic agonist widely used in the prevention of premature labor, did not alter the intervillous and umbilical circulation (60).

FETO-PLACENTAL CIRCULATION

The maternal and fetal circulations, despite their physical separation, influence each other. The feto-placental unit, through regulation of the hormonal milieu, controls the maternal hematologic and cardiovascular adaptions to pregnancy. The fetus, by controlling its own substrate ability, determines its own growth. The umbilical circulation has been studied extensively in the experimental animal with respect to various endogenous or exogenous influences. Very little attention has been given to its influence on fetal growth. In the human, the natural history of an anatomical alteration in the feto-placental circulation is the "common villous district" arteriovenous shunt in twin pregnancy. It may lead to plethora in the recipient and growth retardation and/or death of the donor (61). Some cardiovascular abnormalities (i.e., atrial septal defect) are often associated with intrauterine growth retardation (62). Approximately 25% of newborns with a single umbilical artery weigh less than 2,500 g at birth (63). Ligation of one umbilical artery has also been used to produce intrauterine growth retardation in the experimental animal (64).

Although the umbilical vessels have the capacity to constrict actively after birth, it has generally been assumed that the umbilical-placental circulation is quite passive during intrauterine life. The initial work in this area was accomplished by Cooper and Dawes (65,66) on exteriorized fetal goats or lambs. The first measurements of umbilical blood flow in the fetus *in utero* were made by Meschia et al. (67) using the Fick principle. It measured antipyrine umbilical-venous and umbilical-arterial concentration differences at steady state. This method was quite unreliable in measuring flow changes. The radionuclide labeled microsphere method for measuring the distribution of blood flow in fetal lambs was introduced by Rudolph and Heymann (68). The method is accurate, but has the drawback that only single measurements, representing a short period of time, can be made, and rapid changes in flow cannot be appreciated. In 1976 Rudolph (69) developed a technique for measuring umbilical blood flow continuously in the fetal lamb *in utero* by applying an electromagnetic flow transducer around the common umbilical artery. Values for umbilical-placental blood flow for fetal lambs average 180–200 ml/kg/min during the last third of gestation. The combined ventricular output as measured by the microsphere method averages 450–500 ml/kg/min (70); thus, umbilical blood flow represents 40% of the ventricular output. In animals at mid-gestation, about 45% of the cardiac output is distributed to the placenta. There is a gradual reduction in the fraction of fetal cardiac output supplying the placental circulation with advancing gestation, presumably due to rapid body growth with increasing requirements for blood flow in various organs (69). (These data are summarized in Figs. 7A and 7B.)

Spontaneous changes in heart rate are associated with dramatic changes in umbilical blood flow of similar direction. Fetal respiratory movements cause variable changes in umbilical blood flow, especially large inspiratory efforts > -5 Torr. Even with a considerable increase in mean blood pressure, there is often a fall in the umbilical blood flow when there is associated bradycardia. The concept that the umbilical placental circulation is passive and that flow is determined exclusively by the perfusion pressure cannot be accepted in the presence of variability in heart rate. The classical formula applied to the calculation of vascular resistance is not reliable if there are alterations in heart rate. The long tortuous umbilical-placental circulation presumably exaggerates the factors which contribute to making pulse frequency important in determining flow. Thus, a decrease in umbilical blood flow associated with a decrease in heart rate but no change in blood pressure cannot be interpreted as an increase in umbilical-placental vascular resistance.

The suggestion was made by Longo that the surrounding placental pressure may influence the feto-placental circulation. Rudolph (69) demonstrated that there was a linear relationship between the rise in umbilical venous pressure and percent de-

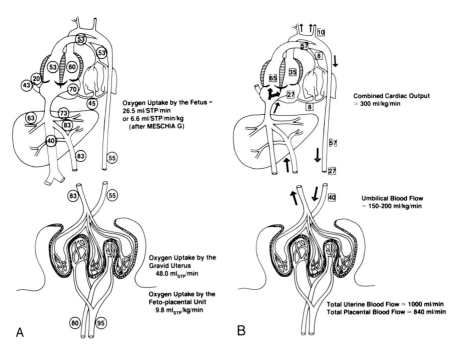

Oxygen Uptake by the Fetus =
26.5 ml/STP/min
or 6.6 ml/STP/min/kg
(after MESCHIA G)

Oxygen Uptake by the
Gravid Uterus
48.0 ml$_{STP}$/min

Oxygen Uptake by the
Feto-placental Unit
9.8 ml$_{STP}$/kg/min

Combined Cardiac Output
= 300 ml/kg/min

Umbilical Blood Flow
= 150-200 ml/kg/min

Total Uterine Blood Flow = 1000 ml/min
Total Placental Blood Flow = 840 ml/min

A   B

FIG. 7. Fetal circulation. **A:** Oxygen saturation (in circles). (From ref. 69.) **B:** Percentage of cardiac output (in squares) and its distribution. (Modified from ref. 68.)

crease in umbilical blood flow. This rise in umbilical venous blood pressure did not alter uterine-placental circulation. This finding was further supported by the observation that graded inflation of a balloon in the fetal descending aorta produced progressive reduction of umbilical arterial pressure and umbilical blood flow, but had no effect on uterine blood flow (69).

Rudolph (69) describes the responses of the umbilical-placental circulation to vasoactive agents. Isoproterenol, dopamine, histamine, tolazoline, and aminophylline have no effect on umbilical blood flow or on vascular pressure when injected directly into the umbilical artery, indicating they do not affect the umbilical-placental vasculature. When the injections are made in the fetal inferior vena cava, both isoproterenol and dopamine produce a small increase in umbilical blood flow, but this is associated with tachycardia. Epinephrine, norepinephrine, and acetylcholine, when injected directly into the umbilical artery, have no effect on the umbilical blood flow. However, when injected directly into the fetal venous system, they cause marked alteration of the umbilical blood flow secondary to their effects on heart rate and/or blood pressure. Acetylcholine decreases umbilical blood flow without changes in vascular umbilical resistance. Norepinephrine or epinephrine produces a sharp increase in fetal arterial blood pressure. This results in reflex bradycardia due to baroreceptor stimulation and umbilical blood flow falls markedly. When atropine is injected into the fetus prior to the injection of catecholamines, no change in umbilical resistance is observed. Prostaglandins E1, E2, F2, angiotensin, and bradykinin all cause a decrease in umbilical blood flow when injected directly into the umbilical circulation or when injected into the inferior vena cava. Fetal arterial pressure increases and heart rate falls (69).

The fetal response to hypoxia (20) results in peripheral vasoconstriction and increased arterial pressure. Reflex bradycardia is observed, but if mild, umbilical blood flow will be maintained due to the increased perfusion pressure. The fetus is able to make circulatory adjustments in response to impaired utero-placental perfusion to preserve coronary and brain flow. This probably explains the "head sparing" that occurs in growth-retarded fetuses, in which the cause is thought to be "placental insufficiency." During acute fetal hemorrhage, fetal bradycardia and decreased arterial blood pressure are observed. The umbilical blood flow is decreased, as well as coronary and brain blood flow (70).

All the animal techniques which I have so far described are extremely invasive and do not have practical applications in human pregnancies. The use of radioactive isotopes carries serious potential hazards. Clinicians have, until recently, relied on indirect tests (cardiotochography, fetal movements, fetal breathing movements) (1). The advent of direct measurement of both fetal and utero-placental blood flow by means of pulsed Doppler ultrasound may in the future allow more precise recognition and management of pregnancies complicated by hypertension and growth retardation. Griffin et al. (57) evaluated the fetal thoracic aorta pulsatility index in pregnancies with severe IUGR. They noted that most of the fetuses had very low end diastolic frequencies, a phenomenon absent in pregnancies with normal fetal development. However, the elevation of the pulsatility index was a late event in IUGR, reflecting an abnormal anatomy of the placenta (56). This is in contrast with the normal decline in pulsatility index with advancing gestation.

MATERNAL MALNUTRITION AND PLACENTAL CIRCULATION

Undernourished women and women living in conditions of poverty have a lower mean placental weight than well-nourished women or women from higher income groups. A decreased number of villi in placentas of malnourished women has also been reported in different studies (71). The reduced villous surface suggests a reduced area for maternal-fetal exchange, a finding that has obvious functional implications on maternal-fetal transfer of nutrients. Measurements of cardiac output and organ blood flow using radioactive microspheres in anesthetized control and food-restricted rats have demonstrated that malnourished mothers do not expand maternal blood volume, cardiac output, and placental blood flow to the same extent as well-fed mothers (72). However, they maintain normal blood flow to the myometrium and to vital organs (74). Thus, the reduced transfer of nutrients found in malnourished mothers may reflect a reduced rate of placental blood flow. This decreased blood flow is probably due to reduced or inadequate blood volume expansion (73). The decreased utero-placental blood flow associated with diet restriction is the result of increased uteroplacental β-adrenergic vasomotor tone (74).

MATERNAL SMOKING AND PLACENTAL BLOOD FLOW

The mean birthweight of infants born to smokers is reduced by 175 to 200 g (75). Mochizvki et al. (76) described significant vascular changes in the placentas of smokers. Pirani (77) has suggested that the mechanism is a dose-dependent decrease in utero-placental flow, due to stimulation of sympathetic neurons by nicotine. Socol et al. (78) found that the fetus of rhesus monkeys shows a decline in arterial PaO_2 when the mother is exposed to passive smoking. The mechanism is probably an increased level of carboxyhemoglobin (levels are increased in smoking mothers and fetal levels are 1.8 times higher). Some authors have found that the intervillous placental blood flow is decreased (79), while others have shown that the umbilical flow changes observed after the mother smoked a single cigarette are insignificant. More studies are needed in order to demonstrate the effect of maternal smoking on utero-placental blood flow (80).

CONCLUSIONS

The last 30 years have seen the accumulation of a plethora of investigations attempting to solve the puzzle of the cause of fetal growth retardation. Most of the recent studies have been performed on animals of different species, involving either the fetal, placental, feto-placental and/or materno-placental unit during the last third of gestation. The techniques used in fetal animal preparations may, due to their invasiveness, induce fetal growth retardation per se. Very few studies have pursued the evaluation of blood flow and fetal growth. Our basic knowledge has, however, progressed markedly in the area of fetal and maternal circulation, leading to promising recent clinical applications which may allow early detection of abnormalities of these circulations, with the possibility of follow-up ad libitum during pregnancy. These techniques still need refinement in the quantification of the measurements of blood flow using Doppler ultrasound, but the placental vessels are now within reach of the clinician. However, the placenta as an area of exchange still belongs to the domain of basic research. The study of placental transport is confounded by species differences, gestational age, and a permanent non-steady state. Measurements of venous and arterial cord blood chemistry are sufficient to distinguish the fraction of nutrient uptake that is dedicated to catabolism from the fraction that is dedicated to fetal growth. These measurements are too invasive to be applied to the human pregnancies, but the development of other techniques, e.g., nuclear magnetic resonance, may one day provide the key to that ephemeral metabolic chamber, the placenta.

REFERENCES

1. Seeds JW. Impaired fetal growth: Definition and clinical diagnosis. Ultrasonic evaluation and clinical management. *Obstet Gynecol* 1984;64:577–83.
2. Usher RH, McLean FH. Normal fetal growth and the significance of fetal growth retardation. In: Davis JA, Dobbins J, eds, *Scientific Foundations of Pediatrics*. London: Heinemann, 1974;69.
3. Butler NR, Alberman ED. *Perinatal problems: The second report of the British Perinatal Mortality Survey*. Edinburgh: Churchill-Livingstone, 1969.
4. Low JA, Pancheim SM, Worthington D, et al. The incidence of fetal asphyxia in 600 high risk monitored pregnancies. *Am J Obstet Gynecol* 1975;121:456–9.
5. Hoffman HJ, Bekketeig LS. Heterogenicity of intrauterine growth retardation and recurrent risk. *Semin Perinatol* 1984;8:15–24.
6. Brosens I, Robertson WB, Dixon HG. The physiological response of the vessels of the placental bed to normal pregnancy. *J Pathol Bacteriol* 1967;93:569–79.
7. MacGillivray I, Rose GA, Rowe B. Blood pressure survey in pregnancy. *Clin Sci* 1969;37:395–407.
8. Boyd JD, Hamilton WT. *The human placenta*. Cambridge: W. Heffer and Sons, 1970;267–74.
9. Silver H, Barnes J, Comline RS, Burton GJ. Placental blood flow: Some fetal and maternal cardiovascular adjustments during gestation. *J Reproduct Fertil* 1982; (Suppl) 31:139–50.
10. Rosenfeld CR, Morriss FH Jr., Makowski EL, et al. Circulatory changes in the reproductive tissues of ewes during pregnancy. *Gynecol Obstet Invest* 1974;5:252–68.
11. Teasdale F. Numerical density of nuclei in the sheep placenta. *Anat Rec* 1976;185:187–96.
12. Teasdale F. Gestational changes in the functional structure of the human placenta in relation to fetal growth: A morphometric study. *Am J Obstet Gynecol* 1980;137:560.
13. Rudolph AM, Heymann MA. The circulation of the fetus in utero. Methods for studying distribution of blood flow, cardiac output, and organ blood flow. *Circ Res* 1967;21:163.
14. Rosenfeld CR. Distribution of cardiac output in ovine pregnancy. *Am J Physiol* 1977;232:231–5.
15. Ehrenkranz RA, Walker AM, Oakes GK, et al. Effect of ritodrine infusion on uterine and umbilical blood flow in pregnant sheep. *Am J Obstet Gynecol* 1976;126:343–9.
16. Wickening RB, Meschia G. Fetal oxygen uptake, oxygenation, and acid-base balance as a function of uterine blood flow. *Am J Physiol* 1983;244:H749–55.
17. Makowski EL, Hertz RH, Meschia GE. Effects of acute maternal hypoxia on the blood flow of the pregnant uterus. *Am J Obstet Gynecol* 1973;115:624–31.

18. Harbert GH. Biorhythms of the pregnant uterus *(Macaca mulatta). Am J Obstet Gynecol* 1977;129:401–8.
19. Beisher NA, Sivasamboo AR, Vohra S, Silpisorn-Kosal S, Reip S. Placental hypertrophy in severe pregnancy anaemia. *J Obstet Gynecol Br Commonw* 1970;77:398–409.
20. Cohn HE, Sacks EJ, Heymann MA, Rudolph AM. Cardiovascular response to hypoxemia and acidemia in fetal lambs. *Am J Obstet Gynecol* 1974;120:817.
21. Dilts PV, Brinkman CR, Kirschbaum TH, Assali NS. Uterine and systemic hemodynamic interrelationship and their response to hypoxia. *Am J Obstet Gynecol* 1969;103:138–57.
22. Karlsson K. The influence of hypoxia on uterine and maternal placental blood flow and the effect of L-adrenergic blockade. *J Perinatol Med* 1974;2:168–76.
23. Walker AM, Oakes GK, Ehrenkranz RA, McLaughlin M, Chez RA. Effects of hypercapnia on uterine and umbilical circulations in conscious pregnant sheep. *J Appl Physiol* 1976;41:727–733.
24. Levinson GS, Shnider M, Delorimer AA, Steffenson JL. Effects of maternal hyperventilation on uterine blood flow and fetal oxygenation and acid base status. *Anesthesiology* 1974;40:340–7.
25. Buss DD, Bisgard GE, Rawlings CA, Rankin THG. Uteroplacental blood flow during alkalosis in the sheep. *Am J Physiol* 1975;228:1497–1500.
26. Ralston DH, Shnider SM, Delorimier AA. Uterine blood flow and fetal acid-base changes after bicarbonate administration to the pregnant ewe. *Anesthesiology* 1974;40:348–53.
27. Elsner R, Hammond DD, Parker HR. Circulatory response to asphyxia in pregnant and fetal animals: a comparative study of Weddel seals and sheep. *Yale J Biol Med* 1970;42:202–17.
28. Rosenfeld CR, Morris FH Jr., Battaglia FC, Makowski EL, Meschia G. Effect of estradiol 17B on blood flow to reproductive and nonreproductive tissues in pregnant ewes. *Am J Obstet Gynecol* 1976;124:618–29.
29. Barton MD, Killam AP, Meschia G. Response of ovine uterine blood flow to epinephrine and norepinephrine. *Proc Soc Exp Biol Med* 1974;145:996–1003.
30. Anderson SG, Still TG, Greiss FC. Differential reactivity of the gravid uterine vasculatures: effects of norepinephrine. *Am J Obstet Gynecol* 1977;129:293–8.
31. Wallenburg HC, Mazer D, Hutchinson DL. Effects of a beta-adrenergic agent (metaproterenol) on utero-placental circulation: an angiographic study in the pregnant Rhesus monkey. *Am J Obstet Gynecol* 1973;117:1067–75.
32. Clark KE, Farley DB, Vanorden DE, Brody MJ. Role of endogenous prostaglandins in regulation of uterine blood flow and adrenergic neurotransmission. *Am J Obstet Gynecol* 1977;127:455–61.
33. McLaughlin MK, Brennan SC, Chez RA. Vasoconstrictive effects of prostaglandins in sheep placental circulations. *Am J Obstet Gynecol* 1978;130:408–13.
34. Gerber JG, Branch RA, Hubbard WC, Nies AS. Indomethacin is a placental vasodilator in the dog: the effect of prostaglandin inhibition. *J Clinc Invest* 1978;62:14–9.
35. Rankin JH. Berssenbrugge GA, Anderson D, Phernetton T. Ovine placental vascular responses to Indomethacin. *Am J Physiol* 1979;236 *(Heart Circ Physiol* 5): H60–4.
36. Chesley LG, Talledo OE, Bohler ES, et al. Vascular reactivity to angiotensin II and norepinephrine in pregnant and non-pregnant women. *Am J Obstet Gynecol* 1965;91:837–42.
37. Gant NF, Daley GL, Chan D, et al. a study of angiotensin II pressor response throughout primigravid pregnancy. *J Clin Invest* 1973;52:2682–9.
38. Rosenfeld CR, Naden RP. Differential responses to infused angiotensin II (AII) in uterine and non-uterine tissues in ovine pregnancy [Abst]. *Society for Gynecologic Investigation* 1983.
39. Leffler CW, Hessler JR, Green RS, Fletcher AM. Effects of sodium chloride on pregnant sheep with reduced uteroplacental perfusion pressure. *Hypertension* 1986;8:62–5.
40. Adham N, Schenk EA. Autonomic inversation of the rat vagina, cervix, and uterus and its cyclic variation. *Am J Obstet Gynecol* 1969;104:508–16.
41. Thorbert G, Alm P, Owman C, et al. Regional distribution of autonomic nerves in guinea pig uterus. *Am J Physiol* 1977;233 *(Cell Physiol* 2):C25–34.
42. Bell C, Malcom SJ. Observations of the loss of cathecholaminea fluorescence during pregnancy in the guinea pig. *J Reprod Fertil* 1978;53:51–8.
43. Falk B, Owman C, Rosengren E, Sjogren NO. Reduction by progesterone of the estrogen-induced increase in transmitter level of the short adrenergic neurons innervating the uterus. *Endocrinology* 1969;84:958–9.
44. Ryan MJ, Clark KE, Brody MJ. Neurogenic and mechanical control of canine uterine vascular resistance. *Am J Physiol* 1974;227:547–55.

45. Ramsey EM, Corner GW Jr, Donner MW. Serial and cineradioangiographic visualization of maternal circulation in the primate (hemochonial) placenta. *Am J Obstet Gynecol* 1963;86:213–25.
46. Wigglesworth JS. Experimental growth retardation in the fetal rat. *J Pathol Bacteriol* 1964;88:1.
47. Dawes GS. The placenta and foetal growth. In: Dawes GS, ed. *Foetal and neonatal physiology.* Chicago: Year Book Medical Publishers, 1968.
48. Creasy RK, Barrett CT, de Swiet M, et al. Experimental intrauterine growth retardation in the sheep. *Am J Obstet Gynecol* 1972;112:566.
49. Dixon HG, Browne JCM, Davey DA. Choriodecidual and myometrial blood flow. *Lancet* 1963; 2:369.
50. Caldero-Barcia R. Fetal malnutrition: The role of maternal blood flow. *Hosp Prac* 1970;43.
51. Brosens I, Dixon HG, Robertson WB. Fetal growth retardation and the arteries of the placental bed. *Br J Obstet Gynecol* 1977;84:656.
52. Theobald GW. Sympathetic nerves and eclampsia. *Br Med J* 1953;1:422.
53. Andrews MC, Jones HW Jr. Impaired reproductive performance of the unicornuate uterus: intrauterine growth retardation, infertility and recurrent abortions in five cases. *Am J Obstet Gynecol* 1982;144:173.
54. Varma TR. Fetal growth. *J Obstet Gynecol Br Commonw* 1973;80:311.
55. Campbell S, Diaz-Recasen SJ, Griffin DR, et al. New Doppler technique for assessing uteroplacental blood flow. *Lancet* 1983;675–7.
56. Griffin, Cohen-Overbee KT, Campbell S. Fetal and uteroplacental blood flow. In: Campbell S, ed. *Clinics in obstetrics and gynecology.* Philadelphia: WB Saunders, 1983;565–602.
57. Fleisher A, Schulman H, et al. Uterine artery Doppler velocimetry in pregnant women with hypertension. *Am J Obstet Gynecol* 1986;154:806–13.
58. Kaar K, Joupilla P, Kuikka J, et al. Intervillous blood flow in normal and complicated late pregnancy measured by means of intravenous 133 XE method. *Acta Obstet Gynecol Scand* 1980;59: 7–10.
59. Lunell NO, Sarby B, Lewander R, Nylund L. Comparison of uteroplacental blood flow in normal and in intrauterine growth-retarded pregnancy. *Gynecol Obstet Invest* 1979;10:106–18.
60. Joupilla P, Kirkinen P, et al. Ritodrine infusion during late pregnancy: effect on fetal and placental blood flow, prostacyclin, and thromboxane. *J Obstet Gynecol* 1985;151:1028–32.
61. Benirschke K. Multiple gestation incidence, etiology, and inheritance in maternal-fetal medicine. Creasy RK, Resnik RR, eds. Philadelphia: WB Saunders, 1986;519–21.
62. Naeye RL. Unsuspected organ abnormalities associated with congenital heart disease. *Am J Pathol* 1965;47:905.
63. Froehlich LA, Fujikura R. Significance of a single umbilical artery. *Am J Obstet Gynecol* 1966;94:274.
64. Emmanouilides GC, Townsend DE, Bauer RA. Effects of single artery ligation in the lamb fetus. *Pediatrics* 1968;42:919.
65. Cooper KE, Greenfield ADM, et al. The umbilical blood flow in the fetal sheep. *J Physiol (London)* 1949;108:160.
66. Dawes GS. The umbilical circulation. *Am J Obstet Gynecol* 1962;84:1634.
67. Meschia G, Cotter JR, Makowski EL, Barron DH. Simultaneous measurement of uterine and umbilical blood flows and oxygen uptake. *Q J Exp Physiol* 1982;52:1.
68. Rudolph AM, Heymann MA. The circulation of the fetus in utero: methods for studying the distribution of blood flow, cardiac output and organ blood flow. *Circ Res* 1967;21:163.
69. Rudolph AM. Factors affecting umbilical blood flow in the lamb in utero. In: Rooth G, Bratteby LE, eds. *Perinatal medicine.* Stockholm: Almguist Wiksell, 1976.
70. Toubas PL, Silverman N, Heymann M, Rudolph AM. Cardiovascular effects of acute hemorrhage in fetal lambs. *Am J Physiol (Heart Circ. Physiol. 9)* 1981;240:H45–8.
71. Aherne W, Dunnill MS. Morphometry of the human placenta. *Br Med Bull* 1966;22:(1)5–12.
72. Ahokas RA, Reynolds SL, Anderson GD, Lipschi J. Maternal organ distribution of cardiac output in the diet-restricted pregnant rat. *J Nutr* 1984;114:2262–8.
73. Goodlin RC, Quaife MA, Dirksen JW. The significance, diagnosis, and treatment of maternal hypovolemia as associated with fetal/maternal illness. *Semin Perinatol* 1981;5:163.
74. Ahokas RA, Reynolds SL, Anderson GD, Lipschi J. Catecholamine-mediated reduction in uteroplacental blood flow in the diet-restricted, term pregnant rat. *J Nutr* 1986;116:412–8.
75. Keirse MJ. Epidemiology and etiology of the growth-retarded baby. *Clin Obstet Gynecol* 1984;11:415–36.

76. Mochizvki M, Marvo T, Musuko K, et al. Effects of smoking on feto-placental maternal system during pregnancy. *Am J Obstet Gynecol* 1984;149:413–20.
77. Pirani B B K. Smoking during pregnancy. *Obstet Gynecol Surg* 1978;33:1–13.
78. Socol ML, Manning FA, et al. Maternal smoking causes fetal hypoxia: Experimental evidence. *Am J Obstet Gynecol* 1982;142:214.
79. Rauramo I, Ilkka, Forss M, et al. Antepartum fetal heart rate variability and intervillous placental blood flow in association with smoking. *Am J Obstet Gynecol* 1983;146:967.
80. Poupilla P, Kirkinen P, et al. Acute effect of maternal smoking on the human fetal blood flow. *Br J Obstet Gynaecol* 1983;90:7–10.

DISCUSSION

Dr. Bossart: My question concerns fetal bradycardia. It seems to me more logical to assume that if you have maternal hypoxia, you should get a fetal *tachycardia* to overcome this situation.

Dr. Toubas: In the adult the response to a low oxygen tension is tachycardia. However, in the fetus the situation is different. If we give the mother a gas mixture containing, say, 9% oxygen to breathe, this results in very severe hypoxia. The fetal pO_2 will go down by about 12 mm Hg, but the fetal response is to redistribute the cardiac output to preserve the placental and brain circulation. As long as the hypoxemia does not become too severe the heart rate changes little. However, if the hypoxia is prolonged and significant, fetal hypoxemia occurs and the next result is that fetal hypertension develops, and when this occurs the result is bradycardia (1).

Dr. Bossart: Are you saying that the bradycardia is mediated through baroreceptors and not through a direct effect of hypoxia on the myocardium? My understanding has been that the first effect of hypoxemia is that it triggers a tachycardia, after which bradycardia occurs through a direct effect on the myocardium, not indirectly through baro- or chemoreceptors.

Dr. Toubas: I have shown that the bradycardia is mediated through baroreceptors and does not appear to be a direct response to hypoxia.

Dr. Senterre: I think this is a very important question. I am not sure that everyone will agree with the explanation that hypoxia leads to fetal bradycardia by a baroreceptor-mediated effect and not by a direct effect on the fetal myocardium.

Dr. Marini: Is this baroreceptor-mediated phenomenon the same at all gestations or is it related to the development of the neurological control of the heart? The reason I ask is that in the human, certain arrhythmias may show different pharmacological responses in the fetus and in the neonate. The sympathetic innervation of the heart is not well developed before 32 weeks gestation, but parasympathetic innervation is. Perhaps there is a different response to hypoxia depending on the development of the autonomic innervation of the heart.

Dr. Toubas: We must differentiate acute from chronic hypoxia. In this workshop, we are discussing intrauterine growth retardation, which is a chronic condition. I agree that in acute conditions changes in heart rate may be mediated in other ways, but in the fetus with intrauterine growth retardation (IUGR), we cannot use heart rate as an indicator of the nutritional status of the baby—it is too imprecise. Doppler ultrasound measurements of uteroplacental blood flow (when the technique will be more advanced) will provide more valuable information.

Dr. Bossart: I should like to know your views on catecholamines and prostaglandins from a clinical point of view. Do you think the dosage of catecholamines used in local anesthesia or that of prostaglandins used to induce labor may be dangerous for the (stressed) fetus?

Dr. Toubas: This really needs to be answered by an obstetrician. However, it is known that lidocaine may be dangerous to the fetus because it has depressant effects on the circulation and may induce seizures (2).

Dr. Chessex: I have a partial answer to Dr. Bossart's question. There was a good review in the *Scientific American* called ''The Stress of Being Born'' which discussed catecholamine excretion, comparing the newborn with stressed adults. At delivery, catecholamine excretion was 20 times higher in the infant than in stressed adults during surgery. I should like to ask Dr. Toubas a question. You showed that catecholamines and prostaglandins affect the placental blood flow. What effect would maternal malnutrition have in relation to the secretion of these hormones?

Dr. Toubas: When a mother is malnourished, she does not expand her blood volume—her total blood volume is in fact reduced. It has been shown that catecholamines are involved in this (3), and urinary excretion of catecholamines is increased. Malnutrition, lack of nutrition, and the search for food lead to permanent anxiety.

Dr. Marini: I was always impressed by the fact that, when you work with sheep, the animals are caged. What is the birthweight of the lambs in these caged animals in comparison with animals which are free? Does the enforced inactivity of the caged animal affect fetal growth?

Dr. Toubas: When we study sheep you must realize that we do many other things apart from restraining them; they have catheters implanted, surgical procedures, etc. Surgery per se has an effect—for example, if we operate on runted animals with a high hematocrit, these animals will die. We have to treat all these pregnant animals, whether sheep, rats, or guinea pigs, with caution. Chronically catheterized sheep are not kept in a cage; more precisely they are restrained in a space of about 6 m² and certainly remain quiet and active. In general they are not stressed by the experimenters. Fetal growth in these animals, from serial measurement of biparietal diameter, is somewhat slower than in the natural state. I think this is likely due to the invasiveness of the preparation and perhaps sepsis as well! Your point about maternal exercise is an interesting one. Experiments have been done in pregnant rats (4) showing that if they are exercised intensively there is a diminution in birthweight and a fair number of pups will die. So I think that intensive maternal work may well play a role in fetal growth retardation.

Dr. Guesry: I think this subject needs a little more discussion. Physical exercise in developing countries is often combined with malnutrition and with long hours of standing, which may also impair the uterine circulation. Do you have any information on sport? In industrialized societies, there are now more pregnant women swimming for long distances, for example, which may divert blood flow from uterus to muscles. Are there any animal experiments on this?

Dr. Toubas: There are some rat data (4). Rats have a gestation period of 21 days. If you exercise pregnant dams quite hard between days 1 and 12 of pregnancy, there is no effect at all. However, if you exercise them throughout pregnancy or between days 12 and 21 there is a decrease in the number of surviving pups. The authors of this work did not study uterine blood flow but they speculated that it decreased during exercise.

Dr. Bossart: It is worth remembering tests which have been used by obstetricians in clinical situations. When fetal heart rate monitoring first became popular, in Eastern European countries obstetricians developed the ''Step Test''! When they were worried about the progress of a pregnancy, especially IUGR, they made the mother step on and off a chair for a minute and then measured fetal heart rate with a stethoscope. If it was slow, they assumed placental insufficiency and delivered the baby.

Dr. Priolisi: Can you give an estimate, even a rough one, of the critical level of umbilical blood flow below which fetal growth starts to falter?

Dr. Toubas: This is a very important question. The total delivery of oxygen which arrives to the fetus is about 25 ml per kg body weight, of which the fetus only consumes about 8 ml per kg. The placenta is a very active metabolic organ and uses about the same amount. The remaining 9 ml or so is surplus to requirements. The placental blood flow has to decrease very markedly indeed in order to impair oxygen delivery to the fetus, certainly below about 500 ml per min. The fetus also has the ability in this situation to extract more oxygen. However, there is a difference between the human and the sheep: the human fetus can achieve a higher extraction than the sheep fetus.

Dr. Canosa: You spoke about blood pressure in the mother in relation to fetal and placental blood flow. It is well known that many mothers in developing countries have hypotension, syptolic, diastolic and mean blood pressure during pregnancy. Could you comment on whether this may be deleterious to fetal growth?

Dr. Toubas: Again, I need an obstetrician's help! I cannot answer this question, but I shall make a general comment about the interpretation of blood pressure. I think we should pay attention not only to systolic and diastolic blood pressure, but to mean blood pressure as well. Also, the technique of measurement is of extreme importance.

Dr. Bossart: I can comment on hypotension. Saling (5) in Berlin did a very good study on this and concluded that it is one of the causes of fetal growth retardation. It is of course well-known that the measurement of blood pressure using the cuff method is not easy to interpret (cuff-effect).

Dr. Marini: I have some data on hypotension from the U.S. collaborative study. Birthweight of the infants increased when maternal diastolic pressure rose from 60 to 90 mmHg. I think this must be related to increasing maternal blood volume. It was also found that women with lower hemoglobin concentrations during the third trimester had larger babies, which would be compatible with hemodilutional "anemia" in women with greater than normal plasma volume expansion.

Dr. Rosso: I should like to comment on some of the hemodynamic changes which occur in relation to maternal nutrition. We need to consider two different kinds of nutritional problems in pregnant women: *acute malnutrition* occurring during gestation and reflected in a low gestational weight gain; and *chronic undernutrition,* where in many cases the woman's growth may have been stunted because of malnutrition during early life. This is common in developing countries, affected women being short and underweight with a ponderal index. In chronic undernutrition, we have found that plasma volume is reduced in proportion to measures of body size, and at the end of pregnancy plasma volume is still reduced. When there is superimposed acute malnutrition it appears that there are two factors operating to put the fetus at risk. On the one hand, there is the low plasma volume, and on the other there is the increased catecholamine secretion which accompanies acute malnutrition and which further reduces placental blood flow. In our rat model which you referred to, we think that the increased catecholamine excretion may have an extremely important role in impairing uterine blood flow, whereas in humans it would only become important if the mother goes through a prolonged period of fasting or very low energy intake.

Dr. Hay: In studies of chronically prepared animals, it appears that reductions in uteroplacental or umbilical blood flow, regardless of how they are measured, have to be of the order of 50% or more before a reduction in transfer of nutrients to the fetus occurs. This suggests that minor reductions in flow may not affect fetal supply. In the second place, I am not aware of any studies which have looked at perfusion of different parts of the placenta. I am concerned that one of the major changes may not be overall flow, but the amount of placental tissue that is perfused. We know quite well that regional variations in perfusion occur in other organs, for example the lung, and I think it possible that portions of the placenta are under-perfused a good part of the time. Many of the changes that we see which might affect trans-port could be a reflection of poor regional perfusion, and an increase in flow to these areas might be expected to improve the transport capacity markedly. Could you discuss these is-sues, and especially in relation to your presentation concerning the pulsatility index? Could this be used to explore the perfusion of parts of the placenta?

Dr. Toubas: I was trying to say that flow is not the whole story, and I am sure you are right in this. The pulsatility index originated from Campbell's team in Great Britain (6,7), arising out of studies of flow in the uterine umbilical arteries and the arcuate vessels using continuous pulsed Doppler techniques. There are problems with such techniques, however; for example, if the probe does not have the correct angle of inclination with respect to the blood vessel the measurement of flow is very difficult. This precludes the use of actual flow values, but it is still possible to construct velocity curves and, by comparing such curves, to derive indices. Work is currently proceeding in baboons to try to validate these indices against actual mea-surements of blood flow using implanted electromagnetic flow probes. However, even with these sophisticated techniques there are problems. For example, the caliber of the vessels changes during pregnancy and an implanted flow probe may create a restriction after a time, which itself will alter flow. New technology will probably overcome these difficulties, but for the moment it is not completely clear what the pulsatility index is measuring.

Dr. Alves Filho: How important is smoking in causing fetal pathology? In Brazil we have a huge problem with smoking, with over 40% of women from the lower socio-economic classes smoking during pregnancy.

Dr. Toubas: We have the same problem in the United States, where about 36% of the pop-ulation smoke. One also has to consider the possible effects of passive smoking (smoke from other people's cigarettes inhaled by the mother). We do not have at the present time good data indicating that smoking has a direct effect on the fetus. The observed effects on fetal growth probably result from indirect actions. I have done some experiments on pregnant sheep where nicotine was directly injected into the fetus, and this had measurable effects on fetal brain function, but to obtain this effect we had to inject a dose of nicotine equivalent to the amount found in one pack of cigarettes. Nevertheless, the implication is that there is probably a direct and harmful effect on the fetus. Smoking may also be implicated in apnea of prematurity and sudden infant death syndrome, since there is a correlation between the duration of apneic epi-sodes and amount of maternal smoking.

REFERENCES

1. Rudolf AM, Heymann MA. *Fetal and neonatal physiology. Proceedings of the Joseph Bancroft Sym-posium.* Cambridge: Cambridge University Press, 1972;89–111.
2. Teramo K, Benowitz N, Heymann MA, Kahanpaa K, Siimes A, Rudolph AM. Effects of lidocaine on heart rate, blood pressure and electrocorticogram in fetal sheep. *Am J Obstet Gynecol* 1974;118:935–49.
3. Ahokas RA, Reynolds SL, Anderson GD, Lipschi J. Catecholamine-mediated reduction in uteropla-cental blood flow in the diet-restricted, term pregnant rat. *J Nutr* 1986;116:412–8.
4. Garris DR, Kasperek GJ, Overton SV, Alligood GR Jr. Effects of excercise on fetal-placental growth and uteroplacental blood flow in the rat. *Biol Neonate* 1985;47:223–9.
5. Saling et al. *Geburtsh Frauenheilk* 1985;45:525–33.
6. Campbell S, Diaz-Recasen SJ, Griffin DR, et al. New Doppler technique for assessing utero-placen-tal blood flow. *Lancet* 1983;2:675–7.
7. Griffin, Cohen-Overbee KT, Campbell S. Fetal and utero-placental blood flow. In: Campbell S, ed. *Clinics in obstetrics and gynecology.* Philadelphia: WB Saunders, 1983:565–602.

Intrauterine Growth Retardation, edited by
Jacques Senterre. Nestlé Nutrition Workshop
Series, Vol. 18. Nestec Ltd., Vevey/Raven Press,
Ltd., New York © 1989.

Hormonal Regulation of Fetal Growth

Jean Girard

*Centre de Recherche sur la Nutrition (CNRS),
92190 Meudon-Bellevue, France*

The regulation of fetal growth is complex and still very poorly understood. It involves genetic factors, maternal nutrition and cardiovascular adaptations, placental growth and function, and to a lesser extent fetal factors, including fetal hormones. The influence of genetic, maternal, and placental factors on fetal growth has been reviewed recently (1) and will not be discussed. The purpose of this chapter is to analyze the specific role of endocrine factors in the determination of fetal growth, assuming that the nutritional supply to the placenta and to the fetus remains unaltered.

The major endocrine factors involved in postnatal growth are: (a) growth hormone (GH) via the secretion of somatomedin; (b) thyroid hormones; (c) cortisol; and (d) sex steroids at puberty (2,3). Insulin is considered to have a merely permissive role in postnatal growth (2,3). In recent years, a body of evidence has accumulated to indicate that the fetus may be less dependent on pituitary and thyroid hormones for growth than the older organism, and more dependent on insulin and tissue growth factors. Studies on the endocrine regulation of fetal growth have involved several major approaches: ablation of fetal endocrine glands; examination of newborns with congenital endocrine deficiencies; treatment of fetuses with hormones; measurement of plasma hormone concentrations and tissue receptor levels during normal or abnormal growth; and *in vitro* studies of hormone effects on fetal tissues. We shall consider principally the changes in fetal body weight in response to variations of fetal endocrine environment. However, it must be remembered that fetal growth also involves changes in body length and in body composition. This is particularly important for the human fetus which accumulates a large amount of fat in the last trimester of pregnancy. In contrast, the fetus from most other species does not accumulate fat before birth (4) (Table 1).

FETAL PITUITARY HORMONES

As maternal growth hormone is not transferred across the placenta, the fetus is entirely dependent on its pituitary gland for GH production. The possible role of GH in fetal growth has been studied in several species by depriving the fetus of its pitu-

TABLE 1. *Body fat content in the newborn of different species*

Species	Body fat (g/100 g body weight)
Human	16
Monkey	2
Pig	1
Sheep	3
Guinea pig	10
Rabbit	6
Rat	2

itary gland *in utero*. The first experiments of this kind were performed on rabbit fetuses by Jost in 1947 (reviewed in 5,6). He deprived rabbit fetuses of their pituitary glands by decapitation *in utero* on day 19 to 23 of gestation (normal term in this species is 32 days) and found that growth of the remaining body was not affected by the lack of pituitary until 28 to 29 days of gestation (Fig. 1). This was confirmed in other species, for example, the rat, mouse, and pig (6,7). In the fetal lamb and monkey, hypophysectomy causes growth retardation (8,9), but pituitary stalk section or encephalectomy is not associated with growth retardation (10,11). As fetal hypophysectomy induces both GH and thyroid hormone deficiency, whereas encephalectomy or pituitary stalk section causes only GH deficiency (12), it has been concluded that growth retardation due to fetal hypophysectomy resulted from thyroid hormone deficiency. In the human, anencephaly and congenital absence of the pituitary, conditions resulting in GH deficiency, are not associated with reduced size and weight at birth (reviewed in 6). Fetal decapitation in the rabbit does not decrease

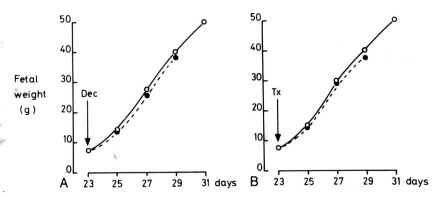

FIG. 1. Effects of fetal decapitation (**A**) or fetal thyroidectomy (**B**) on day 23 of gestation on fetal growth in the rabbit. (Data from refs. 5 and 6.) Dec, decapitation; Tx, thyroidectomy.

fetal weight but increases fetal body lipids (5). Similar observations have been made in the hypophysectomized fetal lamb (8) and in human anencephaly (6).

These studies show that normal fetal growth is possible when GH is lacking or is markedly reduced. GH-dependent growth is not observed until well after birth in most species: 6 months in the human, 3 months in the rabbit, 1 month in the rat, and 1 week in the sheep. The basis for the lack of an effect of GH on fetal growth is not entirely explained, but appears to be due to a lack of GH receptors in fetal tissues as these are important for the production of insulin-like growth factors. In the lamb, hepatic GH receptors are only demonstrated 3 to 6 days after birth (13). In the rat, liver GH receptors are also markedly reduced in early life when compared to adults (14,15).

THYROID HORMONES

Thyroid hormones are not transferred from the mother to the fetus and the fetus is dependent on its own thyroid gland for thyroid hormone production. Fetal thyroidectomy of the rabbit fetus on day 22 or 23 of gestation does not impair normal fetal growth (5,6) (Fig. 1) but results in a 30% increase in body lipids, which are maintained at normal levels by thyroxine injection at the time of thyroidectomy (5).

Thyroidectomy in sheep and monkey fetuses causes a significant inhibition (10% to 30%) of their growth (16,17). In contrast, human newborns suffering of congenital hypothyroidism, or radiothyroidectomized *in utero* by radioactive iodine given inadvisedly to the mother, have a normal size and weight at birth (6,18–21). Thus, thyroid hormones appear to have little effect on fetal growth in most species, but they are essential for normal neural and osseous maturation in sheep and man (20,21).

INSULIN

The concept that insulin might be an important hormone for fetal growth arose primarily from clinical observations associated with insulin excess or insulin deficiency. The infants of diabetic mothers are larger (on average 500 g) and somewhat longer (on average 1.5 cm) than control infants (22), though most of the overweight is due to lipid deposition (23,24). Since the excessive growth becomes obvious after the 28th week (25), at a time where fetal pancreas becomes sensitive to glucose (reviewed in 26), it has been suggested that maternal hyperglycemia is attended by fetal hyperglycemia which in turn stimulates insulin secretion by the fetal pancreas and induces fetal macrosomia (reviewed in 22). In contrast, newborns with pancreatic agenesis have profound intrauterine growth retardation (birthweight: 1.2 to 1.5 kg at term) associated with deficient adipose tissue and a decrease in muscle mass (27,28). Infants with transient neonatal diabetes also have a defect in insulin secretion which is associated with a low birthweight (27,29). These infants have reduced adipose tissue and a stunted muscle mass which undergoes rapid development with

postnatal insulin treatment (30). The birth size of infants born with marked fetal hypoinsulinemia suggests that the human fetus can reach the size of a 30 to 32 week
gestation fetus independently of insulin. This is compatible with the fact that fat deposition in the fetus occurs in the third trimester of pregnancy and is clearly insulin-
dependent. → imp for window of vulnerability

Several studies have recently been performed in animals to analyze the effects of
insulin on fetal growth (Table 2). Injection of large amounts of insulin into the rat
fetus during the last 3 days of gestation increases body weight, total lipids and nitrogen, and the ratio lipids to protein (31). Infusion of insulin (19 U/day) for 28 days
into the fetal rhesus monkey produces a 20% to 30% increase in fetal body weight
(32,33). Infusion of insulin for 14 days in fetal pigs has no effect on fetal weight but
has been shown to cause a significant increase in liver and muscle glycogen levels
and in body fat (34, Table 2). Insulin infusion for 18 days, but at a relatively low
rate, in the fetal lamb has no effect on fetal body weight (35). Thus, most of these
studies suggest that chronic hyperinsulinemia can produce a modest increase in fetal
body weight, mainly due to increase in body fat. However, all these studies have
been performed in species in which fat deposition does not occur before birth (4)
(Table 1). It is obvious that the fetal guinea pig or rabbit, which normally accumulate body fat in late pregnancy (Table 1), should be better experimental models than
the fetal monkey, sheep, pig, or rat to study the effects of insulin on fetal growth
and adiposity.

Experimental fetal hypoinsulinemia has been induced in some studies by the administration of streptozotocin in the fetal rabbit, lamb, or monkey (36–38). Streptozotocin produces fetal growth retardation in those species (36–38) but the data were
difficult to interpret as this drug may have direct toxic effects on tissues other than
the endocrine pancreas. The demonstration that the pancreas is necessary for normal
growth has been made recently in the lamb. Fetal surgical pancreatectomy in the
lamb at 113 to 121 days of gestation is associated with a 25% decrease in body
weight at 139 days gestation (39).

TABLE 2. *Effects of chronic fetal hyperinsulinemia on fetal weight at term*

	Species	Plasma insulin (μU/ml)	Body weight (g)	Body fat (g/100 g body wt)	Reference number
Rat	Control	—	5.83 ± 0.48	2.47 ± 0.27	31
	Insulin	—	6.67 ± 0.30*	2.94 ± 0.07*	
Monkey	Control	28 ± 12	372 ± 54	—	33
	Insulin	340 ± 208*	459 ± 53*	—	
Pig	Control	285 ± 82	829 ± 36	1.05 ± 0.09	34
	Insulin	2,376 ± 576*	855 ± 42	1.25 ± 0.05*	
Sheep	Control	7 ± 1	3,451 ± 194	—	35
	Insulin	31 ± 7*	3,544 ± 203	—	

*$p < 0.05$ when compared with control.

In addition, a positive correlation between fetal plasma insulin level and fetal body weight at term has been reported in the rat, rabbit, and guinea pig (40–42). This suggests that insulin could not only have a permissive role but also a regulatory role in normal fetal growth.

THE INSULIN-LIKE GROWTH FACTORS

The terms somatomedin (SM) and insulin-like growth factors (IGF) are synonymous. Somatomedin A and C are analogous to IGF-I, i.e., a 70 amino acid peptide encoded by a gene on human chromosome 12, whereas multiplication stimulating activity (MSA) discovered in the rat is equivalent to IGF-II, a 67 amino acid peptide encoded by a gene on human chromosome 11. The IGFs share a large structural homology with proinsulin (reviewed in 43).

Plasma Concentrations

IGFs do not cross the placenta (44) and the IGF-I and IGF-II found in fetal plasma in various species are produced by fetal tissues. The concentration of IGF-I is low in fetal plasma in early pregnancy in the sheep, mouse, rat, and human and it increases during gestation (Fig. 2), though it is lower at term than the levels found in the adult (reviewed in 26,45–50). In human infants, the plasma IGF-I concentration is positively correlated with birthweight (51). In the sheep and rat, the concentration of MSA or IGF-II in fetal plasma is higher than during the postnatal period (52,53). In human infants, plasma IGF-II concentration increases during gestation (Fig. 2) and is also positively correlated with birthweight (54).

In plasma, somatomedins (7.5 Kd) are bound to larger carrier proteins (40 and

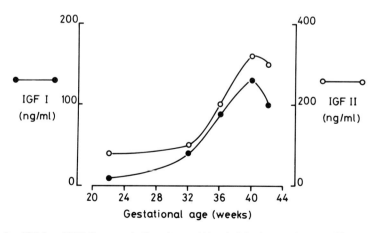

FIG. 2. IGF-I and IGF-II concentrations in cord blood of the human fetuses. (From ref. 54.)

150 Kd) that prevent rapid fluctuations in somatomedin concentrations by prolong-ing their half-life in plasma. This provides a mechanism whereby somatomedin could be delivered continuously to fetal tissues. In the fetus, IGFs circulate primar-ily bound to the 40 Kd carrier protein, whereas in the adult, IGFs circulate bound to the 150 Kd carrier protein. This larger protein is GH-dependent and appears in late gestation or in the postnatal period.

Endocrine Control of IGF Secretion

After birth, the liver is the principal site for IGF-I production and this is under GH control (2,3). In the fetus, IGF-I production is not controlled by GH. Indeed, fetal decapitation, hypophysectomy, or electrocoagulation of the hypothalamus of the lamb or rabbit abolishes GH from the fetal circulation but has no effect on circulat-ing somatomedin or IGF levels (55–58). Moreover, GH fails to stimulate IGF secre-tion by the rat fetus (15) or by cultured fetal rat myoblasts (59). In addition, human anencephalic infants have normal somatomedin levels in cord blood (46,49).

In the fetal lamb, plasma IGF-I concentration is reduced, whereas IGF-II is in-creased after pancreatectomy (60) or streptozotocin administration (37). Infants with transient neonatal diabetes have low levels of IGF-I in cord blood but normal IGF-II levels (61). Insulin infusion in rabbit, pig, or monkey fetuses is associated with increased plasma somatomedin levels (62–64). Moreover, insulin increases IGF-I production by cultured fetal rat myoblasts (65) but is without effect on IGF-II re-lease by cultured fetal rat hepatocytes (66).

Placental lactogen (PL) is produced by the placental trophoblast in some species (human, sheep, rat) and is secreted into the fetal circulation, but at a much lower rate than into the maternal circulation (67). The major physiological role of PL was thought to be the mobilization of maternal energy stores, through its action as an in-sulin antagonist (67), but it is also thought to stimulate maternal IGF secretion (68). More recently, it has been reported that ovine PL stimulates amino acid uptake by fetal rat muscles, glycogen synthesis by fetal rat liver, and IGF-II release by rat fi-broblasts (69–71). Human PL has been shown to stimulate somatomedin release in cultured human fetal myoblasts and fibroblasts (72). However, although the evi-dence that PL has a role in prenatal growth is strong, this hormone is not essential. Indeed, PL is not secreted by the placenta of several species (rabbit, pig, etc.) and infusion of an antiserum to PL for 3 and 6 days in the fetal lamb did not decrease IGF-I or -II concentrations (49). In addition, newborn infants delivered to women devoid of PL are of normal size and weight at birth, even though plasma IGF-I in maternal plasma was very low (73,74).

Paracrine or Autocrine Functions

It has been shown that IGF-I and -II are produced by a large number of fetal tis-sues in rodents (Fig. 3) and humans, and are present in these tissues far in excess of amounts that can be accounted for by contamination from blood (75–77). On the ba-

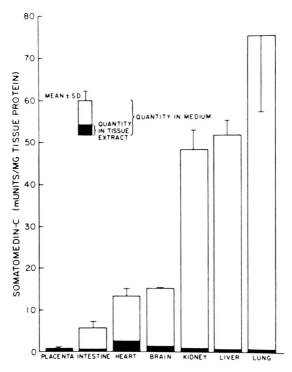

FIG. 3. Somatomedin-C (IGF-I) concentration in extract and in incubation medium of tissues from fetal mouse. (From ref. 76.)

sis of these findings, the classical concept that IGFs could act as endocrine factors, i.e., molecules synthesized and secreted by an organ in the body which pass via the bloodstream to exert their actions distantly, has been progressively abandoned for the concept of paracrine or autocrine function, i.e., molecules synthesized and secreted by an organ and acting at or near their site of production (Fig. 4) (78). As

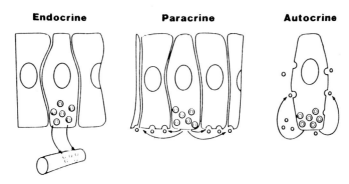

FIG. 4. Schematic view of endocrine, paracrine, and autocrine roles of trophic hormones. (From ref. 3.)

IGF-I and IGF-II stimulate DNA synthesis by human fetal myoblasts, fibroblasts, and chondrocytes (79–81), these locally produced mitogens would be readily available for regulating tissue growth. However, the importance of paracrine/autocrine mechanisms relative to the traditional endocrine actions of IGFs is not clear, and it is possible that IGFs act through all three mechanisms.

REFERENCES

1. Gluckman PD, Liggins GC. Regulation of fetal growth. In: Beard R W, Nathanielsz PW, eds. *Fetal physiology and medicine*. London: WB Saunders, 1984;511–57.
2. Daughaday WH, Herington AC, Phillips LS. The regulation of growth by the endocrines. *Ann Rev Physiol* 1975;37:211–44.
3. Underwood LE, Van Wyk JJ. Normal and aberrant growth. In: Wilson JD, Foster DW, eds. *Textbook of endocrinology*. Philadelphia: WB Saunders, 1985;155–205.
4. Widdowson EM. Chemical composition of newly born mammals. *Nature* 1950;166:626–8.
5. Jost A, Picon L. Hormonal control of fetal development and metabolism. *Adv Metab Dis* 1970;4:123–84.
6. Jost A. Fetal hormones and fetal growth. In: Keller PJ, ed. *Gynecologic and obstetric investigation*. Basel: S. Karger, 1979;1–20.
7. Colenbrander B, Van Rossum-Kok CMJE, Van Straaten HWM, Wensing CJG. The effect of fetal decapitation on the testis and other endocrine organs of the pig. *Biol Reprod* 1979;20:198–204.
8. Liggins GC, Kennedy PC. Effects of electrocoagulation of the foetal lamb hypophysis on growth and development. *J Endocr* 1968;40:371–81.
9. Novy MJ, Aubert ML, Kaplan SL, Grumbach MM. Regulation of placental growth and chorionic somatomammotropin in the Rhesus monkey: effects of protein deprivation, fetal anencephaly, and placental vessel ligations. *Am J Obstet Gynecol* 1981;140:552–62.
10. Liggins GC. The influence of the fetal hypothalamus and pituitary on growth. In: Elliott K, Knight J, eds. *Size at birth*. Ciba Fdn Symp, no. 27. Amsterdam: Elsevier, 1974;165–83.
11. Kittinger GW. Endocrine regulation of fetal development and its relation to parturition in the Rhesus monkey. In: O'Connor M, Knight J, eds. *The fetus and birth*. Ciba Fdn Symp, no. 47. Amsterdam: Elsevier, 1977;235–49.
12. Gluckman PD, Grumbach MM, Kaplan SL. The neuroendocrine regulation and function of growth hormone and prolactin in the mammalian fetus. *Endocrine Rev* 1981;2:363–95.
13. Gluckman PD, Butler J, Elliot T. The ontogeny of somatotropic binding sites in ovine hepatic membranes. *Endocrinology* 1983;112:1607–12.
14. Kelly PA, Posner BI, Tsushima T, Friesen HG. Studies of insulin, growth hormone and prolactin binding: ontogenesis, effects of sex and pregnancy. *Endocrinology* 1974;95:532–9.
15. Flandez B, Alvarez E, Blasquez E. Delayed appearance of liver growth hormone binding sites and of growth hormone-induced somatomedin production during rat development. *Biochem Biophys Res Comm* 1986;136:38–44.
16. Hopkins PS, Thorburn GD. The effects of foetal thyroidectomy on the development of the ovine foetus. *J Endocr* 1972;54:55–66.
17. Kerr GR, Tyson IB, Allen JR, Wallace J, Scheffler G. Deficiency of thyroid hormone and development of the fetal Rhesus monkey. *Biol Neonate* 1972;21:282–95.
18. Anderson HJ. Studies of hypothyroidism in children. *Acta Paediatr Scand* 1961;suppl.125:1–50.
19. Maenpaa J. Congenital hypothyroidism. Aetiology and clinical aspects. *Arch Dis Child* 1972;47:914–23.
20. Thorburn GD. The role of the thyroid gland and kidneys in fetal growth. In: Elliott K, Knight J, eds. *Size at birth*. Ciba Fdn Symp, no. 27. Amsterdam: Elsevier, 1974;185–200.
21. Robinson JS, Kingston EJ, Thorburn GD. Physiological and endocrine factors in human fetal growth. *Postgrad Med J* 1978;54,suppl 1:51–61.
22. Pedersen J. *The pregnant diabetic and her newborn. Problems and management*. Copenhagen: Munksgaard, 1977.
23. Osler M, Pedersen J. The body composition of newborn infants of diabetic mothers. *Pediatrics* 1960;26:985–92.

24. Fee BA, Weil WB. Body composition of infants of diabetic mothers by direct analysis. *Ann NY Acad Sci* 1963;11:869–97.
25. Cardell BS. The infants of diabetic mothers: a morphological study. *J Obstet Gynaecol Br Commonw* 1953;60:834–53.
26. Milner RDG, Hill DJ. Fetal growth control: the role of insulin and related peptides. *Clin Endocrinol* 1984;21:415–33.
27. Hill DE. Effects of insulin on fetal growth. *Sem Perinatol* 1978;2:319–28.
28. Lemons JA, Ridenour R, Orsini EN. Congenital absence of the pancreas and intrauterine growth retardation. *Pediatrics* 1979;64:255–6.
29. Hill DE. Fetal effects of insulin. *Obstet Gynaecol Ann* 1982;11:133–49.
30. Schiff D, Colle E, Stern L. Metabolic and growth patterns in transient neonatal diabetes. *N Engl J Med* 1972;287:119–22.
31. Picon L. Effect of insulin on growth and biochemical composition of the rat fetus. *Endocrinology* 1967;81:1419–21.
32. Susa JB, McCormick KL, Widness JA, et al. Chronic hyperinsulinemia in the fetal rhesus monkey. Effects on fetal growth and composition. *Diabetes* 1979;28:1058–63.
33. Susa JB, Neave C, Sehgal P, Singer DB, Zeller WP, Schwartz R. Chronic hyperinsulinemia in the fetal rhesus monkey. Effects of physiologic hyperinsulinemia on fetal growth and composition. *Diabetes* 1984;33:656–60.
34. Garssen GJ, Spencer GSG, Colenbrander B, MacDonald AA, Hill DJ. Lack of effect of chronic hyperinsulinemia on growth and body composition in the fetal pig. *Biol Neonate* 1983;44:234–42.
35. Milley JR. The effect of chronic hyperinsulinemia on ovine fetal growth. *Growth* 1986;50:390–401.
36. Fletcher JM, Bassett JM. Effects of streptozotocin injection into fetal rabbits on their subsequent growth *in utero*. *Biol Neonate* 1986;49:51–9.
37. Brimsmead MW, Thorburn GD. Effect of streptozotocin on foetal lambs in mid-pregnancy. *Aust J Biol Sci* 1982;35:517–25.
38. Cheek DB, Hill DE. Changes in somatic growth after ablation of maternal or fetal pancreatic beta cells. In: Cheek DB, ed. *Fetal and postnatal cellular growth*. New York: Wiley, 1975;311–21.
39. Fowden AL, Comline RS. The effects of pancreatectomy on the sheep fetus *in utero*. *Q J Exp Physiol* 1984;69:319–30.
40. Girard JR, Rieutort M, Kervran A, Jost A. Hormonal control of fetal growth with particular reference to insulin and growth hormone. In: Rooth G, Bratchy LE, eds. *Perinatal medicine*. Stockholm: Almquist & Wicksell, 1976;197–202.
41. Fletcher JM, Falconer J, Bassett JM. The relationship of body and placental weight to plasma levels of insulin and other hormones during development in fetal rabbit. *Diabetologia* 1982;23:124–30.
42. Jones CT, Lafeber HN, Rolph TP, Frazer-Fellows G. The timing of biochemical changes in development and their alterations by the growth rate of the fetus. In: Salvadori B, Merialdi A, eds. *Fetal medicine*. Rome: Brola Publishers, 1981;86–109.
43. Zapf J, Schmid CH, Froesch ER. Biological and immunological properties of insulin-like growth factors (IGF) I and II. *Clin Endocr Metab* 1984;13:3–30.
44. D'Ercole AJ, Underwood LE. Growth factors in fetal growth and development. In: Nory MJ, Resko JA, eds. *Fetal endocrinology*. New York: Academic Press, 1981;155–82.
45. Brimsmead MW, Liggins GC. Somatomedins and other growth factors in fetal growth. *Rev Perinatal Med* 1979;3:207–42.
46. Hall K, Sara VR. Growth and somatomedins. *Vitam Horm* 1983;40:175–233.
47. Underwood LE, D'Ercole AJ. Insulin and insulin-like growth factors/somatomedins in fetal and neonatal development. *Clin Endocr Metab* 1984;13:69–89.
48. Sara VR, Hall K. The biosynthesis and regulation of fetal somatomedin. In: Ellendorff F, Gluckman PD, Parvizi P, eds. *Fetal neuroendocrinology*. Ithaca: Perinatology Press, 1984:213–29.
49. Gluckman PD. The role of pituitary hormone, growth factors and insulin in the regulation of fetal growth. *Oxford Rev Reprod Biol* 1986;8:1–60.
50. Milner RDG, Hill DJ. Interaction between endocrine and paracrine peptides in prenatal growth control. *Europ J Pediatr* 1987;146:113–22.
51. Gluckman PD, Johnson-Barrett JJ, Butler JM, Edgar B, Gunn TR. Studies on insulin-like growth factor I and II by specific radioligand assays in umbilical cord blood. *Clin Endocr* 1983;19:405–13.

52. Gluckman PD, Butler JH. Parturition-related changes in insulin-like growth factors I and II in the perinatal lamb. *J Endocr* 1983;99:223–32.

53. Moses AC, Nissley SP, Short PA, et al. Increased levels of multiplication stimulating activity, and insulin-like growth factor in fetal rat serum. *Proc Natl Acad Sci USA* 1980;77:3649–53.

54. Bennett A, Wilson DM, Liu F, Nagashma R, Rosenfeld RG, Hintz R. Levels of insulin-like growth factors I and II in human cord blood. *J Clin Endocr Metab* 1983;57:609–12.

55. Hill DJ, Davidson P, Milner RDG. Retention of plasma somatomedin activity in the fetal rabbit following decapitation in utero. *J Endocr* 1979;81:93–102.

56. Brimsmead MW, Liggins GC. Serum somatomedin activity after hypophysectomy and during parturition in fetal lambs. *Endocrinology* 1979;105:297–305.

57. Parkes MJ, Hill DJ. Lack of growth hormone dependent somatomedins or growth retardation in hypophysectomized fetal lambs. *J Endocr* 1985;104:193–9.

58. Gluckman PD, Butler JH. Circulating insulin-like growth factor I and II concentrations are not dependent on pituitary influences in the midgestation fetal lamb. *J Develop Physiol* 1985;7:411–20.

59. Hill DJ, Crace CJ, Fowler L, Holder, Milner RDG. Cultured fetal rat myoblasts release peptide growth factors which are immunologically and biologically similar to somatomedin. *J Cell Physiol* 1984;119:349–58.

60. Gluckman PD, Butler JH, Comline R, Fowden A. The effects of pancreatectomy on the plasma concentrations of insulin-like growth factors I and II in the sheep fetus. *J Develop Physiol* 1987;9:79–88.

61. Blethen SL, White NW, Santiago JV, Daughaday WH. Plasma somatomedins, endogenous insulin secretion and growth in transient neonatal diabetes mellitus. *J Clin Endocr Metab* 1981;52:144–7.

62. Spencer GSG, Hill DJ, Garssen GJ, MacDonald AA, Colenbrander B. Somatomedin activity and growth hormone levels in body fluids of the fetal pig: effects of chronic hyperinsulinemia. *J Endocr* 1983;96:107–14.

63. Hill DJ, Milner RDG. Increased somatomedin and cartilage metabolic activity in rabbit fetuses injected with insulin *in utero*. *Diabetologia* 1980;19:143–7.

64. Susa JB, Widness JA, Hintz R, Liu F, Seghal P, Schwartz R. Somatomedins and insulin in diabetic pregnancies: effects on fetal macrosomia in the human and Rhesus monkey. *J Clin Endocr Metab* 1984;58:1099–105.

65. Crace CJ, Hill DJ, Milner RDG. Mitogenic actions of insulin on fetal and neonatal rat cells *in utero*. *J Endocr* 1985;104:63–8.

66. Richman RA, Benedict MR, Florini JR, Toly BA. Hormonal regulation of somatomedin secretion by fetal rat hepatocytes in primary culture. *Endocrinology* 1985;116:180–8.

67. Grumbach MM, Kaplan SS, Sciarra JJ, Burr IM. Chorionic GH-Prolactin (CGP): secretion, disposition, biologic activity in man and postulated function as the "GH" of the 2nd half of pregnancy. *Ann NY Acad Sci* 1968;148:501–31.

68. Hurley TW, D'Ercole AJ, Handwerger S, Underwood LE, Furlanetto R, Fellows RE. Ovine placental lactogen induces somatomedin: a possible role in fetal growth. *Endocrinology* 1977;101:1635–8.

69. Adams SO, Nissley SP, Handwerger S, Rechler MM. Development pattern of insulin-like growth factor I and II synthesis and regulation in rat fibroblasts. *Nature* 1983;302:150–3.

70. Freemark M, Handwerger S. Ovine placental lactogen, but not growth hormone, stimulates amino acid transport in fetal rat diaphragm. *Endocrinology* 1983;112:402–4.

71. Freemark M, Handwerger S. Ovine placental lactogen stimulates glycogen synthesis in fetal rat hepatocytes. *Am J Physiol* 1984;246:E21–5.

72. Hill DJ, Crace CJ, Milner RDG. Incorporation of [³H] thymidine by isolated fetal myoblasts and fibroblasts in response to human placental lactogen (HPL): possible mediation of HPL action by release of immunoreactive SM-C. *J Cell Physiol* 1985;125:337–44.

73. Nielsen PV, Pedersen H, Kampmann EH. Absence of human placental lactogen in an otherwise eventful pregnancy. *Am J Obstet Gynecol* 1979;135:322–6.

74. Parks JS, Nielsen PV, Sexton LA, Jorgensen EH. An effect of gene dosage on production of human chorionic somatomammotropin. *J Clin Endocr Metab* 1985;60:994–7.

75. Rechler MM, Eisen HJ, Higa OZ, et al. Characterization of a somatomedin (insulin-like growth factor) synthesized by fetal rat liver in organ cultures. *J Biol Chem* 1979;254:7942–50.

76. D'Ercole AJ, Applewhite GT, Underwood LE. Evidence that somatomedin is synthesized by multiple tissues in the fetus. *Develop Biol* 1980;75:315–28.

77. D'Ercole AJ, Hill DJ, Strain AJ, Underwood LE. Tissue and plasma somatomedin-C/IGF I concentrations in the human fetus during the first half of gestation. *Pediatr Res* 1986;20:253–5.
78. Underwood LE, D'Ercole AJ, Clemmons DR, Van Wyk JJ. Paracrine functions of somatomedins. *Clin Endocr Metab* 1986;15:59–77.
79. Conover CA, Rosenfeld RE, Hintz RL. Hormonal control of the replication of human fetal fibroblasts: role of somatomedin-C/IGF I. *J Cell Physiol* 1986;128:47–54.
80. Hill DJ, Crace CJ, Strain AJ, Milner RDG. Regulation of amino acid uptake and DNA synthesis in isolated human fetal fibroblasts and myoblasts: effect of human placental lactogen, somatomedin-C, MSA and insulin. *J Clin Endocr Metab* 1986;62:753–60.
81. Vetter U, Zapf J, Heit W, Helbing G, Heinze E, Froesche ER, Teller WM. Human fetal and adult chondrocytes: effect of IGF I and II, insulin and growth hormone on clonal growth. *J Clin Invest* 1986;77:1903–8.

DISCUSSION

Dr. Bracci: What do you think of the possibility which has been suggested that insulin acts to increase the number of receptors in the tissues? If this is true, it is possible that insulin may moderate the number of receptors during fetal life, which could have important effects on their numbers after birth. This has been suggested, especially in the case of infants of diabetic mothers.

Dr. Girard: The effect of insulin on human fetal growth, and particularly lipid deposition, only appears after about 26 to 27 weeks gestation. Before that time it is not important. It is also clear that during fetal life there is no down-regulation of insulin and insulin-like growth factor (IGF) receptor numbers as occurs during postnatal life, when an excess of insulin results in a decrease in insulin receptor concentration. The lack of this mechanism during fetal life could certainly be an important factor in determining an increase in fetal growth. There are very few studies of IGF receptors during fetal life, but we do know that they exist in most tissues—skeletal muscle, myoblasts, fibroblasts, cartilage, and so on. But there are no studies of change in receptor numbers during maturation, especially during the fetal period, so we don't know to what extent IGF could be implicated. Another factor to consider is the extent to which competition occurs between insulin receptors and IGF receptors. It could be that the extent to which IGF receptors bind to insulin receptors is greater during fetal life, or that insulin receptors bind specifically and mainly to IGF receptors during this period. This is a new field and we do not have the answers yet, but it is a fascinating growth area.

Dr. Bracci: Do you think that other hormones may be important for fetal growth, such as calcitonin or parathyroid hormone (PTH)?

Dr. Girard: It is clear that depriving the pregnant mother of calcitonin or PTH causes a marked reduction in fetal growth, but I think this is more likely to be due to deleterious effects on the mother than to the fetus. When a thyroidectomy is performed on a pregnant rat, the marked effect on fetal growth which occurs is due to metabolic derangement in the mother and not to specific endocrine deficiency in the fetus.

Dr. Toubas: Your very clear presentation gave me the impression that the fetus is in charge of his growth. What is the role of the placenta? It has recently been found that the placenta contains growth factors, such as epidermal growth factor (EGF), and growth factor receptors. Does the placenta control fetal growth?

Dr. Girard: I cannot answer this. I have restricted my talk to the role of fetal endocrine glands in fetal growth, when all is well with the mother, the placenta, and the placental perfusion. Of the various factors influencing fetal growth, it is clear that the fetal endocrine glands are not the most important, and certainly not as important as maternal nutrition, or placental size and blood flow. I have shown you that at worst, when you completely destroy one endocrine gland, you have a reduction in body weight of the fetus of not more than 20% to 30%. So there are much more important factors controlling body weight at term.

Dr. Toubas: What about the possible role of vasoactive intestinal polypeptide (VIP)? This has recently been implicated in the secretion of prolactin. Do you think it may affect fetal growth?

Dr. Girard: If you perform fetal decapitation you deprive the fetus of prolactin, but you do not affect the weight of the fetus at term. Neither do you by administering drugs which inhibit prolactin secretion in the fetus.

Dr. Robyn: However, in 1982, Sinha and Vanderlaan (1) reported that injections of antiprolactin serum in newborn mice were responsible for a high incidence of mortality and generalized developmental abnormalities in the survivors when compared to injections of non-immune serum.

Dr. Girard: The situation is not at all clear. In the rabbit there is definitely no source of prolactin other than in the pituitary, i.e., there is no placental lactogen which provides a source in, say, the sheep fetus. Nevertheless, the decapitated rabbit fetus grows perfectly normally.

Dr. Robyn: In the fetus, there may be sources of prolactin other than the pituitary. Immunoreactive prolactin has been found to be produced by other cells than the lactotrophs of the anterior pituitary gland: the endometrium, the lymphoid tissue, the myometrium, hypothalamic neurons. Immunorective prolactin is present in B-cells of the endocrine pancreas (2). Thus, prolactin may play a significant role in fetal development. Prolactin may even exert paracrine effects.

Dr. Hay: You speak about differences in body weight, but could you also comment on differences in body composition? I refer specifically to fat, which reflects the major difference in body composition between species. In George Alexander's studies (3) on the sheep, he found that hypophysectomized lambs got quite fat, which normally they don't. With growth hormone replacement they did not get fat, which suggests that this hormone has a specific role in the regulation of fat deposition.

Dr. Girard: It is true that when we discuss fetal growth we refer largely to body weight, although growth is clearly also related to length, body composition, and so on. The most interesting effects of hormones on body weight are in relation to their influence on adipose tissue, particularly in humans. Most of the animal experiments, for example, those in the sheep, rat, or rabbit, have been performed in species in which fat accumulation does not normally occur during fetal development, and this is an important limitation. The guinea pig seems to be the only other species in which it is possible to modify body weight composition during the fetal period hormonally. However, it is also true that the decapitated rabbit fetus, while being the same weight as the intact fetus, is also fatter. So it is possible that pituitary hormones may play a role in determining fetal body composition, even if they have no other effects on fetal growth.

Dr. Bossart: Does IGF influence the rate of mitosis or only the weight or size of cells? And does IGF cross the placenta?

Dr. Girard: There are very few experiments with IGF *in vivo*. Purified IGF injected into hypophysectomized rats can cause an increase in growth; and when injected into dwarf mice it will cause an increase in weight. *In vitro* experiments show that it has a major mitogenic effect in a number of different tissues—skeletal muscle, cartilage, fibroblasts, etc. Most of these experiments have been performed in adult tissues, so it would be very interesting to study the effect on fetal tissues as well.

Dr. Cédard: I believe that the fetus is less autonomous than you say. One ought to consider the feto-placental unit as a whole, since the placenta is able to secrete many things, especially EGF and other growth factors, and has receptors for them. It is quite possible that there is an interaction beween the placenta and the fetus. A new placental growth factor has recently been demonstrated in Liège, Belgium (4), which is detectable by specific monoclonal antibodies and which increases in concentration towards the end of pregnancy. This is more likely to be a fetal growth-promoting factor than is placental lactogen, which is found chiefly in the maternal circulation (maternal:fetal plasma ratio = 1,000:1) and probably plays its main role in maternal lipid or glucose metabolism. I should like to see a new concept of IGF in relation to this new growth hormone and to the feto-placental unit as a whole.

Dr. Girard: I restricted my talk to fetal endocrine glands and fetal growth, so I didn't discuss the placenta. It is interesting to me that the placenta contains a large number of insulin receptors, the purpose of which is not known. No one has made a good study of the hormonal controls and other factors involved in placental growth. I believe the size of the placenta to be one of the most important determinants of fetal weight, and a search for the factors which are important for the growth of the placenta would be a very useful exercise.

Dr. Wharton: If you look at placental size in babies with pancreatic hypoplasia or after fetal pancreatectomy, is it reduced or normal?

Dr. Girard: I think it is decreased.

Dr. Wharton: So it is decreased, and yet the primary pathology is in the fetus. That implies to me that it is the fetus that controls the growth of the placenta rather than the other way around. This is not a new concept, of course, but I suggest that the idea of the placenta being all-important may well be wrong. The placenta should be regarded as just another organ of the fetus. Thus, if the fetus does not grow for any reason, be it an endocrine defect, malnutrition, or anything else, then the placenta does not grow either. I believe that the large statistical analysis done on the Dutch famine data (5) suggested that the main determinant of placental growth was the fetus rather than a direct effect of the famine. I think we are attaching too much importance to the placenta.

Dr. Girard: This could be so. It is true that the placenta in diabetic pregnancies is larger, which supports the argument.

Dr. Hay: The other way to look at this issue is to ask whether the fetus can grow independently of the placenta. I do not know of any situation where you can have a large baby and a small placenta.

Dr. Wharton: If we put it the other way, you cannot grow a large placenta unless you have a large fetus, and just as he grows a large leg and a large arm, so he grows a large placenta!

Dr. Marini: I have a couple of comments on what Drs. Hay and Wharton have said. First, Dr. Hay asked about body composition: I think this is very important because, from a clinical point of view, we have two kinds of growth retardation: asymmetrical, such as can be produced by insulin deprivation, and symmetrical, which can follow insults such as malformation syndromes. The experiments Dr. Girard described show that hormonal defects can cause a major influence on weight gain, for example, in the sheep, with little or no influence on length growth. With respect to what Dr. Wharton said about the placenta, this is the same concept as one already proposed by Warshaw (6), which is that intrauterine growth retardation is not a disease but an adaptation, and that neither the fetus nor the placenta grows any more because they do not have the right conditions to do so. There are many clinical implications in these concepts regarding the treatment of mothers with growth-retarded fetuses.

Dr. Rosso: IGF is apparently very important, but depends on insulin secretion, which in turn depends on the amount of glucose available. Thus the fetus is totally dependent on glucose supply. If this is so, I feel that there must be some way in which the fetus can influence what comes across the placenta, by adjusting blood flow, for example. What do you think of this possibility?

Dr. Girard: There is one clear mechanism of control of the flux of glucose from the mother to fetus, and this is that when the blood glucose concentration in the fetus increases, fetal insulin secretion also increases, as does fetal glucose utilization, and you then create a gradient between mother and fetus, allowing an increased glucose flux across the placenta.

Dr. Rosso: My other question relates to IGF release. You showed that it was possible to extract IGF from the placenta but very little is released into the culture medium. The implication of this is that the placenta is not involved in IGF-mediated regulation of fetal growth, since the IGF is apparently not released from the organ. If this is so, then when we see small placentas and small fetuses, there is probably something on the fetal side preventing the placenta from growing.

Dr. Girard: The placenta not only synthesizes IGF-I but will also release it into the culture medium. So the placenta *is* able to secrete and release IGF-I and may well be implicated in fetal growth control. A fascinating new area to explore is the extent to which insulin or other factors may be able to modulate the synthesis and release of IGF-I by specific fetal organs, and to what extent the activity of this IGF is confined to the secreting cell or cells in the immediate neighborhood. I think the autocrine, or paracrine, role of IGF-I is likely to be much more important than its possible endocrine role as a hormone.

Dr. Marini: You said that insulin-like growth factors are controlled by insulin during fetal life, but that after birth they are controlled by growth hormone. What happens in preterm babies? We have recently seen how such infants may develop a lot of fat when fed on the new preterm formulas. Do these infants have an increased production of insulin-like growth factors?

Dr. Girard: One problem is the large amount of glucose which is commonly infused in parenteral nutrition solutions. This stimulates insulin production markedly and leads to increased fat synthesis.

Dr. Senterre: It is not only a question of the type of nutrient—it is a question of overall energy intake and the ratio of protein to energy. If you give too much energy you will cause an increase in fat deposition. Insulin output is increased not only by high carbohydrate but also by high protein intake, since some amino acids are potent insulin stimulants. In our experience, it is possible to mimic intrauterine weight gain composition by giving preterm infants less energy than is usually provided by preterm formulas and by increasing the ratio of protein to fat and carbohydrate (7,8). What influence these manipulations have on insulin, IGF-I, IGF-II, growth hormone, glucagon, and so on is not yet known, but I suspect that effects on all these growth factors will be shown.

Dr. Chessex: I should like to make a further comment on this. We have done a study with total parenteral nutrition in which we compared the effects of isocaloric quantities of glucose and fat at two different levels of intake. We found that plasma insulin was related to the energy intake and not to the composition of the infusion. This supports the view that insulin secretion is more strongly related to the overall energy intake than to the kind of substrate.

Dr. Girard: I do not think these results necessarily mean that insulin is mainly affected by the energy intake. When you give a different mixture of substrates the sensitivity of the tissues will change. Thus, if the plasma concentration of insulin is the same but the tissues are much more sensitive to insulin in one situation than in another, then plasma insulin is not a good indicator of the functional effect of the insulin. When you give a high fat intake the tissues are probably more resistant.

REFERENCES

1. Sinha YN, Vanderlaan WP. Effect on growth of prolactin deficiency induced in infant mice. *Endocrinology* 1982;110:1871–8.
2. Meuris S, Verloes A, Robyn C. Immunocytochemical localization of prolactin-like immunoreactivity in rat pancreatic islets. *Endocrinology* 1983;112:2221–3.
3. Stevens D, Alexander G. Lipid deposition after hypophysectomy and growth hormone treatment in the sheep fetus. *J Develop Physiol* 1986;8:139–45.
4. Hennen G, Frankenne F. Influence des hormones protéiques placentaires sur la physiologie maternelle. *Annales d'endocrinologie*, Paris 1987;48:978–88.
5. Stein Z, Susser M, Saenger G, Marolla G. *Famine and human development: the Dutch hunger winter of 1944–45*. New York: Oxford Univ. Press, 1975;99–104.
6. Warshaw JB. Intrauterine growth retardation: Adaptation or pathology? *Pediatrics* 1985;76:998–9.
7. Putet G, Senterre J, Rigo J, Salle B. Nutrient balance, energy utilization, and composition of weight gain in very-low-birth-weight infants fed pooled human milk or a preterm formula. *J Pediatr* 1984;105:79–85.
8. Putet G, Rigo J, Salle B, Senterre J. Supplementation of pooled human milk with casein hydrolysate: energy and nitrogen balance and weight gain composition in very low birthweight infants. *Pediatr Res* 1987;21:458–61.

Intrauterine Growth Retardation, edited by
Jacques Senterre. Nestlé Nutrition Workshop
Series, Vol. 18. Nestec Ltd., Vevey/Raven Press,
Ltd., New York © 1989.

Fetal Energy and Protein Metabolism

William W. Hay, Jr.

Associate Professor of Pediatrics, Head, Section of Neonatology, Division of Perinatal Medicine, Department of Pediatrics, University of Colorado School of Medicine, Denver, Colorado 80262

The focus of this chapter is fetal energy and protein metabolism. As in postnatal life, energy metabolism and protein metabolism are closely interrelated, based on the contribution of net protein accretion to the energy cost of growth, and on the contribution of protein oxidation, which is influenced by the supply and utilization of nonprotein energy substrates, to the overall metabolic rate.

Knowledge of fetal energy and protein metabolism is essential for understanding intrauterine growth retardation because deficiencies of energy substrate supply or protein supply to the fetus each can lead to reduction in net protein accretion and thus in growth.

FETAL GROWTH: GENERAL CONSIDERATIONS

Fetal energy metabolism has two components: (a) the accretion of organic material (fat, carbohydrate stores, and tissue protein); (b) the oxidation of organic substrates to CO_2 and H_2O, producing chemical energy and eventually heat. The energy requirement of the fetus for each species is dependent on the rate of growth, the composition of new tissue, the relative mix of substrates taken up by the fetus, and the influence of various hormones and cofactors on the rate of oxidation of the organic substrates.

With respect to the rate of growth, Hofman (1) has proposed that among species, the fractional rate of fetal growth is inversely related to fetal size and to gestational length. For example, in late gestation, the mouse fetus grows at 30% per day with a gestation of 18 days, compared with the fetal lamb at 3.5% per day (150 days gestation), and the human at 1.5% per day (280 days gestation) (2). Clearly, data collected from one species must be extrapolated with caution for comparison with another species, and should be expressed by some common factor, such as the fractional rate of growth. For example, the net accretion of protein in the sheep is about twice that of the human (6.9 g/kg-day versus 3.0 g/kg-day) (3,4), but on the basis of the fractional growth rate, the relative net accretions of protein are comparable (6.9/3.5% for the lamb fetus; 3.0/1.5% for the human fetus).

TABLE 1. *Fetal oxygen consumption*

Species	O_2 Consumption $(ml_{STP}/kg\text{-}min)$	Ref.
Horse	7.0	64
Cattle	6.7	65
Sheep	7.0	6
Man	8.0	66
Rhesus monkey	7.0	67
Guinea pig	8.8	68, 69

It also appears that smaller mammals produce comparably smaller young. This would make sense in order to limit the growth demands of the fetus on the mother. However, on closer inspection smaller and smaller mothers produce larger and larger fetuses as a proportion of maternal weight (5). Thus, fetal growth may become even more of a burden on the smaller mother. To balance this demand on maternal metabolism, it appears that fetal weight-specific, resting (basal) metabolic rate does not change with fetal size (Table 1), in contrast to adult organisms in which it is proportional to size (actually metabolic rate/weight$^{0.75}$) (6,7). Thus, the metabolic rate demands of the smaller fetus do not increase on a weight-specific basis as the fetal size decreases. Therefore, a smaller mother can more readily support fetal growth because fetal metabolic rate is relatively less of a burden.

Further complexity is added to the energy requirements of fetal growth when one considers the composition of fetal growth. Table 2 shows the energy value of various tissue components (8). Across species (and also over gestational development in each species) the caloric value of protein and non-fat, non-protein tissues appears relatively constant. Thus, caloric cost of growth can be estimated quite accurately on the basis of relative water, fat, and non-fat dry tissue contents of each fetus. For example, water content at term is about 55% to 60% of body weight in the guinea

TABLE 2. *Energy value of tissue components*

Tissue component	Energy value (kcal/g)
Water	0
Fat	9.45
Non-fat dry weight	4.5 (4.0–4.6)[a]
Carbohydrate	4.15 (3.7–4.2)
Protein	
Calorimetric determination	5.65
In vivo catabolism	4.35

[a]From refs. 3, 9, and 70.
From ref. 8.

pig (9) but about 70% to 75% of body weight in the human (10), and about 80% in the lamb (3). Furthermore, water content decreases markedly over gestation, falling from nearly 90% in early gestation. Thus, metabolic rate in the fetal lamb at 50% of gestation measured in terms of umbilical oxygen uptake per kg of body weight (about 11.0 ml/kg-min), is about 1.6 times as high as at term, but on the basis of dry weight is even higher (102.5 ml/kg dry wt.-min in the early fetus versus 35 ml/kg dry wt.-min in the term fetus) (11).

With respect to fat content, the caloric cost of depositing fat as a part of fetal growth becomes a very large fraction of total caloric growth, given the high caloric value of fat (9.45 kcal/g) relative to non-fat growth (about 4.5 kcal/g dry weight and 0.75 kcal/g wet weight). For example, the human fetus is the fattest of all terrestrial mammals, laying down about 18% of body weight as fat at term (4,10). Figure 1

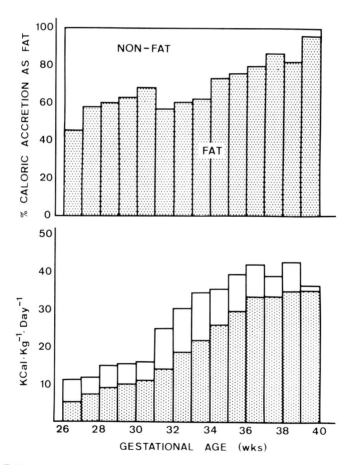

FIG. 1. Estimated caloric accretion in the human fetus during the last 14 weeks of gestation. Upper panel: Fat and non-fat accretion are presented as percent of total caloric accretion. Lower panel: Daily caloric accretion for fat (stippled portion of bar) and non-fat tissue (clear portion of bar). (From ref. 10, with permission of S. Karger AG, Basel.)

shows how significant this fat deposition is with respect to non-fat caloric accretion (10). The next fattest fetus is the guinea pig, with 9% of body weight as fat at term (9). In this species, about 50% of total caloric accretion is accounted for by fat, compared to 70% to 90% in the human. In contrast to these two relatively fatty fetuses, the fetal lamb deposits only about 3% of body weight as fat at term (3). Thus, despite a 50% slower growth rate, the human fetus has a higher caloric accretion rate (40 kcal/kg-day) than the lamb (30 kcal/kg-day).

Finally, within a species, particularly one that is as fat as the human, large variations can occur among fetuses with respect to size, fat content, and total caloric content. Figure 2 shows growth curves for human infants composed by Sparks (12) and

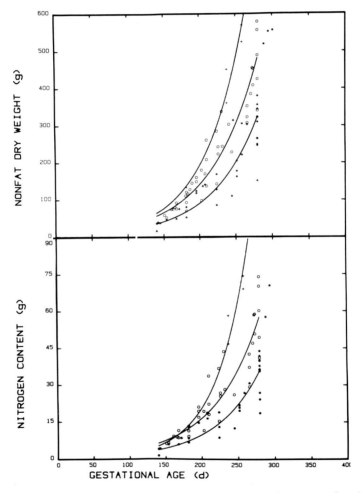

FIG. 2. Mean regression lines for the growth of non-fat dry weight **(upper panel)** and nitrogen content **(lower panel)** over the second half of pregnancy in 97 human fetuses studied at autopsy for tissue contents. * = small for gestational age; o = average for gestational age; + = large for gestational age. (From ref. 12, with permission of Grune & Stratton, Inc.)

based on data from a large number of studies of the weight of human infants at birth at different gestational ages. Since the fat-free and water contents of these fetuses do not differ very much as percentages of body weight, it is clear that a large variation in human fetal caloric accretion depends on body fat content. The causes of such variation in fat content are not known, first because the human fetus cannot be studied *in utero* and second, because there is no convenient animal model for fetal study that produces a comparable amount of fetal fat. Thus, factors regulating fetal fat accretion, such as placental fat transport, the supply of other energy substrates such as glucose and lactate (that can act as fat synthetic precursors), and the effect of hormones such as *insulin* on fat deposition, fat synthesis, and fat breakdown, simply cannot be studied and thus have not been studied. It is also clear from these curves that the fractional rate of growth of small and of large infants is quite similar (i.e., the slopes of the weight gain or nitrogen gain per day are parallel). This observation serves to emphasize that study of fetal growth rate and its determinants may be approached better by interspecies comparisons rather than by trying to dissect out determinants of extremely small changes of growth rate within a species. On the other hand, it is imperative that data collected from one species should be comparable to data from another species. In this regard, many interspecies studies of fetal growth and metabolism are not valid comparative studies, in that different species were studied under very different physiologic states (for example, acute studies carried out under anesthesia and frequently other stresses versus studies in chronic unstressed, conscious animals). Also, data collected in fetuses with very short gestations may reflect dramatic changes in body nutrient pool sizes compared with data from more slowly growing fetuses, if the period of study represents a significant portion of gestation. Thus, emphasis should be placed on carrying out comparative interspecies studies using techniques, such as chronic catheterization in conscious animals, that at least provide data about metabolic processes associated with direct observation of confirmed growth and survival of the fetus (7).

ROLE OF THE PLACENTA

Nutrient supply to the fetus depends upon placental transport. In all species studied, fetal growth is directly related to placental size; that is, large fetuses in a species have large placentas and small fetuses have small placentas. However, a small placenta does not allow the growth of a large fetus. The limitation of placental size on fetal growth has been tested experimentally by animal models that involve a reduction in placental size. For example, Owens and colleagues (13,14) performed uterine carunculectomies in sheep, exploiting a model developed by Alexander (15) that limits the myometrial implantation area and results in placentas significantly reduced in total mass (as well as the number of cotyledons) (Table 3). As a result, fetal weight and fetal nutrient consumption were markedly reduced, nearly proportionate to the placental weight reduction. Of interest is the observation that the weight-specific rates of glucose and oxygen consumption of the growth-retarded (carunculectomy) fetuses were not different from the control fetuses, suggesting that

TABLE 3. *Placental and fetal metabolic results of uterine carunculectomy*
in sheep (mean ± S.D.)

Variable	Control	Carunculectomy
Placental weight (g)	485 ± 105	197 ± 91
Fetal weight (g)	3,720 ± 807	2,198 ± 653
Umbilical blood flow		
(ml/min)	990 ± 345	503 ± 137
(ml/min-kg fetal wt)	268 ± 34	217 ± 46
Fetal O_2 consumption		
(ml/min)	1.208 ± 0.488	0.748 ± 0.215
(ml/min-kg fetal wt)	0.325 ± 0.131	0.340 ± 0.100
Fetal glucose consumption		
(mg/min)	18.4 ± 2.7	11.1 ± 4.3
(ml/min-kg fetal wt)	4.9 ± 0.7	5.1 ± 2.0

[a]From refs. 13 and 14.

there are no fetal or placental compensatory mechanisms to increase fetal nutrient uptake or utilization when nutritional supply is limited by a relatively small placental transport capacity. However, since the fetal weight:placental weight ratio was greater in the carunculectomy (12.6 ± 3.9) than the control group (7.8 ± 1.3), the placenta may have compensatory mechanisms that allow an increased nutrient transport when placental size is restricted. Similarly, in late gestation, fetal growth continues to a greater extent than placental growth, which tends to plateau in weight during the last one-third of gestation (16). In contrast, the functional capacity of the placenta to transport nutrients to the fetus increases significantly during late gestation. Some years ago this fact was demonstrated in the pregnant sheep placenta for growth and urea diffusing capacity (Fig. 3) (17). More recently, also in the sheep model, a similar increase in placental transport capacity has been observed for glucose over the last half of gestation (Fig. 4) (18). Part of this increase in placental glucose transport appears to be the increasing maternal-to-fetal glucose gradient, the result of a progressive decrease in fetal glucose concentration. However, the gestational increase in placental glucose transport is disproportionately large for the increase of the maternal-fetal glucose concentration gradient, suggesting that placental glucose transport capacity increases even more than the gradient. The progressive fall in fetal glucose concentration relative to the maternal glucose concentration, producing the increasing maternal-to-fetal glucose concentration gradient, may suggest an increasing insulin action in the developing fetus over the last half of gestation, or the increasing proportion of fetal "wet" mass that is metabolically active and thus glucose-consuming "dry" tissue. The increasing maternal-to-fetal glucose gradient does not appear to be due to an increasing placental glucose consumption relative to the fetus because the percentage of uterine glucose uptake that is con-

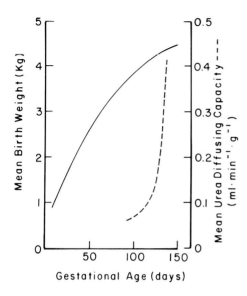

FIG. 3. Mean birthweight (—) and placental urea diffusing capacity (---) for sheep are plotted over gestation, demonstrating the capacity for placental function to increase in late gestation to support fetal growth. (Adapted from data from ref. 17, with permission of the authors.)

sumed by the placenta actually falls over the last half of gestation, from 90% to 72%. Similar changes occur for oxygen. Nevertheless, these data do confirm that the placental metabolic requirements, which are quite large relative to the fetus, markedly affect fetal nutrient supply and that this effect occurs, though changing in magnitude, throughout gestation.

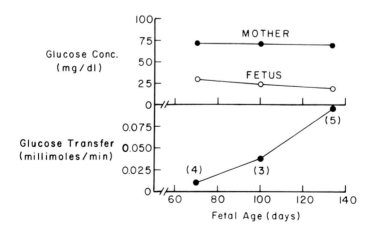

FIG. 4. In pregnant sheep, maternal plasma glucose concentration was fixed for study by intravenous glucose infusion. At advancing gestational age, fetal glucose concentration decreased relative to fixed maternal plasma glucose concentration, and capacity of placenta to transfer glucose to fetus increased dramatically. (*Unpublished data* from Molina, Hay, and Meschia, Division of Perinatal Medicine, University of Colorado School of Medicine.)

The final characteristic of placental function that may affect fetal nutrient supply is regulation of placental nutrient transport by uterine and umbilical blood flow. For highly diffusable substances such as water and oxygen, this relationship is non-linear (19); that is, at moderate to high flows, transfer is regulated by placental and fetal consumption. Thus transport is constant over a wide range of flows (20). At much lower flow rates, transport becomes limited by the supply of the substance, that is, by the blood flow. It is interesting that transport is limited only when flow is reduced to less than half of normal. Recently, Wilkening and colleagues (21) showed that the same phenomenon exists for diffusion-limited substrates, particularly glucose (Fig. 5). As with oxygen (22) and water (19), glucose transport was not affected until flow was reduced to less than 50% of normal. When considered in relation to the experiments which produced small placentas that also had markedly reduced uterine, umbilical, and placental blood flows, the limitation of flow on nutrient transport appears less important than the actual size (transport surface area) of the placenta, at least until very low flow rates are produced. On the other hand, changes of blood flow to an abnormally small placenta or to a functionally compromised placenta may produce more striking changes in placental nutrient transport.

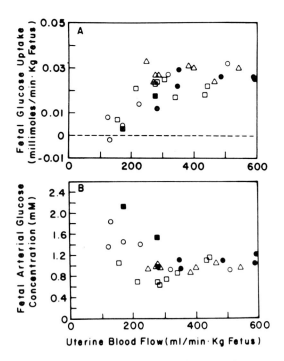

FIG. 5. Fetal glucose uptake from placenta is relatively constant over normal uterine blood flow range but decreases non-linearly as flow falls to less than half normal. Part of decreased glucose transfer is flow-dependent **(panel A, top)** and part is related to progressive fetal hyperglycemia that probably occurs because fetal hypoxemia develops at the same time **(panel B, bottom)**. (From ref. 21, with permission from the *Journal of Developmental Physiology*.)

Such a hypothesis has not been studied adequately, but clearly represents a vital area for investigation with respect to the growth-retarded fetus that already may be limited with respect to nutrient supply.

Clearly such issues relating placental transport capacity and placental nutrient consumption to fetal nutrient supply need further investigation to assess their role and impact with respect to fetal growth and development during gestation. The investigations discussed above involved *in vivo* experiments. It would be helpful, particularly in the human, to perform such studies *in vitro*. Such a study has been performed in term human placentas using a perfusion apparatus (23). This study demonstrated, just as in the sheep, that glucose consumption and glucose transport by the placenta are regulated to a significant degree by the maternal plasma glucose concentration and the maternal-fetal arterial plasma glucose concentration gradient. This study also showed that maximum rates of placental glucose consumption and glucose transport occur in the perfused human placenta, demonstrating saturation kinetics consistent with the model of facilitated diffusion to account for placental glucose metabolism, experimentally determined in animal models such as the sheep (24,25). Such *in vitro* models hold promise also for studying the transport of nutrients other than glucose, such as fats, amino acids, proteins, vitamins, etc., and especially for studying such transport processes over a broad gestational age range to approach issues of developmental regulation of placental transport (as shown for glucose), and among placentas from pregnancies complicated by fetal growth disorders as well as various maternal problems such as diabetes, fasting, hypertension, etc., to study how fetal abnormalities may be produced by placental dysfunction. On the other hand, such *in vitro* models desperately need *in vivo* correlates, primarily to validate the functional capacity of the *in vitro* preparation. This validation can and should be done, at least in part, by using *in vivo* studies in experimental animals, but also now by applying the newer techniques of umbilical vessel blood sampling via fetoscopy and amniocentesis in selected human cases.

FETAL OXYGEN CONSUMPTION AND METABOLIC RATE

Fetal metabolic rate has been measured primarily by indirect calorimetric techniques which involve measurement of fetal oxygen consumption and the caloric equivalents for oxidizable substrates. In the fetal lamb, for example, fetal oxygen consumption is measured by the Fick principle (umbilical blood flow times the umbilical venous-arterial blood oxygen content difference) (26), and because glucose and amino acids are the only oxidized substrates in the fetal lamb, the caloric equivalence of the oxygen consumption is about 4.9 kcal/liter $_{STP}$ O_2. A large number of studies in many laboratories over many years have shown remarkably consistent values for oxygen consumption in the term fetal lamb of about 0.3 mmol/kg-min (about 6.7 ml O_2/kg-min) or about 0.033 kcal/kg-min (about 47 kcal/kg-day). This value is relatively constant and not affected to any major degree ($< \pm 15\%$) by reductions in energy supply or provision of nutrient excess.

On the other hand, as mentioned elsewhere in this chapter, fetal metabolic rate (weight-specific) is much higher in early fetal life, caused in part, perhaps, by the much higher fractional protein synthetic rate in the early fetus compared with the term fetus.

FETAL GLUCOSE METABOLISM

In all species, the major non-protein energy substrate for fetal metabolism is glucose. Initial studies of fetal glucose metabolism established that fetal glucose concentration is directly related to the maternal glucose concentration (although the maternal-to-fetal glucose concentration gradient varies markedly among species with different placental blood flow arrangements; for example, concurrent versus countercurrent, and probably with different rates of placental glucose consumption and transport capacities) (6), and inversely related to the fetal insulin concentration when insulin is infused exogenously (27). These studies also showed that placental-to-fetal glucose transport is directly but non-linearly related to maternal glucose concentration (6,25). Rates of umbilical glucose uptake by the fetus were measured using Fick principle techniques, but when compared with fetal oxygen uptakes were shown to be inadequate to account for all the fetal oxidative metabolism (6,28). Coupled with observations of relatively high fetal urea production rates (29), these results suggest that substrates other than glucose, such as amino acids, contribute to fetal oxidative metabolism and thus to energy production.

More recently, research has focused on the measurement of fetal glucose utilization (as distinct from fetal glucose uptake from the placenta), the regulation of glucose utilization, and the partition of glucose utilization into oxidative and non-oxidative pathways. To measure fetal glucose utilization, radioactive tracers have been infused into the fetus or into the mother and the net uptake of tracer by the fetus determined (30). When the tracer is infused into the mother, net fetal tracer uptake is via the umbilical circulation and is measured by the Fick principle. When the tracer is infused into the fetus, net tracer uptake is determined as the difference between infusion rate and the net loss of tracer by diffusion to the placenta, this diffusional loss being calculated by the Fick principle. Fetal utilization rate is then calculated as the ratio of net fetal tracer uptake divided by fetal arterial specific activity. Both sites of tracer infusion yield statistically comparable utilization rates of glucose (31), which, because they were calculated using *net* fetal tracer uptake, can be compared with the *net* exogenous glucose supply to the fetus, the umbilical glucose uptake rate (32). Using this methodology, fetal glucose utilization rates have been measured in the fetal lamb model. Fetal glucose utilization rate is directly related to maternal glucose concentration and is not different from umbilical glucose uptake over the normal range of maternal glucose levels and rates of umbilical glucose uptake (31). However, as shown in Fig. 6, when umbilical glucose uptake falls to less than half of normal (<2.5 mg/kg-min), glucose utilization begins to exceed umbilical glucose uptake by amounts that must represent another source of glucose

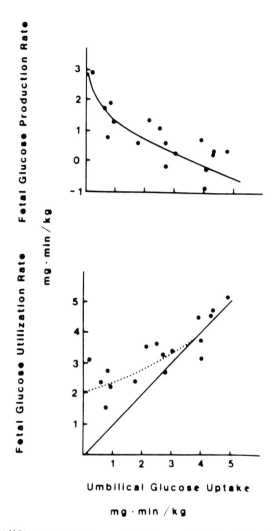

FIG. 6. Using (U-^{14}C)-glucose to measure fetal glucose utilization rate in sheep, fetal endogenous glucose production was calculated as the difference between fetal glucose utilization and fetal umbilical glucose uptake. At umbilical glucose uptake rates less than half normal (less than 2.5 mg/kg-min), fetal glucose production increased progressively, contributing significantly to total fetal glucose utilization. (Data from Hay et al. (31), reproduced with permission from Battaglia and Meschia, Academic Press (8).)

supply to the fetus (31). Direct and indirect data suggest that this additional glucose source represents fetal endogenous glucose production that comes primarily from the fetal liver (33). Because this extra, endogenous supply of glucose persists for days, it appears that gluconeogenesis, the production of new glucose molecules from non-glucose-derived precursors, must play a major role in addition to glycogenolysis as the source of new glucose. Because fetal urea production increases and

fetal growth rate decreases under these same conditions, one mechanism for allowing the fetus to adapt to a decrease in glucose (and thus, energy) supply is to increase protein catabolism and divert certain amino acids to gluconeogenic metabolic
pathways. Because fetal oxygen consumption and thus metabolic rate does not
change in these conditions (34), it appears that fetal adaptation to energy substrate
deficiency involves the protection of fetal metabolic rate at the expense of continued
growth.

Additional evidence to support this hypothesis comes from studies of the metabolic rate of glucose in the fetus. If one collects the labeled CO_2 (e.g., $^{14}CO_2$) exit-
ing from the fetus during a steady-state infusion of a carbon-labeled substrate (e.g.,
[U-^{14}C]-glucose) into the fetus, one can calculate the fraction of substrate that is
converted to CO_2 by oxidation. In the fetus, the labeled CO_2 excretion rate is measured by the Fick principle across the umbilical circulation and is divided by the net
fetal tracer uptake rate to calculate the oxidation fraction. Multiplying this fraction
of oxidation by the substrate utilization rate yields the rate of oxidation of that substrate (35). Using this methodology, glucose oxidation fractions have been calculated in fetal lambs and, when compared with glucose concentration (and thus with
glucose uptake and utilization, which are directly related), it appears that the fraction and rate of glucose oxidation directly increase with glucose supply and utilization (Fig. 7, left) (35). Thus, the amount of oxygen consumption used by glucose

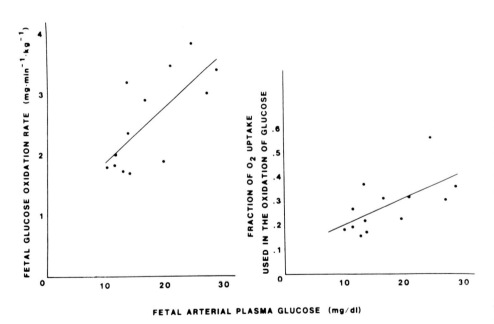

FIG. 7. Fetal glucose oxidation rate (glucose utilization rate times the glucose oxidation fraction) in fetal lambs is directly related to fetal glucose concentration, as is the fraction of fetal oxygen consumption used for glucose oxidation. (From ref. 35, reproduced with permission of the
Society for Experimental Biology and Medicine.)

oxidation varies directly with the supply and utilization of glucose (Fig. 7, right). Clearly, the supply of glucose to the fetus can determine the relative amount of non-glucose oxidative substrates that are oxidized.

Because glucose concentration and insulin concentration are directly related, and both act to increase cellular glucose uptake, it was not clear from these initial studies comparing glucose oxidation with glucose concentration to what extent the increase in glucose oxidation was due to glucose or to insulin. Analysis of this question has been approached using glucose and insulin clamp techniques that allow separate control of glucose and insulin concentrations in fetal plasma. Figure 8 shows the results of such experiments in fetal lambs, in which insulin concentrations above 100 μU/ml (shown previously to result in maximal glucose utilization) were produced by controlled insulin infusions, and glucose was infused to maintain fetal glucose concentration at the control (''normal'') level (36,37). In both control and hyperinsulinemic conditions, glucose utilization rate was equal to the exogenous glucose supply, consisting of the umbilical glucose uptake in the control period and the umbilical glucose uptake plus the exogenous glucose infusion in the hyperinsulinemia period. The results demonstrate that a maximum effect of insulin doubles fetal glucose utilization and also doubles glucose oxidation. Thus, by either means (increased glucose concentration or increased insulin concentration) increased cellular glucose uptake promotes glucose oxidation and so reduces the oxidation of other substrates. Furthermore, as shown in Fig. 9, at these high levels of fetal glucose utilization, fetal oxygen consumption, and therefore metabolic rate, was increased by

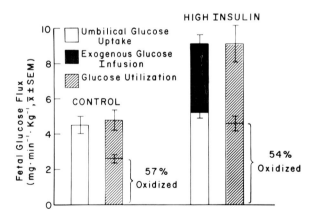

FIG. 8. Glucose utilization rate and oxidation rate in fetal lambs compared with umbilical glucose uptake rate during a control period, and with umbilical glucose uptake and intravenously infused glucose during subsequent insulin clamp experiment, showing that glucose utilization is accounted for by the exogenous glucose supply (umbilical glucose uptake plus infused glucose) and that the fraction of glucose oxidized does not change as glucose utilization increases. These data suggest that increased cellular glucose uptake increasingly displaces other substrates from oxidation and that the contribution of glucose to non-oxidative pathways increases in proportion to glucose oxidation. (From ref. 37, reproduced with permission from the *Quarterly Journal of Experimental Physiology.*)

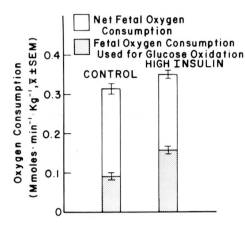

FIG. 9. At maximal insulin-stimulated glucose utilization in fetal lambs, fetal metabolic rate increases by about 15% while the fraction of fetal oxygen consumption used for oxidation of glucose nearly doubles. (From ref. 37, reproduced with permission from the *Quarterly Journal of Experimental Physiology.*)

about 15%. Similar results were observed by Philipps et al. (38) using hyperglycemic glucose infusions in fetal lambs. Thus an increase in energy intake can increase metabolic rate in the fetus but the degree of increase is relatively minor compared to the increase in metabolic rate that occurs with muscle activities (39).

Recently, these studies have been expanded to compare glucose and oxygen metabolism at many different levels of glucose and insulin concentration. Figure 10

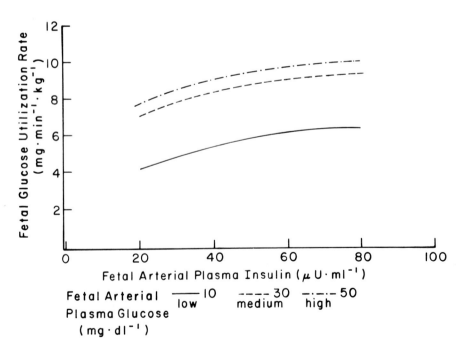

FIG. 10. In fetal lambs, glucose utilization is shown to be a function of both insulin concentration and glucose concentration. (Adapted from Hay WW Jr, ref. 40.)

represents computer-smoothed curves illustrating to what extent glucose and insulin act separately to influence glucose metabolism (40).

Lactate is another carbohydrate that is important as a fetal energy substrate. Lactate has received a bad name with respect to oxidative metabolism because it is common knowledge that lactate production increases during oxygen insufficiency. During pregnancy, however, lactate production by the placenta is a very normal process that occurs in all species studied to date including the human (41–44). Placental lactate production occurs in the presence of normal oxygenation, and in the fetal lamb results in the net delivery of lactate to the fetus at a rate of about half that of glucose (42). Like glucose, lactate is rapidly oxidized, but to an even greater extent than glucose (75% versus 55%) (35). When the sum of fetal glucose and lactate uptake is compared with fetal oxygen consumption, a direct relationship is observed, suggesting that fetal metabolic rate may indeed be regulated by energy substrate supply (45).

FETAL PROTEIN METABOLISM

Protein is supplied to the fetus primarily as amino acids which are actively transported by energy-dependent carriers from the maternal to the fetal plasma (46). Some of the total uterine uptake of amino acids is used also in the placenta for placental growth and peptide hormone production (for example, chorionic gonadotropin and placental lactogen). The magnitude of placental amino acid requirements has not been determined, but because the ratio of umbilical to uterine amino acid extraction is approximately proportional to the ratio of umbilical to uterine blood flows, this amount is likely to be quite small compared to fetal uptake (47). Furthermore, in late gestation, the amino acid requirements for the rapid increase of fetal growth far exceed the requirements for the smaller and more slowly growing placenta.

To date, fetal uptake of amino acids has been measured only in the fetal lamb (47,48). Figure 11 presents data from late-gestation fetal lambs showing that uptake exceeds carcass accretion for the neutral amino acids and equals accretion for the two basic amino acids (histidine and lysine). The two acidic amino acids, glutamate and aspartate, are not supplied to the fetus in any appreciable amount and the fetal supply of these amino acids probably comes from deamination of glutamine and asparagine. There is sufficient uterine and fetal uptake of asparagine to account for both fetal asparagine and aspartate accretion; for glutamate, uterine uptake of glutamine plus the uptake of glutamate from the fetal circulation by the placenta is sufficient to account for the total quantity of glutamine entering the fetus (8). Other amino acid cycles probably exist (for example, between glycine and serine), either in the placenta, the fetal tissues, or both, but there is insufficient information at present to define or quantify such cycles.

Overall, therefore, large amounts of amino acids are taken up by the fetus but do not contribute to protein accretion. Additionally, fetal urea production rate is quite high (0.73 ± 0.05 mg/kg-min for fetal sheep), exceeding neonatal and adult values

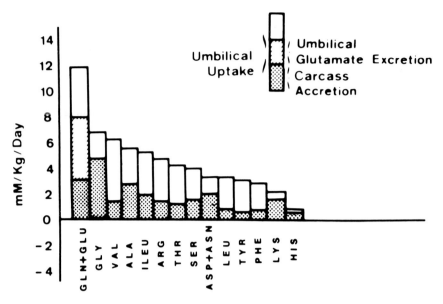

FIG. 11. Comparison of daily net fetal umbilical uptakes of individual amino acids *(entire bar)* with corresponding daily rates of whole body net accretion of amino acids *(stippled portion of bar)* in the fetal lamb. Hatched portion of Gln + Glu bar is umbilical glutamate excretion. (From ref. 47, reproduced with permission from the Society for Experimental Biology and Medicine.)

on a body-weight-specific basis (29). Together these results support the conclusion that, at least in the fetal lamb, there is a considerable rate of oxidation of amino acids. Data from primates suggest that this process may occur in other species as well.

More direct evidence for the contribution of amino acids to fetal oxidative metabolism has come from tracer methodology. Using a model similar to that described for glucose and lactate, ^{14}C-labeled amino acids have been infused into fetal lambs and the rate of $^{14}CO_2$ produced is measured by application of the Fick principle to quantify the $^{14}CO_2$ flux out of the fetus and into the placenta.

For an amino acid that is delivered to the fetus at approximately the same rate as its rate of accretion, its rate of oxidation ought to represent only a small fraction of its utilization rate. For lysine, ^{14}C-lysine infusion yielded an oxidation fraction of about 9%, confirming a relatively low rate of oxidation for this amino acid (49). On the other hand, for leucine, a branched-chain amino acid that is taken up at about twice the rate that is required for accretion (primarily in muscle), similar tracer studies have shown that leucine oxidation in fetal lambs represents about 30% of total leucine utilization, both in mid- as well as late gestation (50,51). Studies of other amino acids have used different experimental models that preclude quantitative comparison with the leucine and lysine data, but active rates of oxidation in fetal lambs have been documented also for alanine (52), glycine (52), and tyrosine (53).

Additional studies with ^{14}C-leucine tracers in fetal lambs have documented that in late gestation, fetal leucine oxidation fraction increases as the leucine concentration in the plasma increases, similar to observations in postnatal animals (8,50). Furthermore, during fasting-induced hypoglycemia and hypoinsulinemia, leucine oxidation increases to nearly twice the fed rate (Fig. 12) (50), which, coupled with the increased fetal urea production rate that occurs under the same conditions, adds support to the concept that fetal protein catabolism is regulated by non-protein substrate supply, and that certain amino acids released by protein catabolism can be oxidized to maintain fetal energy balance at the expense of growth. Furthermore, because the rate of leucine oxidation does not appear to change in the presence of selective hypoinsulinemia (for example, glucose concentration and glucose utilization remain near normal) (54), this regulation of leucine catabolism and oxidation appears to be specific to the intracellular non-protein energy substrate supply rather than hormones such as insulin that may independently affect cellular glucose and amino acid uptake rates.

Several studies have addressed the measurement of fetal protein synthesis rate. In large animals such as the sheep, fractional protein synthesis has been estimated during a constant fetal infusion of labeled amino acid tracer by the ratio of $SA_{pr}/(SA_p \cdot t)$, where SA_{pr} is the specific activity of the traced amino acid in fetal tissue proteins

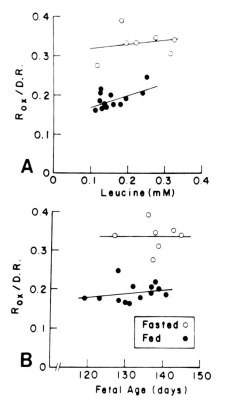

FIG. 12. Plot of fetal leucine oxidation rate/disposal rate ratio versus fetal arterial plasma leucine concentration **(A)** and fetal age **(B)**. Observations in fed ewes are compared with observations in ewes in the fourth to eighth day of fasting. (From ref. 50, reproduced with permission of *Metabolism*.)

(from a whole carcass homogenate), SA_p is the specific activity of the traced amino acid free in plasma (both at steady state), and t is the time of infusion. More precise estimates can be made by knowing the time to reach steady state from the start of infusion and the degree of labeled-carbon recycling from protein degradation of the immediately synthesized proteins that incorporated the labeled amino acid (49). Similar studies have been conducted in small animals using a flooding dose of tracer into the mother that very quickly achieves a maximal labeling of fetal proteins and then calculating the fractional protein synthetic rate from the fetal plasma and protein-specific activities (55).

Actual protein synthesis rates can be measured during a steady-state tracer amino acid infusion if one calculates the net tracer flux into proteins and divides this flux by the steady-state plasma amino acid-specific activity (comparable to calculating the utilization rate of glucose as the net fetal tracer uptake rate divided by the plasma glucose-specific activity). For an amino acid, net tracer uptake by tissue protein is calculated as the tracer infusion rate minus ($^{14}CO_2$ excretion) minus (tracer loss to the placenta).

Not all studies of fetal protein synthesis rate have adhered to the tracer modeling described above, and therefore, differences among studies are quite large. Nevertheless, all of the valid studies have shown that during fetal life, fetal fractional protein synthetic rate decreases with gestational age (Fig. 13) (49). When compared with the fractional rate of growth over the same period of gestation, two important observations can be made. First, protein synthesis proceeds at a much faster rate than growth, supporting the concept that fetal protein turnover rate is high and permits the supply of amino acids for purposes other than growth (for example, oxidation or conversion to other carbon-containing products). Second, the more rapid change (decrease) of protein synthesis over gestation compared to growth suggests considerable remodeling of the relative contribution of those body components, each with markedly different rates of protein synthesis, to overall body protein synthesis (Table 4) (8,55). For example, as shown in Table 4, adult skeletal muscle has

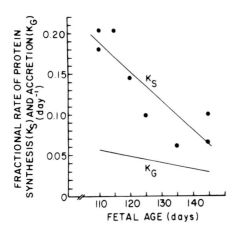

FIG. 13. The fractional rate of protein synthesis (K_s) in fetal lambs is compared with the fractional rate of growth (K_g). (From ref. 49, reproduced with permission from the *American Journal of Physiology*. Data for K_g were originally taken from ref. 3.)

TABLE 4. *Fractional protein synthesis rate (mean ± SEM)*

Organ	Young	Adult
Liver	57 ± 12	54 ± 6
Kidney	50 ± 10	51 ± 7
Brain	17 ± 3	11.3 ± 2.8
Heart	18.5 ± 4	11.0 ± 2.3
Skeletal muscle	15.2 ± 2.8	4.5 ± 0.5

From refs. 8 and 55.

a much lower fractional protein synthesis rate than fetal skeletal muscle. Thus, as the fetus matures, growth of skeletal muscle that increasingly has the lower adult fractional protein synthesis rate will tend to lower the overall body fractional protein synthesis rate. This observation also supports the concept that in late gestation slowing of fetal growth is a normal developmental process and not the result of decreases in placental transport capacity.

Finally, given the high rate of protein synthesis in fetal life, it might seem logical that factors affecting protein synthesis rate might lead to marked changes in fetal growth. Such an attractive hypothesis has been hard to define. First, fetal protein deprivation has been difficult to produce and even when fetal hypoaminoacidemia has been produced experimentally, only a concomitant decrease in fetal non-protein energy supply seems to result in fetal growth retardation (56). Additionally, the studies in fetal lambs using the [1-^{14}C]-leucine tracer described previously in this chapter have shown quite dramatically that a reduction of non-protein energy substrate supply (in this case, fasting-induced hypoglycemia and reduced fetal-umbilical glucose uptake) results in an increase (in fact, a doubling) of leucine oxidation. Thus, a major conclusion to be derived from these studies is that in fetal life (as in postnatal life), changes in body protein accretion, and thus growth, are limited by changes in the rate of protein catabolism, not protein synthesis, and that protein catabolism is regulated to a significant extent by the supply of non-protein energy substrates. In fetal life, because fat is unlikely to be used very much for oxidation, fetal glucose supply may be a key regulator of fetal protein catabolism and growth. Cases of marked fetal growth retardation from fetal pancreatic agenesis or experimentally produced fetal hypoinsulinemia on the one hand and the macrosomia of the hyperglycemic infant of the diabetic mother on the other hand may represent extreme clinical examples of the glucose-regulatory hypothesis.

FETAL FAT METABOLISM

As discussed earlier in this chapter, there is relatively little information about fetal fat metabolism compared with information about fetal glucose and protein metabolism. Thus, while marked differences in fetal fat content at term are present among

TABLE 5. *Fetal fat content (percent of weight) at term*

Species	Fat content
Human	18
Guinea pig	9
Rabbit	5
Rat	1
Mouse	1

From ref. 57.

species (Table 5) (57), the mechanisms responsible for regulation of fetal fat deposition are not precisely known. It is clear that the placentas of some species are more permeable to fat (human, guinea pig, rabbit) and that in these placentas, specific fatty acid transport mechanisms (carriers) are present, along with the capacity to synthesize fatty acids for transport to the fetus (8). Fetal fatty acid synthesis increases with increased glucose supply from the mother (58,59) and appears regulated in some species by the secretion of growth hormone. For example, in the fetal lamb, perirenal fat deposition increases at mid-gestation but then does not progress as growth hormone secretion increases. On the other hand, hypophysectomized, growth-hormone-deficient fetal lambs continue to deposit fat until growth hormone replacement is given (60). In humans, fat deposition is marked in the third trimester when growth hormone secretion is naturally very low (61).

There appears to be very little oxidation of fetal fatty acids. Regulatory mechanisms are not known but low levels of carnitine have been implicated (62). Because rapid fatty acid oxidation can occur in the immediate postnatal period (63) when lipolysis leads to markedly increased plasma fatty acid concentrations but not to increased carnitine concentration, fetal fatty acid oxidation may be dependent on fatty acid concentration as much as or more so than on carnitine concentration.

SUMMARY

In summary, I should like to make several general statements about fetal energy and protein metabolism. First, with advancing gestation, fetal nutrient supply is limited by the overall size of the placenta but enhanced, in normal placentas at least, by increasing placental transport supply. Future research in this area should be focused on factors regulating placental growth and functional maturation as well as on the deficiencies in placental function that may occur in pregnancies that produce significant changes in fetal growth. Second, how fat a fetus becomes appears to be regulated primarily by placental fat transport and secondarily by the supply of glucose for fat synthesis. Future research in this area needs to focus on placental fat transport mechanisms, how fat is synthesized in the fetus, and what regulates fetal fat catabolism and oxidation. Third, an excess of fetal glucose (and perhaps lactate) supply and utilization will lead to a modest increase in fetal metabolic rate as one means of handling nutrient excess, with the balance of the excess supply leading to increased energy stores as glycogen and fat. On the other hand, nutrient deficiency (e.g., with fasting-induced hypoglycemia) does not result in a significant reduction in fetal metabolic rate. Fetal metabolic rate thus seems rather independent of nutrient supply, an essential factor for fetal viability. Fourth, fetal protein synthesis changes during gestation primarily as a result of normal developmental processes such as the remodeling of the relative proportions of tissue components that have different protein synthetic rates. Actual rates of fetal body (and selected fetal tissue or organ) protein synthesis need extensive study and accurate measurement to verify this hypothesis. And last, fetal protein catabolism may be regulated to a large extent by non-protein energy substrate supply. This regulation appears to be mediated by changes in the rate of protein catabolism leading to oxidation directly for some amino acids or indirectly by way of gluconeogenesis for others.

Our data are still patchy, but emerging from these data is an understanding of fetal energy metabolism, protein metabolism, and growth that on the whole is quite rational and consistent with data from growth-after-birth. First, the chief regulator of fetal growth is the dietary nutrient supply. Second, fetal metabolic rate is relatively constant. Third, at adequate levels of protein intake, fetal protein accretion is regulated primarily by protein catabolism rather than by protein synthesis, and this regulation is directly related to non-protein energy supply.

ACKNOWLEDGEMENTS

I wish to express my gratitude to Dr. Donald Barron who started me on my career in fetal and placental physiology, and to Dr. Giacomo Meschia and Dr. Frederick Battaglia who provided the means for me to develop my research. This work was supported in part by NIH grants DK35836, HD20761, and HD00781.

REFERENCES

1. Hofman MA. Evolution of brain size in neonatal and adult placental mammals: a theoretical approach. *J Theor Biol* 1983;105:317–32.
2. Widdowson EM. Changes in body proportions and composition during growth. In: Davis JA, Dobbing J., eds. *Scientific foundations of paediatrics.* Philadelphia: WB Saunders Company, 1974;44–55.
3. Rattray PV, Garret WM, East NE, Hinman N. Growth, development, and composition of the ovine conceptus and mammary gland during pregnancy. *J Anim Sci* 1974;38:613–29.
4. Ziegler EE, O'Donnell AM, Nelson SE, Fomon SJ. Body composition of the reference fetus. *Growth* 1979;40:329–41.
5. Leitch I, Hytten FE, Billewicz WZ. The maternal and neonatal weights of some mammals. *Proc Zoological Soc (Lond)* 1959;133:11–28.
6. Battaglia FC, Meschia G. Principal substrates of fetal metabolism. *Physiol Rev* 1978;58:499–527.
7. Battaglia FC. Commonality and diversity in fetal development: bridging the interspecies gap. *Pediatr Res* 1984;1812:736–45.
8. Battaglia FC, Meschia G. *An introduction to fetal physiology.* Orlando: Academic Press, 1986.
9. Sparks JW, Girard JR, Calikan S, Battaglia FC. Growth of fetal guinea pig: physical and chemical characteristics. *Am J Physiol* 1985;248:E132–9.
10. Sparks JW, Girard JR, Battaglia FC. An estimate of the caloric requirements of the human fetus. *Biol Neonate* 1980;38:113–9.

11. Bell AW, Kennaugh JM, Battaglia FC, Makowski EL, Meschia G. Metabolic and circulatory studies of the fetal lamb at mid gestation. *Am J Physiol* 1986;250:E538–44.
12. Sparks JW. Human intrauterine growth and nutrient accretion. *Sem Perinatol* 1984;8:74–93.
13. Owens JA, Allota E, Falconer J, Robinson JS. Effect of restricted placental growth upon oxygen and glucose delivery to the fetus. In: Jones CT, Nathanielsz PW, eds. *The physiological development of the fetus and newborn*. London: Academic Press, 1985;33–6.
14. Owens JA, Allota E, Falconer J, Robinson JS. Effect of restricted placental growth upon umbilical and uterus blood flows. In: Jones CT, Nathanielsz PW, eds. *The physiological development of the fetus and newborn*. London: Academic Press, 1985;51–4.
15. Alexander G. Studies on the placenta of the sheep (Ovis aries L.). Effect of surgical reduction in the number of caruncles. *J Reprod Fertil* 1964;7:307–22.
16. Alexander G. Birthweight of lambs: influences and consequences. In: Elliott K, Knight J, eds. *Size at birth*, Ciba Foundation Symposium 27. Amsterdam: Elsevier-Excerpta Medica-North-Holland, 1974;215–39.
17. Kulhanek JF, Meschia G, Makowski EL, Battaglia FC. Changes in DNA content and urea permeability of the sheep placenta. *Am J Physiol* 1974;226:1257–63.
18. Molina R, Hay WW, Jr, Meschia G. *Unpublished data*, 1987.
19. Meschia G, Battaglia FC, Bruns PD. Theoretical and experimental study of transplacental diffusion. *J Appl Physiol* 1967;22:1171–8.
20. Wilkening RB, Anderson S, Martensson L., Meschia G. Placental transfer as a function of uterine blood flow. *Am J Physiol* 1982;242:H429–36.
21. Wilkening RB, Battaglia FC, Meschia G. The relationship of umbilical glucose uptake to uterine blood flow. *J Develop Physiol* 1985;7:313–9.
22. Wilkening RB, Meschia G. Fetal oxygen uptake, oxygenation, and acid-base balance as a function of uterine blood flow. *Am J Physiol* 1983;244:H749–55.
23. Hauguel S, Desmaizieres V, Challier JC. Glucose uptake, utilization, and transfer by the human placenta as functions of maternal glucose concentration. *Pediatr Res* 1986;20:269–73.
24. Widdas WF. Inability of diffusion to account for placental glucose transfer in the sheep and consideration of the kinetics of a possible carrier transfer. *J Physiol* 1952;118:23–39.
25. Simmons MA, Battaglia FC, Meschia G. Placental transfer of glucose. *J Develop Physiol* 1979; 1:227–43.
26. Meschia G, Battaglia FC, Hay WW Jr, Sparks JW. Utilization of substrates by the ovine placenta in vivo. *Fed Proc* 1980;39:245–9.
27. Simmons MA, Jones MD Jr, Battaglia FC, Meschia G. Insulin effect on fetal glucose utilization. *Pediatr Res* 1978;12:90–2.
28. Tsoulos NG, Colwill JR, Battaglia FC, Makowski EL, Meschia G. Comparison of glucose, fructose and O_2 uptakes by fetuses of fed and starved ewes. *Am J Physiol* 1971;221:234–7.
29. Gresham EL, James EJ, Raye JR, Battaglia FC, Makowski EL, Meschia G. Production and excretion of urea by the fetal lamb. *Pediatrics* 1972;50:372–9.
30. Hay WW Jr, Sparks JW, Quissell B, Battaglia FC, Meschia G. Simultaneous measurements of umbilical uptake, fetal utilization rate and fetal turnover rate of glucose. *Am J Physiol* 1981;240: E662–8.
31. Hay WW Jr, Sparks JW, Wilkening RB, Battaglia FC, Meschia G. Fetal glucose uptake and utilization as functions of maternal glucose concentration. *Am J Physiol* 1984;246:E237–42.
32. Hay WW Jr, Sparks JW, Battaglia FC, Meschia G. Maternal-fetal glucose exchange: necessity of a 3-pool model. *Am J Physiol* 1984;246:E528–34.
33. Sparks JW, Hay WW Jr, Meschia G, Battaglia FC. Fetal liver metabolism in the unstressed fetal lamb: experience with a chronic indwelling hepatic venous catheter. *Pediatr Res* 1982;1615:265A.
34. Simmons MA, Meschia G, Makowski EL, Battaglia FC. Fetal metabolic response to maternal starvation. *Pediatr Res* 1974;8:830–6.
35. Hay WW Jr, Myers SA, Sparks JW, Wilkening RB, Meschia G, Battaglia FC. Glucose and lactate oxidation rates in the fetal lamb. *Proc Soc Exp Biol Med* 1983;173:553–63.
36. Hay WW Jr, Meznarich HK, Sparks JW, Battaglia FC, Meschia G. Effect of insulin on glucose uptake in near-term fetal lambs (42042). *Proc Soc Exp Biol Med* 1985;178:557–64.
37. Hay WW Jr, Meznarich HK. The effect of hyperinsulinemia on glucose utilization and oxidation and on oxygen consumption in the fetal lamb. *Q J Exp Physiol* 1986;71:689–98.
38. Philipps AF, Dubin JW, Matty PJ, Raye JR. Arterial hypoxemia and hyperinsulinemia in the chronically hyperglycemic fetal lamb. *Pediatr Res* 1982;16:653–8.
39. Rurak DW, Gruber NC. Increased oxygen consumption associated with breathing activity in fetal lambs. *J Appl Physiol* 1983;54:701–7.

40. Hay WW Jr, Meznarich HK, DiGiacomo JE, et al. Effects of insulin and glucose concentrations on glucose utilization in fetal sheep. *Pediatr Res* 1988;23:381–7.
41. Holzman IR, Philipps AF, Battaglia FC. Glucose metabolism and ammonia production by the human placenta in vitro. *Pediatr Res* 1979;13:117–20.
42. Sparks JW, Hay WW Jr, Bonds DR, Meschia G, Battaglia FC. Simultaneous measurements of lactate turnover rate and umbilical lactate uptake in the fetal lamb. *J Clin Invest* 1982;70:179–92.
43. Johnson RL, Gilbert M, Block SM, Battaglia FC. Uterine metabolism of the pregnant rabbit under chronic steady-state conditions. *Am J Obstet Gynecol* 1986;154:1146–51.
44. Sparks JW, Pegorier JP, Girard J, Battaglia FC. Substrate concentration changes during pregnancy in the guinea pig studied under unstressed steady state conditions. *Pediatr Res* 1981;15:1340–4.
45. Sparks JW, Hay WW Jr, Meschia G, Battaglia FC. Partition of maternal nutrients to the placenta and fetus in the sheep. *Europ J Obstet Gynecol Reprod Biol* 1983;14:331–40.
46. Dancis J, Money WL, Springer D, Levitz M. Transport of amino acids by placenta. *Am J Obstet Gynecol* 1968;101:820–9.
47. Meier PR, Teng C, Battaglia FC, Meschia G. The rate of amino acid nitrogen and total nitrogen accumulation in the fetal lamb. *Proc Soc Exp Biol Med* 1981;167:463–8.
48. Lemons JA, Adcock EW III, Jones MD Jr, Naughton MA, Meschia G, Battaglia FC. Umbilical uptake of amino acids in the unstressed fetal lamb. *J Clin Invest* 1976;58:1428–34.
49. Meier PR, Peterson RB, Bonds DR, Meschia G, Battaglia FC. Rates of protein synthesis and turnover in fetal life. *Am J Physiol* 1981;240:E320–4.
50. Van Veen LCP, Teng C, Hay WW Jr, Meschia G, Battaglia FC. Leucine disposal and oxidation rates in the fetal lamb. *Metabolism* 1987;36:48–53.
51. Kennaugh JM, Bell AW, Teng C, et al. Ontogenetic changes in the rates of protein synthesis and leucine oxidation during fetal life. *Pediatr Res* 1987;22:688–92.
52. Hatfield GM, Joyce J, Jeacock MK, Shepherd DAL. The irreversible loss of alanine and of glycine in fetal and sucking lambs. *Br J Nutr* 1984;52:529–43.
53. Schaefer AL, Krishnamurti CR. Whole body and tissue fractional protein synthesis in the ovine fetus in utero. *Br J Nutr* 1984;52:359–69.
54. Hay WW Jr, Kennaugh JM, Loy G. *Unpublished data,* 1989.
55. Waterlow JC, Garlick PJ, Millward DJ. In: *Protein turnover in mammalian tissues and in the whole body.* Amsterdam: Elsevier/North-Holland Biomedical Press, 1978.
56. Domenech M, Gruppuso PA, Nishino VT, Susa JB, Schwartz R. Preserved fetal plasma amino acid concentrations in the presence of maternal hyoaminoacidemia. *Pediatr Res* 1986;20:1071–6.
57. Widdowson E. Chemical composition of newly born animals. *Nature* 1950;166:626–8.
58. Ballard FJ, Hanson RW. Changes in lipid synthesis in rat liver during development. *Biochem J* 1967;102:952–8.
59. Todhunter DA, Scholz RW. *In vivo* incorporation of tritium from ^3H_2O into pulmonary lipids of meal-fed and starved rats. *Am J Physiol* 1980;239:E407–11.
60. Stevens D, Alexander G. Lipid deposition after hypophysectomy and growth hormone treatment in the sheep fetus. *J Develop Physiol* 1986;8:139–45.
61. Jost A. Fetal hormones and fetal growth. *Contrib Gynecol Obstet* 1979;5:1–20.
62. Novak M, Monkus EF, Chung D, Buch M. Carnitine in the perinatal metabolism of lipids. I. Relationship between maternal and fetal plasma levels of carnitine and acylcarnitines. *Pediatrics* 1981;67:95–100.
63. Novak M, Melichar VC, Hahn P, Koklovsky O. Release of free fatty acids from adipose tissue obtained from newborn infants. *J Lipid Res* 1965;6:91–9.
64. Silver M, Comline RS. Fetal and placental O_2 consumption and the uptake of different metabolites in the ruminant and horse during late gestation. In: Reneau DD, Grote J, eds. *Oxygen transport to tissue II—Advances in experimental medicine and biology,* vol. 75. New York: Plenum, 1976; 731–6.
65. Comline RS, Silver M. Some aspects of foetal and utero-placental metabolism in cows with indwelling umbilical and uterine vascular catheters. *J Physiol* 1976;260:571–86.
66. Sandiford I, Wheeler T. The basal metabolism before, during and after pregnancy. *J Biol Chem* 1924;62:329–50.
67. Behrman RE, Lees MH, Peterson EN, DeLannoy CW, Seeds AE. Distribution of the circulation in the normal and asphyxiated fetal primate. *Am J Obstet Gynecol* 1970;108:956–69.
68. Bohr C. Der respiratorische stoffwechsel des sauge-thierembryo. *Skand Arch Physiol* 1900;15:413–24.
69. Moll W, Kunzel W, Ross HG. Gas exchange of the pregnant uterus of anesthetized and unanesthetized guinea pigs. *Respir Physiol* 1970;8:303–18.

70. Etienne M, Henry Y. Influence d l'apport energetique sur l'utilization digestive et metabolique des nutriments, et les performances de reproduction chez la truie gestatte nullipare. *Ann Zootechnologique* 1973;22:311–26.

DISCUSSION

Dr. Pearse: Have you done any work on gluconeogenesis in the growth-retarded fetus?

Dr. Hay: Yes, we are currently using an experimental model similar to the one I have already described, with chronic infusions of insulin into the mother. We are able to restrict the mother's blood glucose concentration to 50% of normal for up to 6 weeks while she continues to eat a normal diet. During this period we can sample fetal blood and perform various physiological studies. Under these conditions we see the same sort of changes in fetal metabolism that I showed you with the fetal hepatic catheterization study, where glucose supply from the liver is greater than the umbilical uptake. We have not carried out enough of these studies to give you quantitative data, but we can say, for example, that under such conditions the conversion of alanine and lactate to glucose is much higher than under control conditions. We have started to look at other amino acids and it looks as though there is an interesting breakdown, with some amino acids such as leucine going directly to oxidation and others, such as alanine and glycine, being converted to glucose.

Dr. Toubas: I have a question about the size of the placenta. I don't want to throw fuel on the flames of the discussion following Dr. Girard's paper, but there have been experiments on removing the placental caruncles which showed that by the end of gestation the fetus achieved a normal weight despite a very much smaller placenta. What do you think about the mechanism for this? There must be a fantastic adaptation if you can remove half the placenta and the fetus can still achieve the same growth as the control.

Dr. Hay: There are many changes in placental functional capacity which are not related to placental weight. This can be shown for glucose and for urea-diffusing capacity. We are approaching a study of amino acid transport using the same kind of model. I think you need to distinguish between placental growth and placental functional capacity before you can talk about the effect of the placenta on fetal growth.

Dr. Senterre: In preterm infants who are deprived of nutrients, protein accretion and protein turnover are decreased, and these changes will cause a reduction in energy expenditure. Have you any animal experience which confirms this?

Dr. Hay: The data I described from the hypoglycemic animal model, where we observe an increase in leucine oxidation, provide one experimental approach to the questions you are asking, namely, what regulates the growth of the fetus, and how can substrates be shunted back and forth from oxidation to growth. When we make an animal hypoglycemic and decrease its glucose utilization rate we see an increase in leucine oxidation, but there is no simultaneous change in protein synthesis rate as measured with the same tracer. So it looks as though glucose entering the cell regulates catabolism and oxidation, whereas the amino acid concentration is the regulator of protein synthesis. We have preliminary data on other experimental situations which support this view. For example, if we eliminate insulin by using a pancreatectomy or streptozotocin model and thus decrease the supply of intracellular glucose by separate means, we can show that protein synthesis does not change when we add glucose back. What does change is the amount of leucine that is oxidized. I therefore feel fairly confident that glucose regulates protein catabolism and oxidation, at least through leucine as the tracer amino acid.

Dr. Marini: I have a question about intrauterine growth retardation. Clinicians always say that if we could increase the supply of nutrients to the fetus, we might manage to improve its growth. What are your comments on this? Is there a critical ratio between oxygen and nutrient supply? And what kind of nutrients are best supplied in a fetus with low oxygen consumption?

Dr. Hay: There are limits to the excess of nutrients that can be provided. As long as you provide sufficient substrate for growth and energy metabolism, providing an excess will not make you grow much faster. In the fetus there is a maximum rate of glucose utilization beyond which the fetus becomes hyperglycemic and acidotic and develops a fatty liver. In postnatal life a number of studies have shown that you can increase growth by providing greater amounts of protein and increasing the energy intake, but you only get to a certain rate of growth, beyond which you start to get the same problems of fatty liver, hyperglycemia, acidosis, and a high blood urea nitrogen. The key is to know the exact amount of nutrients required for normal growth and to provide at least that amount.

Dr. Bossart: Years ago I gave different amounts of glucose to the mother, with and without insulin, during labor, hoping to find a way of giving an increased glucose supply to growth-retarded fetuses. We were surprised how often there was a rapid increase in lactate, so we did not feel that it would be safe to provide such glucose loads blind to a fetus, without being able to monitor acid-base balance.

Dr. Hay: We have seen the same thing in our studies. Lacate production increases in direct proportion to the additional glucose when you provide glucose faster than the rate at which it is immediately metabolized, say 4–6 mg/min per kg in the sheep fetus. I would support your contention that excess glucose has limitations.

Dr. Bossart: Are there any other types of carbohydrate which could be used in this situation without leading to acidemia?

Dr. Hay: Two other carbohydrates have been studied. One is fructose, but this has a very low utilization rate, about one-fifth to one-tenth the rate of glucose, and when provided in excess it merely causes plasma concentrations to rise higher, with potentially serious osmotic effects. It may also produce an acidosis, and it has not been very successful in postnatal studies, either as an enteral nutrient or as part of parenteral nutrition. The other carbohydrate which has been used is galactose, which is of course extremely important in postnatal life, being half of the dietary supply of carbohydrate. I know of no experimental studies in the fetus showing that it can function as a nutrient *in utero*. We have infused galactose in fetal and neonatal lambs and have shown that it is cleared by the liver, but I don't have any information about its nutritional value in this situation.

Dr. Chessex: From your studies, could you suggest any biological markers to differentiate between small normal infants and small-for-gestation (SGA) babies, particularly in relation to plasma amino acid values? We have been comparing amino acid profiles during total parenteral nutrition in appropriate-for-gestation versus small-for-gestation infants and we have used a low overall profile as a marker of the SGA infants. What is your opinion of this?

Dr. Hay: I can only comment about fetal studies, in which there is not a good correlation with intrauterine growth retardation, since the placenta actively transports amino acids to the fetus. If anything, when the fetus is catabolizing protein there is an increase in fetal plasma amino acid concentrations and we see relatively high levels regardless of how we change the rate of oxidation of glucose and amino acids. This changes completely in the postnatal period when dietary supply determines the plasma concentration. Then there is a more direct relationship between plasma concentrations and dietary supply.

Dr. Senterre: I should like to hear some discussion of fat transfer to the fetus. David Hull (1) has shown that placental transport of fatty acids is important, at least for the essential ones, and when you take into account the amount of linoleic acid (C18:2) in fetal adipose tissue you can calculate that about 50% of the fat in the fetus comes directly from transferred fatty acids rather than from endogenous fetal synthesis. I should appreciate your comments about fat transfer and deposition in the fetus.

Dr. Hay: Dr. Hull's work in the rabbit and the human placental perfusion model are the only studies I know of which have looked at placental fat transport. There appear to be specific fatty acid carriers in the placenta and you are right that a large percentage, even the major proportion, of fetal fat deposition is accounted for by transported fats. There appears also to be very little oxidation of fats in fetal tissues, which to me is a bit of a mystery. It has been proposed that this may be due to carnitine deficiency, but the amount of carnitine in the fetus is not particularly small, and in postnatal life the same levels of carnitine appear adequate to support fat oxidation, as shown by the fall in respiratory quotient (RQ) immediately after birth. I have not seen a model testing fat supply to the fetus to see if the RQ will change similarly. There have been a number of recent studies of oral or intravenous supplementation with carnitine in babies fed intravenously with carnitine-deficient regimens. These studies (2,3) have shown that carnitine supplementation increases plasma carnitine in the baby, decreases levels of free fatty acids and triglycerides, and possibly improves nitrogen balance. However, these changes are only of the order of 10%—enough to be statistically significant, but perhaps of doubtful biologic value.

Dr. Bracci: Experiments in dogs have shown that hypoglycemia is advantageous during asphyxia in terms of survival, since it reduces oxygen consumption and the degree of acidosis. What do you think of this idea?

Dr. Hay: I'd be extremely suspicious of interpreting a possible protective effect of reduced plasma glucose in terms of a change in lactate or [H^+]. I'd need an independent study showing what had actually occurred. Also, the dog is not a good model to show changes in neurologic function which are relevant to humans. It is very difficult to show changes in the metabolic rate of neural tissues and to relate them to the production of neurologic injuries. I remain skeptical.

Dr. Marini: There was a study by Myers (4) which showed that if you give an asphyxiated neonate glucose you cause an increase in lactate production and probably reduce the pH in neural tissues. He therefore advised against giving glucose in this situation. Could you tell us how rapidly lactate is metabolized by the fetus?

Dr. Hay: Lactate is metabolized as it is produced, even during ischemia or hypoxemia. We have infused large amounts of lactate into the fetal lamb, up to 10 times the normal utilization rate of 4–5 mg/kg per min, and have barely seen a change in pH; thus lactate is a nutrient that can be well-utilized by fetal tissues. When lactic acidemia occurs on the basis of hypoxia or ischemia, the lactic acid production rate is of course in excess of utilization. The subsequent rate of fall of plasma lactate in this situation depends on how fast you improve the ischemia. Potentially the half-life of lactate is measured in minutes and not hours. A lactate concentration of 30 mM could usually be handled in an hour.

REFERENCES

1. Hull D. Storage and supply of fatty acids before and after birth. *Br Med Bull* 1975;31:32–6.
2. Schimdt-Sommerfeld E, Pen D, Wolf H. Carnitine deficiency in premature infants receiving total parenteral nutrition: effect of L-carnitine supplementation. *J Pediatr* 1983;102:931–5.
3. Helms RA, Whitington PF, Mauer EC, et al. Enhanced lipid utilization in infants receiving oral L-carnitine during long-term parenteral nutrition. *J Pediatr* 1986;109:984–8.
4. Myers RE, Yamaguchi M. Effects of serum glucose concentration on brain response to circulatory arrest. *J Neuropathol Exp Neurol* 1976;35:301.

Intrauterine Growth Retardation, edited by
Jacques Senterre. Nestlé Nutrition Workshop
Series, Vol. 18. Nestec Ltd., Vevey/Raven Press,
Ltd., New York © 1989.

Definitions: Problems and Limitations of Intrauterine Growth Curves

Richard G. Pearse

Neonatal Intensive Care Unit, The Jessop Hospital for Women, Sheffield S3 7RE, England

Although there are numerous problems with "intrauterine" growth curves, they have probably done more to alert obstetricians and pediatricians to the complications of aberrant intrauterine growth than any other single factor. The realization that not all small babies are born prematurely has had important effects on both the search for the etiology of intrauterine growth retardation (IUGR) and on the clinical management of the small baby before and after birth. The problems of the large baby, with the exception of the infant of a diabetic mother, have received less attention.

DEFINITIONS

As yet there is no universally agreed definition of what constitutes abnormal intrauterine growth. To come to agreement it is necessary to define what we are aiming to achieve by fixing the definition. For the obstetrician the purpose of identification may be to alter the intrauterine environment to help the fetus attain an improved rate of growth, to time delivery to minimize the risks to the fetus from prematurity and growth retardation, or at least to deliver the fetus before intrauterine asphyxia causes irreparable damage or death. For the pediatrician, the purpose of identification is to help recognize the baby at risk from such complications of IUGR as postnatal hypoglycemia and to anticipate and prevent their occurrence, and to help him to concentrate his resources on these infants both in the neonatal period and later in the follow-up clinic when looking for long-term complications such as minimal cerebral damage.

It is thus quite possible that a suitable "cutoff" point for an abnormal fetus on a true intrauterine growth chart may be quite different from the suitable cutoff point once the baby has been delivered. For both situations any decision is arbitrary, but its purpose is to attempt to isolate a group containing the maximum number of abnormally grown infants at risk, with as few "normals" as possible.

Ultrasound has been the main method used in recent years to attempt to detect IUGR while the fetus is still *in utero*. Various measurements and calculations have

65

been made such as biparietal diameter (BPD), head:abdomen ratio, total intrauterine volume, thoracic diameter minus BPD, crown-rump length times thoracic area, femur length, and comparison with a "normal ultrasonic fetal weight curve." These have been well-reviewed by Seeds (1). In the published literature none of these methods has shown a sensitivity which is consistently better than 75% (2).

Once the baby is delivered, weight is the traditional measurement by which to judge intrauterine growth and has the great advantage that it is relatively easily and reproducibly measured anywhere in the world. However, it is not a very reliable measure of growth because large variations in body water are present at birth which will alter the results considerably, and because weight cannot be measured *in utero*. Head circumference is a useful measurement but consistent results are more difficult to obtain. It is not a very sensitive predictor of IUGR since brain growth and thus head growth tend to be spared in some cases (see below). Length is a very difficult variable to measure accurately and usually requires two people in attendance as well as special apparatus. Measurement of skinfold thickness is good for diagnosing intrauterine malnutrition but it requires relatively sophisticated apparatus (skinfold caliper) and there is considerable observer variability. Further refinements have been attempted but tend to be complicated and have not received general acceptance. Perhaps the only one to be widely used is the ponderal index (3), in which the formula

$$\frac{\text{birth weight (in grams)} \times 100}{(\text{length in centimeters})^3}$$

is used.

In general, however, we fall back on birthweight as the main variable by which intrauterine growth is assessed.

AIMS

Which Babies Are We Trying to Identify?

If we are trying to identify those babies who have not achieved their true growth potential, how can we do this? We accept that the female fetus is not as large at delivery as the male fetus, i.e., is not as well-grown, and yet if a baby has a trisomy and is small, then we say that he has intrauterine growth retardation. It is obviously ridiculous to say that baby girls are growth-retarded, yet this illustrates how difficult it is to assess growth potential. There have been various attempts to do this, which will be discussed later.

One could say that we are attempting to define those babies in whom intrauterine growth has been less than optimal. However it has been shown in various populations (4,5) that the minimum mortality rate is seen in babies whose birthweight is several hundred grams above the mean, while on the other hand Boersma (6), in studies in Tanzania, has suggested that there may be an advantage in being born mildly growth-retarded in some populations.

Another method, which avoids some of the above difficulties, would be to compare the birthweight of an infant with the average birthweight for that population. This seems simple but Turner (7) showed that 80% of babies with rubella syndrome had a birthweight below the range of variability of their siblings, and yet half of them would not have been identified as small-for-gestational-age (SGA) by standard "intrauterine" growth charts.

It is generally assumed that the range of birthweights will, when plotted, form a Gaussian curve around the mean birthweight for that population. Assuming that the mean birthweight for a population of growth-retarded (SGA) fetuses is, for example, 600 g below the mean for normally grown fetuses appropriate for gestational age (AGA), then it can be seen that a considerable number of the smaller AGA fetuses will have a lower birthweight than the larger SGA fetuses. This may be clinically unimportant for the AGA fetus; however the larger SGA fetuses whose birthweights come within the normal range may thereby not be identified as SGA and yet suffer all the complications of intrauterine growth retardation. There is at present no definition which can separate these two groups of babies, whose birthweights fall in the overlapping range. However Westergaard et al. (8) have suggested that such a separation may be possible by measuring maternal serum concentrations of placental lactogen and Schwangerschaft's protein 1(SP1).

TYPES OF INTRAUTERINE GROWTH RETARDATION

There is now general agreement that in a population of SGA infants there are at least three different clinical types:

(a) The classical type with near-normal skeletal and head growth but with wasted subcutaneous tissue and muscle. This type was originally described by Clifford (9) in 1954 in postmature babies but has subsequently been recognized in babies of all gestations. It is variously known as Clifford's syndrome, disproportionate growth retardation, asymmetric growth retardation, subacute growth retardation, and many other terms. It is generally thought to result from growth retardation which becomes manifest in the latter weeks of the pregnancy, such as is found in preeclamptic toxemia and other conditions (10). These babies seem particularly at-risk from hypoglycemia (11).

(b) The chronic type has a reduction in both soft tissue growth and skeletal and head growth. This is called symmetric or proportionate growth retardation, and it has been suggested that it is this group which is prone to long-term developmental problems (12), but with fewer immediate problems in the neonatal period. The etiology of this form of IUGR includes such serious conditions as intrauterine infections, e.g., the TORCH infections (toxoplasma, rubella, cytomegalovirus, herpes simplex), and chromosomal abnormalities, but of course also includes the normally grown but genetically small baby who may have none of the problems associated with intrauterine growth retardation, either in the short or the long term.

(c) There must also exist a combined type with some features of each of the above and presumably with some of their complications.

The proportion of babies who are born SGA obviously varies depending on the definitions in use, on the particular intrauterine growth charts deployed, and on the population under study. It is often quoted that SGA infants form about one-third of the low birthweight (<2500 g) population in a developed country, the other two-thirds being formed by preterm babies (babies of less than 37 completed weeks of gestation). However, in developing countries the ratios are reversed, with about two-thirds of the babies being SGA and only one-third being preterm (13).

THE SELECTION OF "CUTOFF" CRITERIA TO DETERMINE THE FETUS/INFANT AT RISK

A number of different cutoff points have been advocated. They include: (a) mean ± 2 standard deviations (SD)—equivalent to the 97.5th and 2.5th percentiles (14); and (b) mean ± 1.3 SD—equivalent to the 90th and 10th percentiles (15). Others have recommended the 3rd and 97th percentiles.

It seems that the use of either mean ± 2 SD, which is taken to be the range of normality in many areas of biologic measurement, or the 97th and 3rd percentiles, which encompass a very similar range, can be recommended. The use of the 10th percentile will certainly identify too many babies "at-risk," most of whom will have no problems, and will identify very few genuinely at risk babies not included in the −2 SD or 3rd percentile cutoff point. The babies selected as SGA will vary according to the criteria used. If for example the 10th percentile is used, then 10% of the population will be selected if the intrauterine growth curve is correct for that population. However, this 10% may be made up of different individuals if the 10th percentile for the ponderal index (3) is used. Thus Walther and Raemaekers (16) showed that 23 of 46 consecutive term infants with a weight below the 2.3rd percentile also had a ponderal index below the 2.3rd percentile, but that in 21 of these infants (who were all SGA by weight) the ponderal index was above the 10th percentile. This may partly be explained by the major flaw in the use of the ponderal index as a measure of intrauterine growth, which is the large contribution that head size makes to body weight.

THE PROBLEMS OF EXISTING INTRAUTERINE GROWTH CHARTS

Most charts in current use were constructed from data gathered before 1971 (14,15,17–19). There have been considerable changes in, for example, the socioeconomic status, the proportion of immigrants, and the size of families in many populations since that time. These will all have an influence on the shape of the intrauterine growth curves for that population.

Because most of the curves were constructed before neonatal intensive care became widespread in the developed world, the amount of data on babies of less than 28 weeks gestation is very limited because they were often not recorded as live births (this was as much dependent on the policy of a hospital as on signs of life).

Thus, they either formed samples of very small size (14) or were excluded from the studies (18).

The major problem with existing growth charts is that the estimation of gestational age has been uncertain since it depends almost exclusively on last menstrual period (LMP) calculations and there has been an excess of large "preterm" infants in most studies. This has led to a bimodal distribution of weight at each gestational age and a positive skew which is inversely related to gestation (15,20). It was recognized in several of the studies that errors in the assessment of gestational age were responsible but attempts to correct this have led to even greater difficulties in interpretation. Lubchenco et al. (15) eliminated all babies over the 90th percentile from their study, and Neligan (21) eliminated those at the extremes on a distribution plot. Milner and Richards (22) estimated that about one-third of the babies at each gestational age below 34 weeks had been wrongly assessed, causing a second peak usually representing term babies whose gestation had been underestimated by up to 12 weeks.

There have been two major developments which have taken away most of the uncertainty from the estimation of gestational age since data for the early charts were gathered. Firstly, in 1970 Dubowitz and her co-workers (23) described the method of gestational age assessment which bears her name and which has become widespread. Secondly, during the 1970s ultrasound scanning of the fetus became common and early ultrasound assessment of pregnancy reduced any doubts in those cases where the duration of gestation was uncertain. Intrauterine growth curves constructed from data gathered after these two refinements in the assessment of gestational age do not show the biomodality seen in earlier studies (24).

So called "intrauterine" growth charts are constructed from the recorded birthweights of babies born at various gestational ages; thus they are all constructed from cross-sectional data. There are a number of problems inherent in the interpretation of cross-sectional data. The preterm infant is by definition abnormal and therefore does not necessarily reflect the growth and development of the normal fetus who remains *in utero* at that gestation. It has been shown that the birthweight of the extremely preterm infant correlates well with the weight of fetuses delivered by therapeutic abortion for social reasons (25). However, this method of comparison is not available for gestational ages greater than the legal limit for therapeutic termination and could still be criticized in that the social and emotional stresses in the period leading up to the operation could alter fetal growth. Preterm live births above 22 weeks gestation but below 28 weeks tend to be heavier than the therapeutic and spontaneous abortion groups (25), which offers some support for this criticism. On the other hand, this may also be interpreted to mean either that large fetuses at this low gestation are more able to survive labor or (more probably) that there is bias in recording the data, whereby the larger baby is more likely to be considered viable, recorded as a live birth, and offered intensive care. The smaller baby of the same gestation may often be thought to be non-viable and recorded as a miscarriage in an attempt to spare the parents' emotions.

Keirse (26) showed that, if a baby is defined as being growth-retarded when birth weight is 2 SD below the mean for local "intrauterine" growth charts, then to be considered growth-retarded at 30 weeks gestation, the baby would have to weigh below 1,023 g in Montreal, below 640 g in Baltimore but below 300 g in Britain. Keirse (27) has also shown, using the 10th percentile derived from the data of the 1970 British Births Survey, that a baby who completely stops growing at 38 weeks gestation while AGA but just above the 10th percentile becomes SGA if delivered within the next four weeks but "is cured" and becomes AGA again if not delivered until after the 42nd week, without any change in the baby's weight.

All intrauterine growth charts have shown a tailing off in weight gain as term is approached but it is still not clear whether this effect is real or artifactual. It is probable that the placenta becomes relatively less efficient towards the end of pregnancy, thus constraining fetal growth, but since all the curves originate from cross-sectional data we cannot prove this. It is equally possible that this shape of curve is obtained because bigger babies are born sooner while smaller ones remain *in utero* to be delivered later, thus reducing the slope of the curve near to term and even causing a fall in apparent birthweight after 41 weeks, as is seen in the 10th percentile of the 1970 British Births Survey.

SELECTION OF POPULATION

Given all the problems with existing intrauterine growth curves, it would seem sensible that such curves should be calculated for the population in question. Given the wide availability of computers, this is not such an onerous task. However, there are major decisions to be made as to how this is done, particularly with regard to inclusion and exclusion criteria.

The factors which are known to have a major effect on fetal growth are:

Birth order	Maternal nutrition
Sex of infant	Smoking/alcohol
Maternal height	Hypertension
Ethnic origin	Placental insufficiency
Plurality	Diabetes
Altitude	Anemia
Social class	Fetal malformations
Fetal disease	

Should allowance be made for any or all of these? I think that some of the "biologic" factors should be taken into account, and in this group I would include birth order, sex of infant, and possibly maternal height. However, there is some evidence that much of the variation in birthweight with maternal height is due to environmental factors (28) and thus should not be included. There are also practical difficulties in taking maternal size into account, as there seems no simple way of doing this (29) (although allowance for maternal height was included in the data published by Thomson, Billewicz, and Hytten (30)).

While it is generally accepted that birth order has a marked effect on birthweight, it has of course nothing to do with genetic growth potential and must be the result of altered environmental constraint with successive pregnancies. There is therefore a strong argument for excluding first born infants from intrauterine growth charts, or making separate charts (30).

Ethnic effects may also be largely environmental. Wharton (31) has shown a secular trend to increase in the birthweight of Asian babies in Birmingham, UK. His studies also suggest that small Asian babies have anthropometric, biochemical, and immunologic evidence that their lack of growth is pathologic and not normal. Furthermore, he makes the important point that if we had separate growth charts for each race in each geographic location, then we would have almost as many charts as babies. Miller (32) reviewed six American birthweight standards and showed the difficulties in comparing one with another, their data being so different. One excluded 30 growth-retarding factors, one allowed for parity, two excluded toxemia, two excluded major anomalies, and two corrected for the infant's sex. Four of the standards made allowances for ethnic origin but none for maternal height. Other charts have been derived differently. Some give mean values but others give median values, and as already discussed the measures of dispersion, e.g., standard deviation or percentiles, are different. A growth chart for Japanese babies (32a) calculated standard deviation at 36 weeks and then applied it to all gestations. This was not done in most other studies but the fact that the standard deviation lines in these studies run nearly parallel to the mean at lower gestations (and therefore birthweights) indicates, at least in part, the increasingly small numbers in the groups at lower gestational ages.

As a result of these variations in methodology it is almost impossible to compare one intrauterine growth chart with another. There seem to be two ways to improve this situation. First, it is important that agreement is reached on the criteria for inclusion and exclusion of data used to compile each growth chart. The format in which these data are presented must be standardized. Second, it is necessary to define an international reference chart for intrauterine growth so that the local growth charts can be compared with the standard and decisions made about whether intervention is indicated. As Wharton (31) points out, this chart does not imply a standard of excellence but only a standard for reference. In this regard the approach of Dunn (33,34) has great advantages as his reference curves are calculated from a study of various intrauterine growth charts. He has shown that the slope of incremental weight gain with gestation is remarkably constant and is effectively linear between 28 and 38 weeks gestation. In the period between 38 weeks and term, and in the immediate postnatal period, there is a flattening of the curve but the slope is regained soon afterwards and maintained until 18 weeks post delivery.

CONCLUSION

In spite of the limitations of so called "intrauterine" growth curves as they exist at present, they remain the major method for identifying the baby whose growth has deviated from the normal. Standardization of the methods of data collection and of the construction of growth curves will allow comparison between curves for the local population and an international reference curve. This will aid the identification of the infant at risk and indicate when and how intervention may be necessary.

REFERENCES

1. Seeds JW. Impaired fetal growth. ultrasonic evaluation and clinical management. *Obstet Gynecol* 1984;64:577–84.
2. Ott WJ, Doyle S. Ultrasonic diagnosis of altered fetal growth by use of a normal ultrasonic fetal weight curve. *Obstet Gynecol* 1984;63:201–4.
3. Rohrer F. Der Index der Körperfülle als Mass des Ernährungszustandes. *Münchener Medizinische Wochenscrift* 1921;68:580–2.
4. Karn MN, Penrose LS. Birthweight and gestation time in relation to maternal age, parity and infant survival. *Ann Eugen* 1951;16:147–64.
5. Wilcox AJ, Russell IT. Birthweight and perinatal mortality: II. On weight specific mortality. *Int J Epidemiol* 1983;12:319–25.
6. Boersma ER. *Perinatal circumstances in Dar es Salaam, Tanzania.* Thesis for the degree of Doctor of Medicine of Erasmus University, Rotterdam. 1979; 114, and personal communication.
7. Turner G. Recognition of intrauterine growth retardation by considering comparative birth-weights. *Lancet* 1971;2:1123–4.
8. Westergaard JG, Teisner B, Hau J, Grudzinskas JG, Chard T. Placental function studies in low birthweight infants with and without dysmaturity. *Clin Obstet Gynecol* 1985;65:316–8.
9. Clifford SH. Postmaturity with placental dysfunction. *J Pediatr* 1954;44:1–13.
10. Campbell S. Fetal growth. *Clin Obstet Gynecol* 1974;1:41–65.
11. Jarai I, Mestyan J, Schultz K, et al. Body size and neonatal hypoglycaemia in intrauterine growth retardation. *Early Hum Devel* 1977;1:25–38.
12. Taylor DJ. Low birthweight and neurodevelopmental handicap. *Clin Obstet Gynecol* 1984;11:525–42.
13. Rudolph AJ. Failure to thrive in the perinatal period. *Acta Paediatr Scand* 1985;Suppl. 319:55–61.
14. Usher R, McLean F. Intrauterine growth of live-born caucasian infants at sea level: standards obtained from measurements in 7 dimensions of infants born between 25 and 44 weeks of gestation. *J Pediatr* 1969;74:901–10.
15. Lubchenco L, Hansman C, Dressler M, Boyd E. Intrauterine growth as estimated from liveborn birthweight data at 24 to 42 weeks gestation. *Pediatrics* 1963;32:793–800.
16. Walther FJ, Ramaekers LHJ. Neonatal morbidity of SGA infants in relation to their nutritional status at birth. *Acta Paediatr Scand* 1982;71:437–40.
17. Tanner JM, Thomson AM. Standards for birthweight at gestation periods from 32 to 42 weeks, allowing for maternal height and weight. *Arch Dis Child* 1970;45:566–9.
18. Babson S, Behrman R, Lessel R. Fetal growth. Liveborn birthweights for gestational age of white middle class infants. *Pediatrics* 1970;45:937–44.
19. Gairdner D, Pearson J. A growth chart for premature and other infants. *Arch Dis Child* 1971;46:783–7.
20. Butler N, Alberman E. *Perinatal problems.* 2nd report of the 1958 British Perinatal Mortality Study. London: Churchill Livingstone, 1969.
21. Neligan G. A community study of the relationship between birthweight and gestational age. In: Dawkins M, MacGregor B, eds. Gestational age, size and maturity. *Clin Devel Med* 1965;19:28–32.
22. Milner RDG, Richards B. An analysis of birthweight by gestational age of infants born in England and Wales 1967 to 1971. *J Obstet Gynaecol Br Cwlth* 1974;81:956–67.
23. Dubowitz LMS, Dubowitz V, Goldberg C. Clinical assessment of gestational age in the newborn infant. *J Pediatr* 1970;77:1.
24. Keen DV, Pearse RG. Intrauterine growth curves: problems and limitations. *Acta Paediatr Scand* 1985; Suppl. 319:52–4.
25. Keen DV, Pearse RG. Birthweight between 14 and 42 weeks gestation. *Arch Dis Child* 1985;60:440–6.
26. Keirse MJNC. Aetiology of intrauterine growth retardation. In: Van Assche FA, Robertson WB, eds. *Fetal growth retardation.* Edinburgh: Churchill Livingstone, 1981;37–56.

27. Keirse MJNC. Epidemiology and aetiology of the growth-retarded baby. *Clin Obstet Gynecol* 1984;11:415–36.
28. Naeye RL, Tafari N. Biologic bases for international growth curves. *Acta Paediatr Scand* 1985; Suppl. 319:164–9.
29. Carr-Hill RA, Pritchard CW. Reviewing birthweight standards. *Br J Obstet Gynaecol* 1983;90:718–25.
30. Thomson AM, Billewicz WZ, Hytten FE. The assessment of fetal growth. *J Obstet Gynaecol Br Cwlth* 1968;75:903–16.
31. Wharton BA. Sorrento studies of birthweight. Case for international reference data. *Acta Paediatr Scand* 1985; Suppl. 319:170–9.
32. Miller HC. Intrauterine growth retardation. An unmet challenge. *Am J Dis Child* 1981;133:944–8.
32a.Funakawa H. Statistical observations of low birthweight newborns and standards of birthweight and length according to gestational age. *Jpn J Ped* 1964;17:872 (in Japanese).
33. Dunn PM. The gestogram—a new standard perinatal growth chart. Proceedings 3rd German Congress of Perinatal Medicine. Stuttgart: Thieme Verlag 1972;242–7.
34. Dunn PM. The perinatal growth chart for international reference. *Acta Paediatr Scand* 1985; Suppl. 319:180–7.

DISCUSSION

Dr. Villar: Do you think we should classify babies as having intrauterine growth retardation (IUGR) if they have a low ponderal index, even if their birthweights are above the 10th percentile for the population?

Dr. Pearse: Yes I think that you should, if you are convinced that the ponderal index is a good way to measure it. I think there are probably better ways of recognizing intrauterine malnutrition.

Dr. Villar: Do you think the cubic power of length should be used in deriving a ponderal index?

Dr. Pearse: Length is a difficult measurement to make in the neonate anyway, and using cubic length makes it even more inaccurate. It would be nice to get away from length altogether because the reproducibility of the measurement is so uncertain.

Dr. Wharton: My question relates to symmetric versus asymmetric growth retardation. We accept that symmetric growth retardation probably reflects an early pregnancy problem, and asymmetric growth retardation a late one, but I know that when I go around the nursery looking at babies who are light-for-gestational age I do not always find it very easy to differentiate them in this way. For example, I know that I see babies whose mothers had severe pre-eclampsia who appear to have symmetric growth retardation, despite the fact that they should be asymmetric! The ponderal index was supposed to differentiate between these types of IUGR, but in fact you don't get a bimodal distribution as you should if the concept were correct. I just wonder if we are trying to force the facts into the concept rather than the other way round.

Dr. Pearse: That is why I included a ''mixed'' group and why I did not specify proportions in the various groups.

Dr. Villar: We try to divide infants into symmetric and asymmetric growth retardation based on an instrument which is not really adequate. I think we should go back to the original concept of the fetus receiving insults at different stages of pregnancy. The timing of the insult is the central concept and the problem at the moment is that our instruments for measuring it *in utero* are not good enough. The timing is crucial because it will determine the outcome in terms of physical growth, and even more in terms of mental development. I think we should be trying to improve our ability to measure the outcome, but also to consider more carefully when the fetus is insulted, in relation to the physiology of growth and development at that particular time.

Dr. Pearse: I quite agree with this. However, the point that Dr. Wharton was making was that you may think you know when the insult occurred quite precisely, but when you examine the baby he does not fit the clinical category he ought to. It seems that the baby has not read the books!

Dr. Villar: We have seen that the proportion of the IUGR subgroups you have described (symmetric, asymmetric, and mixed) is not fixed but variable, depending on the population. In developed countries, for example, there is likely to be a low proportion of symmetric SGA infants. In developing countries, on the other hand, there is a very high proportion of symmetric IUGR. We must be very careful when comparing IUGR incidence in the different populations.

Dr. Canosa: If we are to follow your suggestions, we must make intrauterine growth charts for every different population—perhaps six or seven charts for the United Kingdom, 10 or 15 for Spain, and maybe 30 to 50 for India! What are your specific recommendations for a given country, taking into account three limiting factors: maternal height, baby's sex, and parity or birth order? My second question is, What do you suggest we should take as the international reference standard? And what specific measurements do you suggest we do to differentiate small appropriate-for-gestational-age (AGA) infants from large SGA infants?

Dr. Pearse: I believe we should have measurement charts specific to each region. This does not mean that these represent the ideal growth curves, but at least they take into account specific regional differences which affect birth size. For example, there is not much point in using birthweight of the Denver population born 5,000 ft high as your standard if you happen to work in Los Angeles. Denver babies cannot be expected to achieve the same birthweight as babies born at sea level. It is also very important to exclude smokers from standards. Most standard charts include smoking mothers, and this is bound to give misleading information. As to what international reference standard to use, I do not think this matters very much, so long as everyone is in agreement about it although the Gestogram has much to recommend it. If your babies are so many standard deviations below or above the reference standard, you can start to ask why. Are you a race of pygmies, or are your mothers smoking too much, or aren't they eating properly? Or if you are Swedish and your babies are above the standard percentiles, is this because your mothers are taller? As far as measurements go, I think at the moment the three basic measurements (weight, length, and head circumference) still seem to be as good as any, even though length measurements are not very easy and head circumference is not as simple as it sometimes seems.

Dr. Priolisi: I think that in the clinical practice we should have only one reliable reference standard, so that we can describe our population in comparable terms everywhere the standard is used.

Dr. Pearse: I agree, so long as the reference standard is constructed from appropriate and reliable data—sea level, non-smokers, and so on. But I still think that it is useful to compare your population with the reference standard as well as individual babies. That is why I think that it is worthwhile constructing growth curves for your own population.

Dr. Marini: The real problem is what to do clinically. If the obstetrician is faced with retarded fetal growth, what should he do? Should he act on his assessment of fetal weight, or should he be looking at biochemical changes in the fetus to guide him?

Dr. Pearse: I don't think obstetricians are good enough at judging weight *in utero* to use this assessment in making clinical decisions. I think judgments have to be made on the basis of gestation, neonatal mortality and morbidity rates in your neonatal unit, and the balance of risks in leaving the baby undelivered. This is bound to be better than making a guess that the weight of a baby is, say, 800 g and then finding it is 500 g, which is the kind of error which does not infrequently occur.

Dr. Belizan: Getting back to reference standards, I think you must include something about the validation of gestational age in your recommendations about the construction of such charts.

Dr. Pearse: It is impossible to construct such a chart unless you know the gestation. Ideally, you need early ultrasound confirmation, and it is preferable only to use data where obstetric history, ultrasound, and pediatric findings all agree.

Dr. Guesry: Tanner and others have shown that growth velocity is more informative than attained size at any particular time. Is there any work that has been done on the velocity of various measurements of fetal growth during pregnancy?

Dr. Bracci: I agree that growth velocity is certainly very important. Don't you think that serial ultrasound measurements can yield useful velocity data? For example, what about charts of crown-rump length, humerus length, femoral length, head diameter, and so on?

Dr. Pearse: I thought when ultrasound first started in obstetrics that we should be able to get good longitudinal data, but I now think ultrasound has been a little disappointing. None of the measurements is easy enough to give really accurate reproducible longitudinal data.

Dr. Bossart: That is a revealing comment. It is certainly true that people tend to believe in figures when they are written down on paper. What measurements do you think are the best for clinical use?

Dr. Pearse: The one we use most is the biparietal diameter, which has major limitations in the diagnosis of asymmetric growth retardation. It is also not particularly easy to get right if the baby is lying in an awkward position or if there is oligohydramnios, which of course is a clinical situation where it is particularly important to know about fetal growth. We also use crown-rump length and femur length and abdominal girth, but I have not been particularly impressed with these measurements. However, I should say that on the whole the more measurements you use the better the prediction. There is no one perfect measurement.

Dr. Bossart: From an obstetrician's point of view, I should say first that we like to make measurements on several occasions and not just once; and second, that crown-rump length is very difficult to get right because of variations in intrauterine lie. Biparietal diameter is relatively easy to measure as well as the length of the major bones, such as the humerus and the femur, and finally abdominal circumference at the level of the umbilical insertion.

Dr. Villar: When you read the literature on the value of ultrasound in monitoring fetal growth it seems to me somehow disappointing. I think that if one wants to use it, one should include a measure of linear growth, such as femur length, and abdominal or trunk circumference. If you do not use combinations of measurements, the published data suggest that the predictability of abnormal fetal growth is very low.

Dr. Canosa: Postnatally, chest circumference is one of the best predictors of gestational age. A multinational study has shown that its correlation with birthweight is better than head circumference, crown-heel length, arm length, etc. It can easily be performed by primary health workers.

Dr. Pearse: What does it tell you, other than the fact that the birthweight is low or high?

Dr. Canosa: It is a good surrogate for birthweight, which could be important for developing countries.

Dr. Priolisi: I have some data on correlations between four indicators of intrauterine growth, measured at birth, for single (n = 8,736) and multiple (n = 208) births, as shown in Table 1. The correlation between pairs of the four indicators included in this study is higher

TABLE 1. *Product moment correlation coefficient. Single births (above diagonal)
and multiple births (below diagonal)*

Attribute	Birthweight	Birth length	Head circumference	Gestational age
Birthweight	1.00	0.87	0.84	0.38
Birth length	0.84	1.00	0.69	0.27
Head circumference	0.85	0.86	1.00	0.20
Gestational age	0.67	0.62	0.63	1.00

for multiple births. The analysis of the frequency distribution of the 8,736 single births for the above four indicators showed, in both histogram and in cumulative sample form, that the shape of these distributors suggests that more than one normal or Gaussian component may be present. A mixture of two normal distributions was fitted to the data for single births and the results are shown in Table 2. The approach adopted to the representation of distribution of birthweight, birth length, head circumference, and gestational age reflects the presence of a mixture of two distributions superimposed one to another. Each distribution can be described in terms of mean and standard deviation, with higher accuracy for the primary distribution. For each of the four indicators the mean of the primary distribution is higher, and the standard deviation is lower. The reverse occurs for the secondary distribution where a lower mean corresponds to a higher standard deviation, indicating a greater variability around the mean. Birthweight-specific neonatal mortality rates computed separately for the two components show a wide gap, being much lower for the primary than for the secondary distribution. Low birthweight (<2,500 g) does contribute heavily to mortality, but this effect is very much stronger in the secondary distribution. To work out health policies, the fraction of the population belonging to this secondary distribution needs to be known for defined geographical

TABLE 2. *Palermo live single births. Results of fitting mixtures to normal distributions
(and standard error)*

	Distribution				% in primary distribution
	Primary		Secondary		
Attribute	Mean	Standard deviation	Mean	Standard deviation	
Birthweight (g)	3,350	470	2,796	1,040	87.4
	(7.0)	(7.0)	(6.1)	(3.8)	(1.4)
Birth length (cm)	49.3	1.7	43.8	5.2	92.8
	(0.02)	(0.02)	(0.4)	(0.2)	(0.5)
Head circumference (cm)	34.0	1.4	29.5	3.8	95.7
	(0.02)	(0.02)	(0.5)	(0.2)	(0.6)
Gestational age (days)	280	9.2	259	32	84.8
	(0.1)	(0.1)	(1.2)	(0.7)	(0.7)

areas. On general grounds, it might be anticipated that the majority of single births would correspond to a normal pattern of fetal growth and would collectively form the primary distribution. A minority of pregnancies would belong to the secondary distribution and would represent some kind of fetal impairment and vulnerability.

REFERENCES

1. Dunn PM. The gestogram—a new standard perinatal growth chart. Proceedings 3rd German Congress of Perinatal Medicine. Stuttgart: Thieme Verlag 1972;242–7.
2. Dunn PM. The perinatal growth chart for international reference. *Acta Paediatr Scand* 1985; Suppl. 319:180–7.
3. Priolisi A, Pomilia ML, Ashford JR. Descriptive analysis of intrauterine growth indicators. *Acta Med Auxol* 1986;18:141–8.

Intrauterine Growth Retardation, edited by
Jacques Senterre. Nestlé Nutrition Workshop
Series, Vol. 18. Nestec Ltd., Vevey/Raven Press,
Ltd., New York © 1989.

Sonographic Evaluation of Fetal Growth and Well-Being

John W. Seeds

*The Department of Obstetrics and Gynecology, University of North Carolina at Chapel Hill,
Chapel Hill, North Carolina 27514*

INTRAUTERINE GROWTH RETARDATION

Intrauterine growth retardation (IUGR) is not itself a discrete disease process but an abnormality of fetal growth common to a variety of different conditions (1–4). The clinical significance of IUGR is well-established, but variation in definition, applicable birthweight (BW) standards, and primary etiologies of strikingly different significance can make it difficult to discuss IUGR with practical clarity (1). The most commonly used definition is a birthweight less than the tenth percentile for gestational age (1,5). By definition, therefore, the incidence of the condition is 10%. Affected infants face a 30% to 50% likelihood of intrapartum hypoxic distress and a 50% risk of neonatal complications that may include hypoglycemia, meconium aspiration pneumonia, or long-term growth impairment (6–10). Although inconsistency in the definition of IUGR chosen by individual investigators and variability of birthweight standards used to judge growth lead to a measure of confusion in reported clinical data on growth retardation, the greatest source of difficulty when comparing the outcomes of growth retarded infants is the variability of etiology of IUGR (5,11,12).

IUGR (BW below 10th percentile) may be the result of (a) constitutional influences (40%), (b) environmental factors (10%), (c) specific genetic disorders (10%), or (d) utero-placental insufficiency (40%) (Fig. 1) (1–3,12–20). Each of these categories of fetal growth impairment shows a typical anthropomorphic pattern as well as characteristic outcome. Furthermore, within each of these broad categories of etiology, there are many different specific disorders, each with a different long-term prognosis.

Etiology

Inevitably, the natural frequency distribution of birthweight will result in a group of babies small-by-weight standards who are not diseased or in danger, but rather

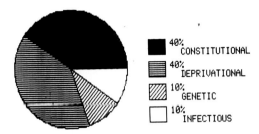

40% CONSTITUTIONAL
40% DEPRIVATIONAL
10% GENETIC
10% INFECTIOUS

FIG. 1. IUGR (BW below the 10th percentile) may be the result of several broad categories of etiology.

are simply small because of constitutional influences, such as familial growth patterns (11). Such infants do not necessarily face long-term developmental problems. Another group of babies are small because of toxic environmental factors such as maternal alcohol abuse (17,18). Evidence suggests that such infants do show long-term growth and neurobehavioral abnormalities, but the impact of obstetrical management on these problems is limited. IUGR on the basis of specific genetic abnormalities such as renal agenesis or trisomies is of minor importance when compared to the serious implications of the primary condition (16,20). Finally, IUGR resulting from utero-placental deprivation occurs most often with an otherwise normal fetus. Long-term follow-up has shown that the single perinatal factor most closely associated with later development is the presence or absence of perinatal asphyxia (7,10,21). Prenatal detection of fetal growth impairment offers the opportunity to apply methods of perinatal intensive care and possibly to prevent asphyxia. Furthermore, when Kurjak (22) studied 260 IUGR infants, he found that perinatal mortality was three-fold higher in cases where the diagnosis of IUGR was not made prior to labor. It is these normal infants, growth-retarded on a deprivational basis, who are most likely to benefit from prenatal diagnosis and intensive perinatal care.

Prenatal Sonographic Diagnosis

The sonographic evaluation of fetal growth and well-being is based on simple empirical observations. The larger the fetus, the larger will be the sonographic dimensions. Using this principle, fetal growth standards may be established from uncomplicated pregnancies, and these standards may be used to judge the quality of fetal growth in the individual case (22,23). The comparison of dimensions from the same fetus allows evaluation of the symmetry of growth, and the integration of selected dimensions may be used to estimate fetal weight *in utero* (24–27). The observation of dynamic events on real-time ultrasound offers important information about fetal well-being (28). Finally, deep Doppler ultrasound techniques, which are capable of evaluating fetal cardiovascular dynamics, seem able to identify those fetuses who are reacting to acute deprivation (29–31).

Fetal Adaptions

In the study of fetal biometry, it should be remembered that an important fetal mechanism for coping with acute and chronic deprivation is redistribution of cardiac output (32,33). The fetus responds to deprivational insults with vasoconstriction in most visceral and musculoskeletal beds in order to maintain flow to the cerebral, coronary, and adrenal circulations. The result is fetal hypertension, slowing of the heart rate (at least temporarily), the maintenance of brain growth, and therefore, cranial growth well into any deprivational sequence. This preferential redistribution on a chronic basis leads to an asymmetry of growth favoring cranial growth and delaying abdominal growth (22,25). Furthermore, hemodynamic flow characteristics are altered, including maximum blood flow rate, diastolic flow, and mean flow velocity in those vessels serving vasoconstricted vascular beds (29,30).

In this chapter, I shall briefly discuss the efficacy of clinical methods for the diagnosis of IUGR and the possible role of routine early pregnancy ultrasound examinations in screening for altered fetal growth. I shall evaluate the utility of static dimensions both individually and in combination to judge the quality and the symmetry of fetal growth and to estimate fetal weight. Important real-time observations related to monitoring fetal well-being, and Doppler techniques reflecting the status of fetal hemodynamics, will then be examined.

CLINICAL DIAGNOSIS OF IUGR

The clinical diagnosis of fetal growth retardation is typically expected to have a sensitivity of about 50% and may also have an accuracy of only 50% (34,35). Clinical diagnosis is based on both the serial measurement of uterine growth and on a high index of suspicion for IUGR in pregnancies complicated by maternal conditions known to be associated with impaired fetal growth (36). Although clinical methods are relatively imprecise, the only alternative to clinical screening of low-risk pregnancies as a basis for referral for more sophisticated and expensive technical evaluations is the routine serial sonographic evaluation of all pregnancies. Although routine ultrasound screening is practiced in many parts of the world, it is not part of standard care in the United States.

Fundal Growth

The uterus measured from the pubic symphysis to the top of the fundus between 20 and 34 weeks gestation is about equal in centimeters to the gestational age in weeks. Belizan (37–39) and other investigators have found that with a reasonable attention to consistency, determination of this index of growth may identify IUGR with 60% to 89% sensitivity. These observers have reported that the tenth percentile for fundal growth is approximately 4 cm less than the gestational age in weeks. Fundal growth delay in the low-risk prenatal population may therefore be a good clinical screening test for impaired fetal growth and should offer the possibility of detecting at least two-thirds of the affected infants in this group. It is estimated that one-third of the babies whose birthweight is below the tenth percentile come from the 65% of pregnancies that are otherwise low-risk (3,40).

TABLE 1. *Maternal risk factors for IUGR*

Previous history of growth retarded infant
Chronic or acute hypertension
Congenital or acquired heart disease
Chronic renal disease
Prepregnancy weight below 45 kg
Total pregnancy weight gain under 5 kg
Severe anemia
Advanced maternal age
Alcohol abuse
Heavy smoking

IUGR, intrauterine growth retardation.

Maternal High Risk Factors

The family of historical and clinical factors known to be associated with an increased risk of the birth of a growth-retarded infant (Table 1) includes maternal conditions associated with constitutional, deprivational, environmental, and genetic growth delay (3,40,41).

Low prepregnancy maternal weight and low weight gain certainly identify pregnancies that include a large number of constitutionally small infants (3,40). A large proportion of those women delivering successive pregnancies with IUGR are also only expressing familial tendencies. Acute and chronic maternal hypertension, maternal heart disease, and maternal renal disease are more often associated with deprivational fetal growth delay because of relative utero-placental insufficiency (41–43). Increased maternal age is associated with an increase in the likelihood of aneuploidy, which is associated with fetal growth retardation. The presence of any of these historical or clinical factors is sufficient indication for early ultrasound referral to establish or confirm gestational age and generate dimensional data as the basis for future evaluation of growth. Up to two-thirds of growth-retarded infants are born to the one-third of patients with one or more of these high-risk factors (40).

SONOGRAPHIC EVALUATION OF FETAL GROWTH

Sonographic tracking of fetal growth is based on two possible normative standards. First, an accurate knowledge of gestational age, either from an accurate history of the last menstrual period or early sonographic confirmation of gestational age, allows the comparison of fetal dimensions at one ultrasound examination to the expected values, so that diagnostic conclusions may be drawn regarding growth. But if early confirmation of gestational age was not accomplished or accurate menstrual data are not available, then sonographic information must be recorded at two examinations no closer than two weeks apart. The growth rate may then be evaluated. During the interval between examinations, ultrasonic or electronic fetal heart rate monitoring should be used to monitor fetal well-being.

TABLE 2. *Sonographic methods: diagnosis of IUGR*

Fetal dimensions alone
  BPD
  AC

Analysis of symmetry
   HC/AC
   AC/FL

Estimation of fetal weight
  From AC alone
  From BPD and AC
  From BPD, AC, and FL

IUGR, intrauterine growth retardation; BPD, biparietal diameter; AC, abdominal circumference; HC, head circumference; FL, femur length.

The sonographic indices of growth include individual fetal dimensions (22,23), comparison of selected dimensions intended to evaluate symmetry of growth (25,44), and the integration of certain dimensions in the estimation of fetal weight (Table 2) (26,27).

Fetal Dimensions

The widely varying accuracy and sensitivity in the detection of IUGR shown by several investigators (Table 3) for biparietal diameter by itself, serial biparietal diameter (BPD), abdominal circumference (AC), and head circumference (HC) to abdominal circumference ratio, probably reflect the variability in the growth characteristics of infants who are small because of deprivation compared to those who are small for constitutional reasons (22,45–47).

Asymmetrical growth is typical of deprivational growth retardation (44). In the deprivationally small infant, the biparietal diameter alone is not sensitive to the condition because of the sparing of brain growth secondary to redistribution of blood flow. It appears that abdominal circumference, both alone and in combination with

TABLE 3. *Relative sensitivity[a]*

Dimension	Sensitivity (%)
Single BPD	49
Serial BPD	50
AC	83
HC/AC ratio	80

[a]See Table 2 for explanation of abbreviations.

head circumference, offers the greatest sensitivity for diagnosing IUGR (22,47). Since the liver at the level where AC is measured constitutes about two-thirds of the area of the trunk image at that level, it is no surprise that this dimension appears to be a sensitive measure of the quality of fetal growth. The fetal liver is affected early and severely in cases of fetal deprivation. Furthermore, the AC will also be small in IUGR occurring on the basis of consitutional, genetic, and toxic factors, and is thus a valuable measurement in symmetric as well as in asymmetric IUGR. Mean abdominal diameter (MAD), as a fixed relative of abdominal circumference, may be substituted in most methodologies where AC is used.

Symmetry

The ratio of HC to AC in normal pregnancies follows a pattern which illustrates the gradually changing relationship of the head to the body (25). Normally the fetal head circumference in early gestation is larger than the abdominal circumference. The ratio slowly decreases until about 36 weeks gestation when the circumferences are approximately equal. Near to term the abdominal circumference becomes larger (Table 4).

An abnormality of this ratio suggests an abnormality of growth (25,44). An increased HC:AC ratio would suggest growth delay. A decreased ratio would be consistant with increased growth or macrosomia. Even in the case of deprivation, however, head growth will eventually be affected, and greater apparent symmetry will be noted late in the deprivational sequence (48).

In addition to the symmetry of growth of the fetal head and abdomen, a study of the comparative growth of the abdomen and the femur appears to offer possibilities in the diagnosis of IUGR (49,50). Vintzileos (49) and Seeds (50) have both reported that aberrations in the ratio of the abdominal circumference to femur length (FL), or of the mean abdominal diameter to femur length, can identify the IUGR infant with a sensitivity of about 80% (Figure 2 shows MAD:FL in graphic form, while Table 5 shows AC:FL in tabular form.).

More important is the observation that these ratios appear to detect selectively the

TABLE 4. *Head circumference/abdominal circumference*

Gestational age	− 2 SD	Mean	+ 2 SD
28	0.99	1.08	1.18
30	0.97	1.07	1.16
32	0.95	1.05	1.14
34	0.94	1.03	1.13
36	0.92	1.01	1.11
38	0.90	1.00	1.09
40	0.89	0.98	1.08

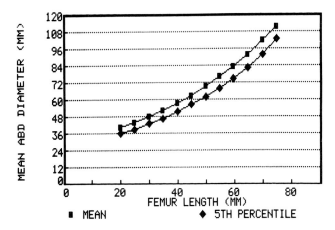

FIG. 2. Mean abdominal diameter in relation to femur length.

fetus with deprivational growth impairment. This suggests that in the intrinsically normal infant suffering only from nutritionally inadequate circumstances, the liver mass and therefore abdominal circumference will show growth impairment be-fore—and to a greater extent than—the femur. Furthermore, the detection of an anomaly of this relationship does not require accurate knowledge of gestational age since the data are not indexed to gestational age.

Estimation of Fetal Weight

The essential clinical measurement of IUGR is birthweight. An accurate knowl-edge of fetal weight, therefore, would be an ideal element of the accurate diagnosis.

TABLE 5. *Abdominal circumference (AC)/femur length (FL)*

FL (mm)	AC	
	Mean (cm)	5th percentile (cm)
20	12.9	11.3
25	14.0	12.3
30	15.1	13.5
35	16.5	14.8
40	18.2	16.3
45	19.8	17.9
50	22.0	19.6
55	24.0	21.4
60	26.2	23.6
65	28.9	26.1
70	32.0	28.9
75	35.2	32.4

TABLE 6. *Formulas for estimation of fetal weight*

1. $\log(BW) = 1.599 + 0.144(BPD) + 0.032(AC) - 0.111(BPD^2 \times AC)/1,000$
2. $BW = -299.076 + 9.337(BPD \times AC)$ (under 34 weeks only)
3. $BW = 10.1(AC \times BPD) - 481$ (under 2000 g only)

BW, birthweight; BPD, biparietal diameter; AC, abdominal circumference.

A wide variety of sonographic systems for the estimation of fetal weight have been reported since 1977 (Table 6) (26,27). These methods rely on the proportional growth of the fetus. Investigators simply determine selected dimensions of a group of fetuses shortly before birth and draw regression relationships between the selected dimensions and the recorded birthweight. Published systems include both simple linear relationships and logarithmic transformations (51,52).

Single dimension methods have used fetal abdominal circumference, while multiple dimension systems have shown improved accuracy using at least two dimensions, most often abdominal circumference and biparietal diameter (26). Other observers claim greater accuracy with at least three dimensions including AC, BPD, and femur length (53).

Clearly, differences in fetal proportionality will contribute to inaccuracy in estimation of fetal weight derived from only a limited number of dimensions. Furthermore, disproportionality is more often characteristic of the IUGR infant. It might thus be expected that these popular techniques would fall short in detection of growth impairment. Ott (54), however, in studying estimated fetal weight (EFW) methods in the care of pregnancies at risk of IUGR, found a sensitivity of 89%. He used his own normal fetal estimated weight data and the tenth percentile to achieve this level of detection (Table 7) (27). There was a false positive rate of 40%.

The sonographic dimensions used for the estimation of fetal weight are measured in a standard way. The BPD is the same BPD as that used for estimating gestational age, and the AC is also determined at the same level and with the same methods as

TABLE 7. *Mean estimated fetal weight and expected gain*

Gestational age (weeks)	Mean EFW (g)	5th percentile (g)	Expected gain in 2 weeks (g)
28	1,130	918	305
30	1,435	1,166	333
32	1,768	1,436	343
34	2,111	1,715	329
36	2,440	1,982	286
38	2,726	2,211	213
40	2,939	2,377	—

EFW, estimated fetal weight.

for gestational dating. The BPD is the largest diameter of the fetal cranium, outer edge to inner edge. This dimension is most often obtained at the level of the thalami. The AC is measured from a transverse image of the fetal trunk at the level of the umbilical vein within the liver mass. This is one of the most variable of fetal dimensions and requires considerable care in producing an image as close as possible to perpendicular to the fetal trunk (55). Once the correct image is generated at the level of the fetal liver, at right angles to the fetal spine, the circumference may be measured in two ways. Most modern ultrasound equipment offers electronic perimeter measurement systems. Infidelity to the true fetal skin curvature, however, introduces a positive error of up to 3% and the possibility of increased variability based on this error (56). The determination of two perpendicular diameters, and the estimation of circumference from the average diameter avoids much of this potential error.

From the normal estimated fetal weight data, expected growth rates may be derived, and at any given weight an expected weight gain in two weeks can be calculated (27). This manipulation gives the opportunity in the pregnancy of unknown gestational age to track fetal weight gain over the minimal two-week interval (Table 7) (54,55).

Amniotic Fluid Volume

The blood flow redistribution already mentioned that characterizes the fetal response to utero-placental insufficiency can, if sustained and severe enough, lead to reduced amniotic fluid volume because of reduced renal cortical flow and reduced fetal urine output.

Manning and others (57) reported that severe oligohydramnios itself suggests an element of immediate fetal distress, since they found perinatal mortality to be increased tenfold when IUGR was combined with greatly reduced amniotic fluid (a pocket less than 1 cm in greatest dimension). There may be difficulty in discriminating IUGR with severe oligohydramnios from IUGR with renal agenesis in the case of a patient first seen late in gestation. Careful anatomic examination may clarify the case, but can be difficult because image clarity is diminished by oligohydramnios. Maternal furosemide treatment might produce a fetal diuresis and establish the presence of a fetal urinary tract (58), but failure to produce a diuresis does not prove absence of fetal kidneys (59).

Routine Screening

Since imprecision in clinical assessment of gestational age or even complete absence of reliable clinical data complicates and compromises the diagnosis of IUGR, several investigations have focused on the efficacy of routine sonographic screening for IUGR. Warsof et al. (60) reported an 85% sensitivity and accuracy using a two-stage screen. Their approach utilized an early examination to establish or confirm gestational age, followed by a second examination at 32 weeks to evaluate fetal growth.

Doppler Evaluation

Sound echoes originating from a moving object have a higher frequency if the object is moving toward the observer and a lower frequency if the object is moving away. This is the Doppler effect. If either a pulse-echo or continuous wave ultrasound beam is directed at blood within a vessel, the frequency shift of the echoes reflected from moving red cells is proportional to the velocity of the cells, and inversely related to the beam angle (29). Computer analysis of the frequency shift results in a spectrum of individual data points, since individual echoes from blood cells of differing velocities will produce a spectrum of related proportional Doppler shifts and not a single uniform shift (29). The shape of the maximum velocity profile offers important information about the vascular resistance of the circulation served by the vessel studied. The ratio of systolic peak velocity (S) to the diastolic minimum (D) is proportional to resistance. The beam angle does not directly influence this ratio, but if the angle is not sufficiently acute, technical measurement error has a greater relative impact on the result.

Pulse Doppler systems built into real-time sector machines as well as independent continuous wave (CW) Doppler devices both seem to provide adequate data for resistance measurements, but there are important differences in cost and in the acoustic power used. Duplex pulse Doppler systems range in cost up to $70,000.00, compared to continuous wave Doppler machines, which cost less than $15,000.00. Duplex pulse Doppler may require a temporal peak/spatial peak intensity of 1,000 mw/cm^2 to produce useful data, compared to the typical continuous wave intensity of 1 mw/cm^2. There are no reported adverse effects of the higher intensity of pulsed Doppler energy, but the significant difference in both cost and power may result in greater application of the CW types of systems.

Shulman (29) has studied the Doppler S:D ratio from fetal umbilical vessels using continuous wave equipment in both the normal and the IUGR pregnancy and found that in the normal case, the S:D ratio averages 2.8 at 25 weeks, dropping to 2.2 at term. In IUGR, the ratio was found to average 3.8 at 29 weeks and drop to 3.0 at term. Diagnostic sensitivity and power of discrimination are yet to be clearly established for Doppler methods, but this technique does offer insight into the fetal physiological response to stress and may prove to be a useful adjunct to the other methods presented.

Summary

Careful evaluation of these many points allows the conclusion that with careful clinical monitoring of low-risk pregnancies, including measurement of fundal height and ultrasonic evaluation of pregnancies with uncertain dating or fundal growth discrepancies, and with sonographic evaluation of high risk pregnancies, up to 90% of IUGR infants may be detected prior to labor (55). Such examinations should include BPD, AC, and FL, as well as estimation of fetal weight and amniotic fluid volume. The false positive rate may approach 40%, but if intensive perinatal surveillance is the appropriate response to such a diagnosis, sensitivity is the more valuable result. Neither routine ultrasonic screening of all pregancies nor Doppler methods have yet shown a higher rate of diagnostic sensitivity than this, although Doppler studies do offer a greater understanding of the pathophysiology of the condition.

SONOGRAPHIC EVALUATION OF FETAL WELL-BEING

The surveillance of fetal condition is an integral feature of the care of the pregnancy at risk for IUGR or one in which the diagnosis is already made. The diagnosis of IUGR is by itself insufficient to justify the delivery of a premature infant (55), and evidence of immediate fetal distress is the additional element necessary to proceed to delivery. Electronic fetal heart rate monitoring, in the form of the non-stress test (NST) and the contraction stress test (CST), is the standard approach to this surveillance (61–63). These tests record fetal heart rate without (NST) and with (CST) uterine contractions using Doppler techniques for detecting fetal heart movement. Heart rate accelerations indicate normal fetal midbrain function and well-being, while absence of these accelerations suggests compromise. Uterine contractions can be spontaneous and of sufficient frequency (3 per 10 min) to constitute a contraction stress test. Alternatively, dilute pitocin or nipple stimulation may be required to stimulate contractions. Late decelerations after two or three contractions during a CST suggest fetal hypoxia (64).

Non-stress tests demonstrate a low false negative rate, but a high rate of false positive results. The risk of fetal death within one week of a reactive (normal) non-stress test is as low as 3:1,000 in a high-risk population, but if the test is abnormal (non-reactive), as it is in up to 18% of tested cases, only 3% to 5% of these are truly in danger, either judged by the results of a contraction stress test or behavior in labor (61). A normal CST also has a good record of predicting a normal outcome, but a 50% false positive rate if abnormal, judged by labor performance (64).

Biophysical Profile

The empirical observation that a higher rate of fetal or perinatal death was seen in pregancies demonstrating decreased fetal breathing movements led to the development of a combination of dynamic observation on real-time ultrasound in addition to the NST, to produce a scoring system called the biophysical profile (28). The biophysical profile uses fetal breathing movements, trunk movements, limb movements, amniotic fluid volume, and the results of a non-stress test (Table 8).

Each normal observation allows 2 points, while absence results in 0 points. A re-

TABLE 8. *Biophysical profile*

Observation	Score	
	2 Points	0 Points
Fetal breathing	30 sec/30 min	Absent
Trunk movements	3/30 min	Absent
Limb movements	3/30 min	Absent
Heart rate acceleration on NST	15 BPM × 15 sec × 2/40 min	Absent
Amniotic fluid	One pocket 1 × 1 cm	Absent

NST, non-stress test; BPM, beats per minute.

active NST gives 2 points, while a non-reactive result gives 0 points. A score of 8 to 10 is normal. A score of 4 to 6 requires re-evaluation within 24 hr, and a score under 4 suggests the need for delivery.

Careful randomized comparison between the biophysical profile and the non-stress test in large series of high-risk pregnancies shows that the NST and the BPD are comparable in predicting a normal outcome, but that the BPD is significantly superior in the prediction of the compromised fetus (28). These results indicate that the NST remains a reasonable primary surveillance tool, and that the BPD, together with the contraction stress test, is useful in the case of the abnormal NST.

REFERENCES

1. Seeds JW. Impaired fetal growth: definition and clinical diagnosis. *Obstet Gynecol* 1984;64:303.
2. Daikoku NH, Johnson JWC, Graf C, et al. Patterns of intrauterine growth retardation. *Am J Obstet Gynecol* 1979;133:281.
3. Resnik R. Maternal diseases associated with abnormal fetal growth. *J Reprod Med* 1978;21:315.
4. Battaglia FG. Intrauterine growth retardation. *Am J Obstet Gynecol* 1970;106:1103.
5. Battaglia FG, Lubchenco LO. A practical classification of newborn infants by weight and gestational age. *J Pediatr* 1967;71:159.
6. Dobson PC, Abell DA, Beischer NA. Mortality and morbidity of fetal growth retardation. *Aust NZ J Obstet Gynaecol* 1981;21:69.
7. Koops BL. Neurologic sequelae in infants with intrauterine growth retardation. *J Reprod Med* 1978;21:335.
8. Chandra RK. Fetal malnutrition and postnatal immunocompetence. *Am J Dis Child* 1975;129:450.
9. Manara LR. Intrapartum fetal morbidity and mortality in intrauterine growth-retarded infants. *J Am Osteopath Assoc* 1980;80:101.
10. Low JA, Karchmar J, Broekhoven L, et al. The probability of fetal metabolic acidosis during labor in a population at risk as determined by clinical factors. *Am J Obstet Gynecol* 1981;141:941.
11. Brenner WE, Edelman DA, Hendricks CH. A standard of fetal growth for the United States of America. *Am J Obstet Gynecol* 1976;126:555.
12. Gruenwald P. Growth of the human fetus—I. Normal growth and its variation. *Am J Obstet Gynecol* 1966;94:1112.
13. Bosely ARJ, Sibert JR, Newcombe RG. Effects of maternal smoking on fetal growth and nutrition. *Arch Dis Child* 1981;56:727.
14. Jones KL, Chernoff GF. Drugs and chemicals associated with intrauterine growth deficiency. *J Reprod Med* 1978;21:365.

15. Knox GE. Influence of infection on fetal growth and development. *J Reprod Med* 1978;21:352.
16. Johnson TRB, Corson VL, Payne PA, et al. Late prenatal diagnosis of fetal trisomy 18 associated with severe intrauterine growth retardation. *Johns Hopkins Med J* 1982;151:242.
17. Kuzma JW, Sokol RJ. Maternal drinking behavior and decreased intrauterine growth. *Alcoholism* 1982;6:396.
18. Little RE, Streissguth AP, Barr HM, et al. Decreased birthweight in infants of alcoholic women who abstained during pregnancy. *J Pediatr* 1980;96:974.
19. Andreasson B, Svenningsen NW, Nordenfelt E. Screening for viral infections in infants with poor intrauterine growth. *Acta Paediatr Scand* 1981;70:673.
20. Kurjak A, Kirkinen P. Ultrasonic growth pattern of fetuses with chromosomal aberrations. *Acta Obstet Gynecol Scand* 1982;61:223.
21. Starfield B, Shapiro S, McCormick M, et al. Mortality and morbidity in infants with intrauterine growth retardation. *J Pediatr* 1982;101:978.
22. Kurjak A, Kirkinen P, Latin V. Biometric and dynamic ultrasound assessment of small-for-dates infants: report of 260 cases. *Obstet Gynecol* 1980;56:281.
23. Little D, Campbell S. Ultrasound evaluation of intrauterine growth retardation. *Radiol Clin North Am* 1982;20:335.
24. Hadlock FP, Deter RL, Roecker E, et al. Relation of fetal femur length to neonatal crown-heel length. *J Ultrasound Med* 1984;3:1.
25. Campbell S, Thoms A. Ultrasound measurement of the fetal head to abdomen circumference ratio in the assessment of growth retardation. *Br J Obstet Gynaecol* 1977;84:165.
26. Warsof SL, Gohari P, Berkowitz RL, et al. The estimation of fetal weight by computer assisted analysis. *Am J Obstet Gynecol* 1977;128:881.
27. Ott WJ, Doyle S. Normal ultrasonic fetal weight curve. *Obstet Gynecol* 1982;59:603.
28. Manning FA, Baskett TF, Morrison I, et al. Fetal biophysical profile scoring—a prospective study in 1184 high-risk patients. *Am J Obstet Gynecol* 1981;140:289.
29. Schulman H, Fleischer A, Stern W, et al. Umbilical velocity wave ratios in human pregnancy. *Am J Obstet Gynecol* 1984;148:985.
30. Kurjak A, Rajhvajn B. Ultrasonic measurements of umbilical blood flow in normal and complicated pregnancies. *J Perinat Med* 1982;10:3.
31. Bracero L, Schulman H, Fleischer A, et al. Umbilical artery velocimetry in diabetes and pregnancy. *Obstet Gynecol* 1986;68:654.
32. Meschia G. Supply of oxygen to the fetus. *J Reprod Med* 1979;23:160.
33. Evans MI, Mukherjee AB, Schulman JD. Animal models of intrauterine growth retardation. *Obstet Gynecol Surv* 1983;38:183.
34. Arias F. The diagnosis and management of intrauterine growth retardation. *Obstet Gynecol* 1977;49:293.
35. Rosenberg K, Grant J, Hepburn M. Antenatal detection of growth retardation—actual practice in a large maternity hospital. *Br J Obstet Gynaecol* 1982;89:12.
36. Scott A, Moar V, Ounsted M. The relative contributions of different maternal factors in small-for-gestational-age pregnancies. *Eur J Obstet Gynecol Reprod Biol* 1981;12:157.
37. Belizan J, Villar J, Nardin JC, et al. Diagnosis of intrauterine growth retardation by a simple clinical method-measurement of uterine height. *Am J Obstet Gynecol* 1978;131:643.
38. Calvert JP, Crean EE, Newcombe RG, et al. Antenatal screening by measurement of symphysis-fundus height. *Br Med J* 1982;285:846.
39. Rosenberg K, Grant J, Tweedie I, et al. Measurement of fundal height as a screening test for fetal growth retardation. *Br J Obstet Gynaecol* 1982;89:447.
40. Galbraith RS, Karchmar EJ, Piercy WN, et al. The clinical prediction of intrauterine growth retardation. *Am J Obstet Gynecol* 1979;133:281.
41. Long PA, Abell DA, Beischer NA. Fetal growth retardation and preeclampsia. *Br J Obstet Gynaecol* 1980;87:13.
42. Breart G, Rabarison Y, Plouin PF, et al. Risk of fetal growth retardation as a result of maternal hypertension. *Dev Pharmacol Ther* 1982;4:116.
43. Lunell NO, Sarby B, Lewander R, et al. Comparison of uteroplacental blood flow in normal and in intrauterine growth-retarded pregnancy. *Gynecol Obstet Invest* 1979;10:106.
44. Crane JP, Kopka MM. Prediction of intrauterine growth retardation via ultrasonically measured head/abdomen circumference ratios. *Obstet Gynecol* 1979;54:597.
45. Duff GB, Evans LJ. Measurement of the fetal biparietal diameter by ultrasound is not an accurate method of detecting fetal growth retardation. *NZ Med J* 1981;94:312.

46. Sabbagha RE. Intrauterine growth retardation—antenatal diagnosis by ultrasound. *Obstet Gynecol* 1978;52:252.
47. Wittmann BK, Robinson HP, Aitchison T, et al. The value of diagnostic ultrasound as a screening test for intrauterine growth retardation: comparison of nine parameters. *Am J Obstet Gynecol* 1979;134:30.
48. Crane JP, Kopka MM. Comparative newborn anthropometric data in symmetric versus asymmetric intrauterine growth retardation. *Am J Obstet Gynecol* 1980;138:518.
49. Vintzileos AM, Lodeiro JG, Feinstein SJ, et al. Value of fetal ponderal index in predicting growth retardation. *Obstet Gynecol* 1986;67:584.
50. Seeds JW, Egley CC, Katz VL, Cefalo RC. The relationship between mean abdominal diameter and femur length in normal and impaired fetal growth. *Am J Perinatol* 1986;3:245.
51. Thurnau GR, Tamura RK, Sabbagha R. A simple estimated fetal weight based on realtime ultrasound measurements of fetuses less than 34 weeks' gestation. *Am J Obstet Gynecol* 1983;145:557.
52. Weinberger E, Cyr DR, Hirsh JH, et al. Estimating fetal weights less than 2000 grams: an accurate and simple method. *Am J Radiol* 1984;141:973.
53. Woo JSK, Wan CW, Cho KM. Computer assisted evaluation of fetal weight prediction using multiple regression equations with and without fetal femur length. *J Ultrasound Med* 1985;4:65.
54. Ott WJ, Doyle S. Ultrasonic diagnosis of altered fetal growth by use of a normal ultrasonic fetal weight curve. *Obstet Gynecol* 1984;63:201.
55. Seeds JW. Impaired fetal growth: ultrasonic evaluation and clinical management. *Obstet Gynecol* 1984;64:577.
56. Tamura RK, Sabbagha RE, Pan WH, Vaisrub N. Ultrasonic fetal abdominal circumference: comparison of direct versus calculated measurement. *Obstet Gynecol* 1986;67:833.
57. Manning FA, Hill LM, Platt LD. Qualitative amniotic fluid volume determination by ultrasound-antepartum detection of intrauterine growth retardation. *Am J Obstet Gynecol* 1981;139:254.
58. Wladimiroff J. Effect of furosemide on fetal urine production. *Br J Obstet Gynaecol* 1975;82:221.
59. Romero R, Cullen M, Grannum P, et al. Antenatal diagnosis of renal anomalies with ultrasound: III. Bilateral renal agenesis. *Am J Obstet Gynecol* 1985;151:33.
60. Warsof SL, Cooper DJ, Little D, Campbell S. Routine ultrasound screening for antenatal detection of intrauterine growth retardation. *Obstet Gynecol* 1986;67:33.
61. Flynn AM, Kelly J, O'Conor M. Unstressed antepartum cardiotocography in the management of the fetus suspected of growth retardation. *Br J Obstet Gynaecol* 1979;86:106.
62. Baskett TF, Sandy EA. The oxytocin challenge test—an ominous pattern associated with severe fetal growth retardation. *Obstet Gynecol* 1979;54:365.
63. Kariniemi V, Ammala P. Short-term variability of fetal heart rate during pregnancies with normal and insufficient placental function. *Am J Obstet Gynecol* 1981;140:289.
64. Odendaal JH. The fetal and labor outcome of 102 positive contraction stress tests. *S Afr Med J* 1981;60:782.

DISCUSSION

Dr. Toubas: I would just like to comment how things are changing. Ten years ago, when attending deliveries, neonatologists used to make jokes about how obstetricians predicted birthweight. Weight discrepancies between predicted weight and birthweight were sometimes enormous. Neonatologists nowadays do not laugh anymore. Due to technical advances in ultrasound imaging, such discrepancies are now rare when pregnant women receive regular prenatal care from well-equipped centers with qualified staff.

Dr. Bossart: When there is very little amniotic fluid, what is its specific gravity? Do you think it may be necessary under some circumstances (for example, if the baby has a severe degree of hemoconcentration for some reason) that less fluid of high specific gravity may maintain the fetus's internal milieu? In other words, production is low to maintain its specific gravity and osmotic pressure.

Dr. Seeds: It sounds logical that this would be the situation in pre-renal azotemia, for example, but I cannot comment further.

Dr. Chessex: Your biophysical scoring system is interesting, but aren't you being rather over-restrictive in your assessment of fetal breathing movements by only looking at them for 30 min? I have heard recently that there can be periods of up to 4 hr with no breathing movements at all in an absolutely normal fetus. I suppose you restrict your observation period on grounds of practicality?

Dr. Seeds: I agree that you could clearly have a false positive biophysical profile if you were to look at breathing movements alone, but if you have a non-compromised fetus who is simply taking a nap then the other measures of our 5-point scale will be normal (reactive non-stress test, good amniotic fluid volume, and so on). We do not use the biophysical profile for primary surveillance in high-risk pregnancies because it is far too labor-intensive. The non-stress test alone is an adequate discriminator of the normal or not immediately threatened high-risk pregnancy. We use the profile as a back-up to the non-stress test, and then we go on to ultrasound, and even then we will not normally deliver a preterm baby on this evidence alone without a contraction stress test.

Dr. Kuletharn: What is the significance of fetal gasping movements which you sometimes see?

Dr. Seeds: I don't know what their significance is in the absence of other indications of fetal distress, though during fetal distress they may clearly result in meconium being drawn deeper into the tracheo-bronchial tree, which makes the obstetrician gasp too. Gasping can be confused with gagging sometimes. A fetus with nasopharyngeal anomalies can be seen gagging when he tries to swallow amniotic fluid. We saw this clearly on real-time ultrasound in a fetus with a pedunculated meningomyelocele.

Dr. Toubas: In animal experiments it has been shown that one isolated gasp or deep breath of -20 cm H_2O is of no significance, but when there is repetitious gasping it usually means there is some degree of asphyxia (1,2).

Dr. Wharton: What proportion of growth-retarded fetuses with non-reactive cardiotocography would be regarded as normal or not at immediate risk after doing your biophysical profile?

Dr. Seeds: Around 15% to 18% of non-stress tests will be unreactive in our high-risk obstetric population, and in about one-third of these the fetus will turn out to be in serious difficulty. The biophysical profile is capable of picking up the vast majority of these.

REFERENCES

1. D.G.R.S.T. Colloque de Port Bail. Toubas PL, Monset M, Couchard M, Dumez Y, Vigia P. Effet du Clampage du Cordon in Utero sur les Mouvements Respiratoires Foetaux. Progres scientifique, numéro special, Fev. 1979.
2. Tchobroutsky C, Toubas PL. Effect of cord clamping on fetal breathing. [Abstr.] Fifth conference on fetal breathing. June 1979. Nijmegen (Netherlands).

Intrauterine Growth Retardation, edited by
Jacques Senterre. Nestlé Nutrition Workshop
Series, Vol. 18. Nestec Ltd., Vevey/Raven Press,
Ltd., New York © 1989.

Endocrine Assessment of Feto-Placental Growth

L. Cédard, J. Leblond, and G. Tanguy

*Unité 166 INSERM et Laboratoire de Chimie Hormonale, Maternité Baudelocque,
75014 Paris, France*

Intrauterine growth retardation (IUGR) accounts for increased perinatal morbidity and mortality, and the early identification of the growth-retarded fetus remains a key factor in achieving the most favorable outcome for the infant and the mother.

IUGR implies the operation of certain factors (such as hypertension, toxemia, and infection) which inhibit the achievement of the full genetic potential of the fetus. It is necessary to consider what reduction in the potential weight of the full-term fetus can be described as pathological. On the basis of a study on the siblings of small-for-gestational age (SGA) babies, this reduction has been estimated at 653 g (1), but it is evident that there is an overlap between SGA and normal or appropriate birth-weight for gestation age (AGA).

It thus appears that the diagnosis of IUGR is difficult. However, in this situation hormonal assays will be useful because they allow us to perform longitudinal studies in patients who are considered by conventional risk factors to be at high risk.

This chapter will describe some of the biochemical indices which have been developed to overcome the inadequacy of clinical diagnosis and to establish a strategy for use when the fetus is considered to be at risk.

There is good evidence from hemodynamic studies that the blood supply to the feto-placental unit is impaired in most pregnancies with IUGR, even when they are not associated with hypertensive disorders of pregnancy. Gross and microscopic examination of placentas from SGA pregnancies shows diverse abnormalities; villous dysmaturity, abnormal configurations, widespread subchorionic thrombosis, and infarction. The functioning mass in terms of parenchymal and cellular content is markedly decreased in the small placenta of the SGA infant (2). This may account for the high incidence of fetal distress during the intrapartum period in pregnancies complicated by fetal growth retardation and for the low hormonal levels in the maternal blood.

HUMAN PLACENTAL LACTOGEN

Human placental lactogen (hPL), also called chorionic somatomammotrophic hormone (hCS), is a peptide produced in large amounts by the placenta (approximately 2 g/day) and secreted mainly into the maternal circulation. Its short half-life (15–25 min) and ease of analysis (usually by radioimmunoassay) explain why the determination of hPL has commonly been used for routine screening in pregnancy. Another advantage of hPL measurement is the absence of a diurnal variation in plasma levels. Serum samples also retain hPL activity for up to 3 days at ambient temperature, allowing central collection and assay. When frozen, activity remains for at least 6 months. Synthesis of hPL is related to placental mass and so a correlation is to be expected between hPL levels and placental weight. Most researchers have also shown a significant correlation between hPL and birthweight (3). An association between low maternal hPL levels and low birthweight in IUGR has been reported as early as 28 to 32 weeks gestation and has been found even more frequently after 36 weeks. Spellacy et al. (4) suggested that hPL might be a useful measurement for detection of the fetus at risk, and subsequently suggested that hPL concentration should be greater than 4 μg/ml after 30 weeks gestation (Fig. 1); the area below this on a plot of hPL against gestational age was called the "fetal danger zone." In a retrospective analysis of hPL measurement in 2,318 high risk pregnancies, Spellacy et al. (5) have been able to relate perinatal mortality after 30 weeks to hPL values in the fetal danger zone. There were 71 fetal deaths, and in 36 of these hPL was in the danger zone. However, low hPL was found in only 20% of women whose infants died in the neonatal period, and hPL in the danger zone was observed more frequently in patients with severe toxemia.

In a 3-year prospective study, these authors (5) included all high-risk patients, who were divided into two groups: one in which the hPL values were not reported, and delivery was planned when the clinician thought appropriate by other criteria; and the second in which hPL values less than 4 μg/ml were specially reported. If it was considered that the fetus might be mature, amniocentesis was performed and delivery was carried out if the lecithin/sphingomyelin ratio was mature. Of the 2,733 patients, 230 had hPL in the fetal danger zone; the perinatal death rate was significantly lower in the treatment group than in the control group (15% versus 3.4%) (Table 1).

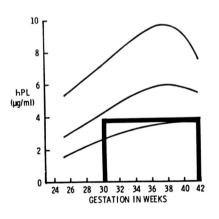

FIG. 1. Fetal danger zone for hPL concentrations. (From ref. 4.)

TABLE 1. *Human placental lactogen in fetal danger zone in 230 patients*

	Unreported group (%)	Treatment group (%)
Proportion of group in fetal danger zone	8.2	8.6
Fetal death rate	14.2	2.6 ($p < 0.003$)
Perinatal death rate	15.0	3.4 ($p < 0.005$)
Neonatal death rate	0.9	0.9 NS

From ref. 5.

Our first study in 1974 concerned 123 women in whom fundal height was less than would be expected for gestational age at two consecutive antenatal visits (6). After delivery, birthweight percentiles were calculated from Lubchenco's data (7), infants having a birthweight below the 10th percentile being classified as small for gestation (SGA). This corresponds approximately to the 3rd percentile in Paris, thus giving a high-risk newborn population. Most of the mothers were normotensive and without associated pathology. One-third of their infants (39/123) were SGA and two-thirds (84/123) were appropriate-weight-for-gestation (AGA). We excluded from this study diabetic and multiple pregnancies because in such cases the hPL levels are higher than in normal singleton pregnancies (8). In the study pregnancies, the mean values of hPL were lower than in normal pregnancies in both the SGA and the AGA groups, but the mean hPL value plateaued at 4 μg/ml at 28 to 30 weeks in the SGA pregnancies, whereas it continued to increase in the AGA group until the 39th week. Most of the values were lower than the mean for normal pregnancies; in 38 assays from the SGA pregnancies (70%) the values fell between the mean and the minus 1 SD level. We therefore felt that fetal growth retardation was unlikely when hPL values were higher than the population mean.

We observed a correlation between birthweight and the hPL value obtained between 4 weeks and 5 days before delivery. In 11 assays performed in women who delivered a newborn weighing less than 1,800 g after 35 weeks, hPL values were lower than 3 μg/ml. There was also a correlation between hPL and placental weight; all hPL values >4 μg/ml, except for one, corresponded to a placental weight of >400 g.

These results are similar to those reported by other workers (3–5) who have observed a significant trend toward low mean hPL values in IUGR pregnancies, and have found it possible to differentiate AGA from SGA pregnancies as early as 33 weeks gestation. However, many authors have pointed out that there is a considerable false positive rate; for example, Letchworth et al. (9) found a normal outcome in as many as 57% of pregnancies with hPL levels below 4.3 μg/ml. In a study by Morrison et al. (10), on the other hand, there was a high false negative rate, with only 41% of the cases of growth retardation being predicted by low hPL values. These workers concluded that hPL would appear to have a limited role in antepartum evaluation, and that screening should be limited to pregnancies associated with hypertension, to help reduce the risk of stillbirth and fetal distress occurring specifically in the IUGR fetus.

Recently Obiekwe et al. (11) measured hPL in serial blood samples obtained from 663 women at weekly intervals from 30 to 40 weeks gestation, including 231 with preeclampsia. The hPL levels were significantly lower in pregnancies associated with fetal growth retardation, but the clinical value of this observation appeared to be greater in multigravidae than in primigravidae, suggesting that in the latter group maternal hPL levels reflected both the pathology of the disease and the condition of the fetus, and that in primigravidae with preeclampsia the cutoff point between normality and abnormality should be slightly raised.

In IUGR pregnancies, measurements of mRNA sequence coding for hPL with an hPL complementary probe have indicated that the hPL mRNA concentrations are similar to normal pregnancies and that low hormonal levels associated with growth-retarded fetuses can be explained by their lower placental weights, which correlate with their total RNA content. The total capacity of *in vitro* hPL production per placenta is significantly lower than normal, but without basic intracellular disturbance in hPL synthesis (12).

It is interesting to note that normal pregnancies associated with partial or complete absence of hPL have been described. This abnormality is extremely rare and is due to gene deletion (13).

Other protein specific for pregnancy, such as alpha-feto-protein (AFP), which is a major constituent of the circulating proteins in early fetal life, and pregnancy-specific β-glycoprotein SP_1, have also been assayed in IUGR but their predictive value remains to be established.

ESTROGENS

The measurement of estrogens in pregnancy has largely been employed as an index of feto-placental function to identify the fetus at risk. The basic physiology underlying this practical application is the concept of the feto-placental unit described several years ago (14).

Estrogen, and chiefly estriol (E_3), is secreted by the placenta from androgenic precursors initially synthesized in the fetal adrenal gland and then further processed by the fetal liver. Estrogen production in pregnancy has frequently been measured in 24-hr urine collection and it is generally necessary to control for the completeness of the collection by simultaneously estimating creatinine. In most routine laboratories, estrogen is measured by the Brown colorimetric method (15) or by fluorometry (16).

The normal limits for estrogen excretion in the second half of pregnancy have been defined. Between 30 and 40 weeks the lower limit can adequately be described by a straight line joining 8 and 12 mg/24 hr, and this defines a zone of fetal risk (17). Estrogen excretion is very variable, both between women and daily in the same woman. Many factors are known to influence the urinary excretion of estrogens, some of which greatly reduce the value of this estimation in clinical practice. Nevertheless, many researchers have observed a correlation between urinary estrogen excretion (E_{ur}) and birthweight, and have claimed that the test is a useful one.

We have assayed urinary estrogen by the Ittrich method (16) in 123 women with suspected IUGR who delivered 39 SGA and 84 AGA infants (18). In women who delivered infants of normal birthweight, the urinary estrogen excretion was within the normal range. In the group delivering SGA infants, the mean urinary estrogen values were lower, with a plateau after the 32nd week instead of the normal increase, a phenomenon previously described by Klopper (19).

Beisher et al. (20) measured urinary estrogen excretion in 597 women; they reported that the perinatal mortality was 4.4% in the low estrogen group (<10th percentile) compared to 0.4% in the group with normal estrogens, and that birthweight was significantly reduced in the low estrogen group. The low estrogen group contained 21.2% infants with IUGR compared to 3.1% in the group with normal estrogens. However, only 54% of growth-retarded fetuses were detected by measurement of urinary estrogens in this study. False positive (low) results have been observed, particularly in preeclampsia, indicating that when estrogen excretion is low the clinical problem is usually obvious.

Advances in radioimmunoassay techniques have facilitated routine determination of unconjugated (E_3) or total estriol (E_3T) in plasma, and the ease of blood sample collections compared with 24-hr urine collection has led to increased interest in the clinical use of estrogen measurements. However, differences in methods for measurement of E_3, together with the extent of diurnal and random fluctuations in plasma E_3 concentrations, as well as the limited extent of current appraisal of fetal outcome have obscured the value of this method as an aid in the management of complicated pregnancies. Few data have been analyzed appropriately to evaluate whether the test contributes any useful clinical information, and it has never been established whether it is more valuable to determine the unconjugated estriol fraction (E_3) or the total plasma estriol (E_3T), which is ten times higher. Both have similar individual and diurnal variations.

We have been performing routine assays of E_3T since 1977, using an RIA kit (IM 82) at the Radiochemical Centre (Amersham, England), and we shall report here some characteristic observations, together with those results that have been subjected to computer analysis (21).

We have established E_3T levels for normal pregnancies from longitudinal values obtained in 88 patients who were judged to be free of complications, as determined by the course of pregnancy and delivery of a term singleton infant of normal birthweight, who did well during labor and the neonatal period. In the same group of women we also measured total estrogens in urine and hPL in plasma. We then studied 141 high-risk pregnancies between 31 and 39 weeks of gestation, complicated by idiopathic IUGR or with arterial hypertension and various other disorders or factors predisposing to fetal growth retardation. Fetal distress was confirmed in 15 suspected cases (11%). Total plasma estriol and 24-hr urinary estriol (expressed as mg estrogen/g creatinine) were correlated with each other when the samples were collected on the same day, and the results have been grouped into 3-week periods. It appears from Table 2 that the correlations are highly significant between E_3T and E_{ur} in all the groups except in preeclampsia. The general shape of the curves obtained by sequential determination of E_{ur} and E_3T is similar. This similarity holds true for the increasing levels observed in high-risk patients where pregnancy was normal, as well as for the sustained falls corresponding to *in utero* deaths in severe hypertension or preeclampsia.

In cases of fetal distress the estrogen values were lower than normal, but were not significantly different from those of the high-risk group without fetal distress. It therefore appears that the same information can be derived from E_3T plasma assays as from urinary estrogen analysis, but that a single determination could not give unequivocal information on the state of the fetus, better information being provided by sequential determination of estrogens, either in serum or urine.

The predictive value of estrogen measurements in cases of suspected IUGR seems to be better. In a group of 222 patients who delivered of 152 AGA infants and 70 SGA infants (mean birthweight 2,002 g at 37.8 weeks), there appeared to be a significant difference between the two populations for both variables except at the end of pregnancy in the case of E_3T (Table 3).

It should be noted that while 53% to 82% of E_3T values were low in SGA pregnancies, 28% to 41% of the values in AGA pregnancies were also low. The predictive value of a low E_3T was 41% to 45% according to the gestational age. The predictive value of E_{ur} was lower at 37% to 41%.

We were interested to see whether the combination of the two variables increased the precision of the diagnosis. We did not observe any SGA infants with normal E_3T and E_{ur}, or with low E_3T and normal E_{ur}. Fetal growth retardation was most likely to result when both of the tests were low at the same time, but the combination of E_3T and E_{ur} did not improve the predictive value, demonstrating once again that the same

TABLE 2. *Correlation between total plasma estriol (E_3T) and 24-hr urinary estrogen (E_{ur})*
(expressed as mg/g creatinine)

| | | Weeks of pregnancy | | | | | |
| | | 34–36 | | | 37–39 | | |
	No. of patients	No. of paired samples[a]	r	p	No. of paired samples[a]	r	p
Hypertension	33	6	0.85	< 0.05	49	0.31	< 0.05
Toxemia	8	6	0.49	NS	—	—	—
Hypertension + IUGR	21	15	0.58	< 0.05	22	0.68	< 0.001
IUGR	22	28	0.67	< 0.001	18	0.52	< 0.05

IUGR, intrauterine growth retardation.
[a]Paired samples E_3T/E_{ur}.
From ref. 21.

TABLE 3. *Percentage of normal and low plasma total estriol and urinary estrogens in suspected intrauterine growth retardation with (SGA) and without (AGA) birth of small-for-age neonate*

	Weeks of pregnancy					
	31–33		34–36		37–39	
	AGA	SGA	AGA	SGA	AGA	SGA
E_3T	n = 40	n = 11	n = 58	n = 23	n = 47	n = 17
Normal ($\geq$ 10th percentile)	72	18	59	26	72	47
	$p < 0.01$		$p < 0.01$		NS	
Low ($<$ 10th percentile)	28	82	41	74	28	53
E_{ur}	n = 59	n = 31	n = 85	n = 49	n = 73	n = 38
Normal ($\geq$ 50% of mean)	76	58	69	41	67	47
	NS		$p < 0.01$		$p < 0.05$	
Low ($<$ 50% of mean)	24	42	31	53	33	53

SGA, small for gestational age; AGA, appropriate for gestational age; E_3T, total plasma estriol; E_{ur}, 24-hr urinary estrogens.
Boxed numbers, %.
From ref. 21.

information can be derived from E_3T plasma assays as from the urinary estrogen analysis (21).

In a prospective study of 1,042 women with singleton pregnancies and known length of gestation, Nielsen (22) has tried to determine the prognostic value of E_3T. In high risk pregnancies, a low E_3T value ($<$2.5th percentile) was associated with a 42% risk of delivery of an infant with perinatal complications and a 17% risk of an SGA infant. Perinatal complications had been forecast or detected in 7% of these infants and fetal growth retardation in 19% by routine clinical screening. In a subgroup of 800 pregnancies considered normal according to given criteria, a low E_3T level involved a 17% risk of perinatal complications and a 15% risk of an SGA infant. In this group, 4% and 14%, respectively, had been detected by routine screening. He concluded that there should be a low threshold for measuring E_3T levels, but that the test was of limited value in pregnancies that are clinically quite normal.

Evans et al. (23) have carried out a prospective study of the clinical usefulness of plasma estriol determinations in predicting ''light-for-date'' infants before birth. Maternal estriols were measured at 35 to 36 weeks of gestation and the 10th percentile for E_3T and unconjugated E_3 values were used as cutoff points. Low estriol values were identified in less than a third of all low weight babies, and less than a third of pregnancies with low estriol values were associated with birth of light-for-date infants.

Chard et al. (24) have compared hPL and unconjugated E_3 in the prediction of IUGR. They measured hPL and E_3 in 392 women at weekly intervals from 36 to 40 weeks of gestation and found reduced levels of both in subjects delivering an SGA infant. The clinical significance of this observation was similar for the two compounds, with a marginal advantage to hPL. There was a higher incidence of falling levels of hPL and E_3 in cases of growth retardation. However, the findings had very little predictive value in the individual patient. In a further publication (25), these authors discuss the evidence that maternal E_3 levels are related to fetal growth and well-being, and conclude that this is likely to be a reflection of placental function, which is the final and probably rate-limiting step in the synthetic pathways from fetal precursors. This explains why measurements of E_3 seem remarkably similar to those of placental products such as hPL.

We should not forget the possible occurrence of sulfatase deficiency (26) in the case of very low levels of plasma or urinary estrogen. This is an interesting anomaly of placental steroidogenesis observed only in the male fetus, indicating that this deficiency is under control of a sex-linked recessive character (27). *In vivo* loading tests with dehydroepiandrosterone sulfate (DHA-S) allow an antenatal diagnosis of this condition, which may be confirmed by *in vitro* experiments showing zero or virtually zero placental sulfatase activity toward $\triangle_5$-pregnenolone or DHA-S.

We shall not dwell on the various general mechanisms which may result in a decrease of plasma or urinary levels of estrogen, such as antibiotics (e.g., ampicillin) which disturb intestinal glycuroconjugation or corticosteroids which inhibit the adrenal secretion of C_{19} steroids, but we wish to mention our personal observation of a significant decrease of unconjugated estradiol (E_2) and E_3T in plasma, and of E_{ur}, in patients treated with oral chlormadinone acetate for threatened premature labor. This phenomenon is due to a temporary inhibition of placental sulfatase by the synthetic steroid agent, without any noticeable fetal effects (28).

Metabolic Clearance of DHA-S

Measurements of metabolic clearance rate of DHA-S suggest that decreased utero-placental blood flow is the main factor contributing to reduced estrogen production and to prolonged DHA-S half-life (29). The *in vivo* placental clearance of DHA-S through E_2 is especially flow-dependent (30). There has been some controversy about the use of the DHA-S loading test (DLT) as described by Lauritzen (31) for the diagnosis of IUGR. We have studied the half-life of injected DHA-S and have found this variable to be more reliable than estrogen determinations in the diagnosis of IUGR (32). The half-life of DHA-S (50 mg intravenously) (DHA-S t 1/2) was calculated by least square analysis in the plot of log DHA-S concentration versus time at several intervals. We performed 102 tests in pregnant women between 30 and 41 weeks of gestation (Table 4).

We then compared the predictive value of (a) plasma E_3T, (b) the maximal E_2 increase after DLT (E_2), (c) its rate of increase per minute during the first 15 min after DLT (V E_2) (33), and (d) that DHA-S is the main precursor of estrogens in pregnancy. DHA-S first undergoes 16α-hydroxylation in the fetal liver, then in the placenta a conversion to estriol DHA-S t 1/2. As shown in Table 4, the maximal E_2 was similar in the control and the AGA groups, but was significantly lower in SGA pregnancies. V E_2 was also similar in control and AGA groups and significantly lower in

TABLE 4. *Results of dehydroepiandrosterone sulfate (DHA-S) loading test in suspected intrauterine growth retardation and controls*

	Control	AGA	SGA
Number of cases	43	39	20
Birthweight			
(g) (mean ± SEM)	3,066 ± 65	2,730 ± 68	1,881 ± 89
Maximal E_2 increase			
(ng/ml) (mean ± SEM)	34.4 ± 2.45	33.7 ± 2.9	19.5 ± 1.92
	(36)[a]	(26)	(17), $p < 0.001$[b]
Rate of increase of			
E_2 (ng/ml) (mean ± SEM)	1.86 ± 0.21	1.73 ± 0.20	1.08 ± 0.15
	(30)	(26)	(16), $p < 0.02$
DHA-S t½			
(hr) (mean ± SEM)	2.90 ± 0.12	3.24 ± 0.12	5.05 ± 0.20
	(43)	(39)	(20), $p < 0.001$

AGA, appropriate for gestational age; SGA, small for gestational age; E_2, maximum increase in plasma estrogen after DHA-S loading test.
[a]The numbers of assays in each category are given in parentheses.
[b]Student's t-tests were used to compute the significance of the difference between the AGA and SGA group.

fetal growth retardation. The mean value of DHA-S t 1/2 was similar in control and AGA groups. In SGA pregnancies the DHA-S t 1/2 was longer and the difference between AGA and SGA groups was highly significant. All the SGA babies except one had DHA-S t 1/2 >4.29 and most of the normal babies had values lower than this. A value lower than 3.75 always corresponded to normal birthweight for gestational age.

The E_3T was not a good criterion, as previously described. A low level was observed in 50% of the cases with normal birthweight. An E_2 value lower than 25 ng/ml was observed in 15 out of 17 cases of fetal growth retardation versus 7 out of 26 AGA pregnancies and 11 out of 37 control pregnancies. V E_2 was less discriminant, but had a high sensitivity: 13 of 16 determinations were <1.50 ng/ml per min in SGA pregnancies. However, the specificity was low, a slow increase being observed in 50% of AGA pregnancies and 36% of controls.

In a complementary approach we performed sequential assays of steroid intermediates after DLT in clinically suspected cases of IUGR. We observed that plasma levels of Δ_4-androstenedione and testosterone were significantly increased and remained elevated for 2 to 3 hr in SGA pregnancies whereas in the AGA group these values were increased only for a short period of time after the injection (34). *In vitro* perfusions of the delivered placentas of those patients given DHA-S have shown that a low estrogen production coincides with an accumulation of neutral steroids in the perfusate and it appears that the placental conversion of DHA-S into estrogen may be slowed at the aromatization step in some case of IUGR (35). This phenomenon is independent of the placental blood flow, since each perfusion is performed under standardized conditions of pressure and flow. It suggests that an impairment of placental metabolism could be superimposed on the hemodynamic alteration.

PREDICTIVE VALUES OF THE ENDOCRINE ASSESSMENT OF FETOPLACENTAL GROWTH

Echographic measurements of fetal development have been steadily improving over several years. Nevertheless, attempts are still being made to define the clinical usefulness of estriol assay for diagnosing fetal growth retardation (23) and to determine cutoff points which discriminate between normal and abnormal hPL values in the prediction of IUGR. For example, Litford et al. (36) determined the effects of changing the cutoff points on the sensitivity, specificity, and predictive value of the test. When the 10th percentile of hPL values was used, 29% of all growth-retarded fetuses were identified and 91% of all normal fetuses were excluded. The 15th and 25th percentiles yielded improved sensitivities of 37% and 50%, respectively, but specificity was reduced. They proposed the 10th percentile as the best compromise between sensitivity on the one hand, and predictive value on the other, and suggested that this concept can also be applied to other biochemical or non-biochemical tests of fetal well-being.

Aickin et al. (37) analyzed urine and plasma E_3 data obtained during 608 pregnancies together with plasma progesterone, hPL, SP_1, β-glycoprotein, and serum cystyl aminopeptidase. The predictive accuracy of low values for the identification of SGA infants was assessed for each test at various gestation ages. Dates were analyzed to obtain 10th to 90th percentile values for each test from 28 weeks to delivery. Groups with values under different percentile levels were compared; those under the lower percentiles had higher proportions, but smaller absolute numbers of SGA infants than those under higher percentiles. No test was superior to the others at all percentiles and gestations, and it was concluded that biochemical screening of pregnant populations to identify women requiring intensive monitoring has limited potential.

The problem is complicated by the fact that racial differences may interfere with the determination of reference standards of intrauterine growth. It has been shown that Asian mothers have higher hPL levels between 28 and 38 weeks than European mothers, and in IUGR their hPL levels were only low in the last trimester, and urinary estriol excretion was normal (38).

Two years ago we tried to define a strategy for the use of the biochemical assays (hPL, E_3T, E_{ur}, and E_2 increase and DHA-S t 1/2 after loading test), based on a study of 178 women admitted to hospital for suspected IUGR during a period of two years, and who had also ultrasonic determination of biparietal and transverse abdominal diameters between 27 and 40 weeks of gestation (*unpublished observations*).

These women delivered 52 SGA infants (29%), indicating a high risk of fetal hypotrophy in the group. Table 5 shows that four measurements had diagnostic value:

TABLE 5. *Distribution of echographic variables and hormonal estimations in suspected intrauterine growth retardation (SGA) and control (AGA) groups*

| | SGA | | AGA | | |
	n	%	n	%	p
Biparietal diameter					
> 10th percentile	26	50	92	73	< 0.01
≤ 10th percentile	26	50	34	27	
Transverse abdominal diameter					
> 10th percentile	21	42	86	69	< 0.001
≤ 10th percentile	29	58	38	31	
hPL					
Normal	15	31	66	53	
Low	34	69	58	47	< 0.01
E_3T					
> 10th percentile	28	56	78	61	NS
≤ 10th percentile	22	44	49	39	
E_{ur}					
Normal	12	36	49	51	NS
Low	21	64	48	49	
DHA-S t½					
< 4.29 hr	23	45	91	71	< 0.01
> 4.29 hr	28	55	37	29	

SGA, small for gestational age; AGA, appropriate for gestational age; hPL, human placental lactogen; E_3T, total plasma estriol; E_{ur}, 24-hr urinary estriol excretion; DHA-S t½, half life of dehydroepiandrosterone sulfate after 50 mg loading dose.
Boxed numbers, %.

biparietal and abdominal diameters, hPL and DHA-S t 1/2. Biparietal diameter had the highest specificity and hPL the highest sensitivity. The predictive value of these two criteria was identical.

In an attempt to choose the best cutoff point for DHA-S t 1/2 we determined the sensitivity and the specificity for different values. It appears that the value 4.29 hr, which had previously been chosen, is a good compromise, the sensitivity being 54.9%, and the specificity being 71%. The two echographic variables (biparietal and abdominal diameters) both had a sensitivity of 76%, using the 10th percentile as cutoff point, and a specificity of 68%. Due to the low cost of hPL versus DHA-S t 1/2, we consider that the former is a better complementary biochemical variable.

In a more theoretical study we integrated these results to establish the predictive value of the different tests for screening a general population where the prevalence of IUGR is 5%, and a high-risk population with a prevalence of 20%. Whatever the a priori risk of IUGR (5% or 20%), the presence of at least two abnormal results gives a high probability of identifying fetal growth retardation (between 36% and 92%).

It thus appears that in the low-risk population it is not necessary to undertake

TABLE 6. *Probability of small-for-gestational-age (SGA) infants in a population having a low risk of fetal growth retardation (5%)*

Transverse abdominal diameter		n	Probability (%)
< 10th percentile	hPL low	294	68
	hPL normal	945	11
≥ 10th percentile	hPL low	1,000	15
	hPL normal	7,761	1

hPL, human placental lactogen.

DHA-S t 1/2 determination when transverse abdominal diameter and hPL are both normal or both low, and that this latter screening procedure allows us to isolate a group including 3% of the population in which the risk of fetal growth retardation is high (68%) and a group at very low risk (<1%) which includes 78% of the population (Table 6).

Since 1983 we have also observed in our hormone laboratory, as in others, that there are important correlations between various biochemical indices in high-risk pregnancies and the non-invasive determination of utero-placental blood flow using either 113 indium and a computer-linked gamma camera (39) or, more commonly, blood velocity measured by the Doppler effect on ultrasound (40), both of which are capable of predicting the severity of fetal growth retardation.

Nevertheless, it is evident that assays of hPL, and to a lesser extent estrogens, may have a place in the prediction of IUGR, especially if used in conjuction with ultrasonography, providing that they can be repeated at least twice between the 30th and the 36th week of pregnancy to detect stationary or falling levels.

REFERENCES

1. Ounsted M, Ounsted C. *On fetal growth rate*. Clinics in Developmental Medicine, n° 46, Spastics International Medical Publications. London: Heinemann, 1973.
2. Teasdale F. Morphological and functional aspects of placental dysfunction. *Contrib Gynec Obstet* 1982;9:17–28.
3. Letchworth AT. Human placental lactogen assay as a guide to fetal well-being. In: Klopper A, ed. *Plasma hormone assays in evaluation of fetal well-being*. Edinburgh: Churchill Livingstone, 1976;147–73.
4. Spellacy WN, Teoh ES, Buhi WC. Human chorionic somatomammotrophin (hCS) levels prior to fetal death in high risk pregnancies. *Obstet Gynecol* 1970;35:685–9.
5. Spellacy WN, Buhi WC, Birk SA. The effectiveness of human placental lactogen measurements as an adjunct in decreasing perinatal deaths. Results of a retrospective and a randomized controlled prospective study. *Am J Obstet Gynecol* 1975;121:835–44.
6. Cedard L, Hubert CH, Legraverand M, Laurent A, Tanguy G, Henrion R. Intérêt des dosages hormonaux urinaires et plasmatiques pour la surveillance des femmes enceintes présentant un retard du développement utérin. In: Sholler R, ed. *Exploration hormonale de la grossesse*. Paris: Sepe, 1974;487–509.

7. Lubchenco LO, Hansman C, Pressler M, Boyd E. Intrauterine growth as estimated from liveborn birthweight data at 24 to 42 weeks of gestation. *Pediatrics* 1963;32:793 800.
8. Ursell W, Brudenell M, Chard T. Placental lactogen levels in diabetic pregnancy. *Br Med J* 1973;20:80–2.
9. Letchworth AJ, Slattery M, Dennis KJ. Clinical application of human placental lactogen values in late pregnancy. *Lancet* 1978;1:955–7.
10. Morrison I, Green P, Oomen B. The role of human placental lactogen assays in antepartum fetal assessment. *Am J Obstet Gynecol* 1980;136:1055–60.
11. Obiekwe BC, Sturdee D, Cockrill BL, Chard T. Human placental lactogen in preeclampsia. *Br J Obstet Gynaecol* 1984;91:1077–80.
12. Hubert CH, Mondon F, Cedard L. Biologic activity and quantification of messenger RNA coding for human chorionic somatomammotropin in normal and intrauterine growth retarded pregnancies. *Am J Obstet Gynecol* 1982;144:722–5.
13. Wurzel JM, Parks JS, Hera JE, Nielsen PV. A gene deletion is responsible for absence of human chorionic somatomammotropin. *DNA* 1982;1:251–7.
14. Diczfalusy E. Steroid metabolism in the foeto-placental unit. In: Peale A, Finzi C, eds. *The foeto-placental unit*. Amsterdam: Excerpta Medica Foundation, 1969;65–109.
15. Brown JB, MacLeod , MacNaughton C, Smith MA, Smyth B. A rapid method for estimating estrogens in urine using a semi-automatic extractor. *J Endocrinol* 1968;42:5–15.
16. Ittrich G. Eine neue methode zur chemischen bestimmung der ostrogenen hormone in harn. *Hoppe-Seylers Z Physiol Chem* 1958;31:1–14.
17. Beisher NA, Brown JB. Current status of estrogen assays in obstetrics and gynecology. Part 2, Estrogen assays in late pregnancy. *Obstet Gynecol Survey* 1972;27:303–43.
18. Cedard L, Tanguy G, Leblond J, Kaminsky M. Intérêt du dosage des oestrogènes plasmatiques dans la surveillance biologique des grossesses à risque. In: Cedard L, Sureau C, eds. *Endocrinologie prénatale et parturition*. Paris: Colloque Inserm 1978;77:149–68.
19. Klopper A. Assays of urinary oestriol as a measure of placental function. In: Cataldo C, ed. *Research on steroids,* vol 2. Rome: Il pensiero scientifico, 1966;63–83.
20. Beisher NA, Bhargava VL, Brown JB, Smith MA. The incidence and significance of low estriol excretion in an obstetric population. *J Obstet Gynaecol Br Cwlth* 1968;75:1024–33.
21. Cedard L, Bedin M, Leblond J, Tanguy G. Maternal plasma total estriol and DHAS loading test as indicators of feto-placental function or placental sulfatase deficiency. *J Steroid Biochem* 1979; 11:501–7.
22. Nielsen PV. Estriol screening in pregnancy: prognostic value of total estriol in serum in an obstetrical population. *Acta Obstet Gynecol Scand* 1983;62:1–4.
23. Evans JJ, Wilkinson AR, Aickin DR. Clinical usefulness of estriol assay for predicting light for date infants. *Clin Chem* 1984;30:138–40.
24. Chard T, Sturdee J, Cockrill B, Obiekwe BC. Which is the best placental function test? A comparison of placental lactogen and unconjugated estriol in the prediction of intrauterine growth retardation. *Europ J Obstet Gynecol Reprod Biol* 1985;19:13–7.
25. Perry L, Hickson R, Obiekwe BC, Chard T. Maternal estriol levels reflect placental function rather than foetal function. *Acta Endocrinol* 1986;111:563–6.
26. France JT, Liggins GC. Placental sulfatase deficiency. *J Clin Endocrinol Metab* 1969;36:1–9.
27. Bedin M, Weil D, Fournier T, Cedard L, Frezal J. Biochemical evidence for the non-inactivation of the steroid sulfatase locus in human placenta and fibroblast. *Hum Genet* 1981;59:256–8.
28. Bedin M, Fournier T, Tanguy G, Cedard L, Zorn JR, Sureau C. *In vivo* and *vitro* study of the mechanism of action of a synthetic progestin in lowering unconjugated E_2 and total E_3 in plasma during normal pregnancy. *Am J Obstet Gynecol* 1983;145:373–4.
29. Gant NF, Hutchinson HT, Siiteri PK, MacDonald PC. Studies of the metabolic clearance rate of dehydroepiandrosterone sulfate in pregnancy. *Am J Obstet Gynecol* 1971;111:555–61.
30. Everett RB, Porter JC, MacDonald PC, Gant NF. Relationship of maternal placental blood flow to the placental clearance of maternal plasma dehydroepiandrosterone sulfate through estradiol formation. *Am J Obstet Gynecol* 1980;136:435–9.
31. Lauritzen C, Strecker J, Lehmann WD. Dynamic tests of placental function. In: Klopper A, ed. *Plasma hormone assays in evaluation of fetal well-being,* London: Churchill Livingstone, 1976; 113–23.
32. Tanguy G, Zorn JR, Sureau C, Cedard L. Exogenous DHAS half life: a good index of intrauterine growth retardation. *Gynecol Obstet Invest* 1980;11:170–3.

33. Tanguy G, Thoumsin HJ, Zorn JR, Cedard L. Clinical values of DHAS half life during loading test in cases of intrauterine growth retardation. In: Klopper A, Genazzani A, Crosignani PG, eds. *The human placenta*. Serono Symposium no. 35. London: Academic Press, 1980;225–9.
34. Tanguy G, Thoumsin HJ, Zorn JR, Cedard L. DHEAS loading test in cases of intrauterine growth retardation: relationship between the pattern of the maternal plasma metabolites and the fetoplacental dysfunction. *Gynecol Obstet Invest* 1981;12:305–6.
35. Thoumsin HJ, Alsat E, Cedard L. In vitro aromatization of androgens into estrogens in placental insufficiency. *Gynecol Obstet Invest* 1982;13:37–42.
36. Lilford RJ, Obiekwe BC, Chard T. Maternal blood levels of human placental lactogen in the prediction of fetal growth retardation: choosing a cut-off point between normal and abnormal. *Br J Obstet Gynaecol* 1983;90:511–5.
37. Aickin DR, Duff GB, Evans JJ. Antenatal biochemical screening to predict low birth weight infants. *Br J Obstet Gynaecol* 1983;90:129–33.
38. Bissenden JG, Scott PH, Hallum J, Mansfield HN, Scott P, Wharton BA. Racial variations in tests of fetoplacental function. *Br J Obstet Gynaecol* 1983;90:109–14.
39. Nylund L, Lunell NO, Lewander R, Sarby B. Utero-placental blood flow index in intrauterine growth retardation of fetal or maternal origin. *Br J Obstet Gynaecol* 1983;90:16–20.
40. Soothill PW, Bilardo CM, Nicolaides KH, Campbell S. Relation of fetal hypoxia in growth retardation to mean blood velocity in the fetal aorta. *Lancet* 1986;2:1118–9.

DISCUSSION

Dr. Bossart: When you did the loading test did you only look at estriol or did you look at other hormones such as estrone? When we looked at estrone with the same loading test we found it gave more significant results than estriol. And what about Schwangershaft's protein 1 (SP 1, a placental glycoprotein specific for pregnancy), oxytocinase, and so on? Are they as good as human placental lactogen (hPL), or better?

Dr. Cédard: We did not look at estrone, but I believe the results would be the same. With regard to the second question, we have done some SP1 assays which seem to give the same results as hPL. However, it is possible that some countries might be more interested in SP1 because it can be used throughout the course of pregnancy. This would have obvious advantages in terms of the cost of analytic equipment, since it could replace two assays (human chorionic gonadotropin (hCG) estimations at the beginning of pregnancy and hPL towards the end).

Dr. Seeds: Do you think any of these hormonal tests are likely to be useful for the detection of high-risk groups in developing countries? What do you think of the possible use of hPL or serum estriol as screening tests in such areas?

Dr. Cédard: I think hPL is the more robust test because there is no diurnal variation and because the gestational increase in values is less than for estriol. It is thus possible to define an absolute fetal danger zone, which can be set at 4 μg per ml irrespective of definite knowledge of gestation. I think values below that level will define most cases of severe IUGR.

Dr. Marini: I know two factors which support your view that hPL is better than estriol. First, there has been a recent study from Padua in which it was demonstrated that hPL was a good predictor of IUGR; and second, we know that estriol is unreliable when the mother is given steroids to prevent hyaline membrane disease in the baby. This causes a large fall in estriol.

Dr. Cédard: It is true that estriol values are modified by many substances, and especially corticoids. hPL, on the other hand, is not subject to hormonal regulation and remains very stable, with little diurnal variation.

Dr. Wharton: Do you find that the etiology of IUGR has different effects on the biochemical measurements? In our population in Birmingham, the indigenous white mothers have conventional reasons for IUGR, such as smoking, preeclampsia, and so on (with a large number of "unknowns"), and in these both estriol and hPL are reasonably predictive—not very good but reasonable. On the other hand, in our large Asian population, where we think malnutrition is the major cause of IUGR, estriol has no predictive value at all, though hPL is still useful (1).

Dr. Cédard: We have not shown a difference between different populations in estriol measurements. But we do find that hPL is more predictive for the whole population. The main problem arises when you are dealing with a fetus with a malformation syndrome. In these babies the hPL may be normal in spite of pronounced IUGR. Thus, where there is a discrepancy between ultrasound findings and hPL values, we suspect fetal malformation.

Dr. Wharton: Does hPL tell us anything about the function of the placenta or is the level in the plasma simply proportional to placental size?

Dr. Cédard: It is related to functional placental mass.

Dr. Wharton: I believe there has been some recent work suggesting that hPL measured early in pregnancy is highly correlated with postconceptional age and so could be used as a substitute for ultrasound in developing countries to confirm the length of gestation. Could you comment on this?

Dr. Cédard: I know that this has been done but cannot comment on its reliability.

Dr. Dias-Correa: In my city it is extremely difficult to get women to do complete 24 hr urine collections. Do you also find this difficulty?

Dr. Cédard: I agree there are considerable difficulties. This is why tests relying on urine collection are generally bad. There are too many sources of error.

Dr. Dias-Correa: What about a random urine sample related to creatinine?

Dr. Cédard: I don't think a random sample is reliable, even if related to creatinine excretion. Correction using creatinine may be useful if you suspect that a 24 hr collection is not complete but not if there is preeclampsia or hypertension, which affect the degree of creatininuria. Personally, I think that the results obtained using plasma estrogen measurements are the same as using urinary estrogens, so you might as well take the plasma sample and avoid the uncertainty of incomplete urine collections.

Dr. Belizan: My advice is that, if you want to detect or monitor IUGR, you should not bother with any of these hormonal measurements. You are wasting time and money, and maybe even life. This is not only my experience but the experience of a large body of published work. I have used these tests for 10 years but I have now abandoned them because they do not help.

Dr. Cédard: I must disagree. I think they do work, especially hPL, which is more robust than estriol for various reasons I have already discussed.

REFERENCES

1. Bissenden JG, Scott PH, Hallum J, Mansfield HN, Scott P, Wharton BA. Racial variation in tests of fetoplacental function. *Br J Obstet Gynaecol* 1981;88:109–14.

Intrauterine Growth Retardation, edited by
Jacques Senterre. Nestlé Nutrition Workshop
Series, Vol. 18. Nestec Ltd., Vevey/Raven Press,
Ltd., New York © 1989.

Intrauterine Growth Retardation: Management of Delivery

Hans Bossart

*Département de gynécologie-obstétrique, Centre Hospitalier Universitaire Vaudois,
1011 Lausanne, Switzerland*

MANAGEMENT OF DELIVERY

"Management" of delivery means observing and taking stock of a great number of factors concerning the mother and infant. It is therefore not only a scientific approach, but a practical one based on personal knowledge and experience. It is impossible to cover all aspects of delivery or review the great number of papers published on the subject in recent years. It is much easier to deal with single subjects such as biometry by ultrasound, placental enzymes, hormones, or other well-defined items.

It may be very difficult to determine the optimal time for delivery, in the light of the possible combinations of maternal, placental, and fetal pathology. Racial, social, and traditional factors may also be important, as well as medical practice. My suggestions and opinions are therefore only partially based on hard scientific facts. They are also based on how obstetrics is done in my country and in my department. My considerations should provide the basis for a discussion and, I would hope, lead to some acceptable conclusions. To illustrate my way of thinking, I would like to recall a problem which I had when I was the co-editor of an obstetric textbook. We were quite unable to handle the management of breech presentation in a standard way, since certain Canadian colleagues absolutely refused to consider vaginal delivery. Their attitude was based not only on statistics but also on malpractice problems in their country. On this side of the Atlantic Ocean, vaginal delivery of breech presentation is still routinely done under certain conditions. Policy on the handling of growth-retarded fetuses might be subject to similar difficulties.

Intrauterine growth retardation (IUGR) fetuses should be delivered whenever the intrauterine conditions for fetal survival seem less favorable than the ones offered in extrauterine life. It is quite clear that these extrauterine conditions depend not only on medical knowledge and equipment, but also on socio-economic and other factors. The three main questions that follow must therefore be adapted to the medical environment to a major degree.

As soon as IUGR is suspected, the following questions must be asked:

(1) *Where* should the baby be delivered?
(2) *When* should the baby be delivered?
(3) *How* should the baby be delivered?

Where?

As soon as intrauterine growth retardation is suspected clinically, the responsible doctor will have to answer the following questions:

Is my suspicion accurate? After careful history taking, consultation of earlier pregnancy records (particularly ultrasound measurements), and clinical examination for signs of intrauterine growth retardation, the suspicion will be more or less confirmed.

Do I have additional means of confirming the diagnosis? Various facilities are necessary: biometry with adequate ultrasonic equipment; laboratory facilities for determination of placental indices; and the possibility of admitting the patient to hospital for monitoring of fetal growth and well-being (by analysis of fetal movements, breathing, heart rate, and amniotic fluid volume).

In cases of early and very severe growth retardation, can I get information about genetic aspects, major malformations, infectious diseases? Can I do placental biopsies, Doppler flow studies, etc.?

If the answer to these questions is yes, then delivery can be managed satisfactorily.

If the answer is no, the patient must be transferred to a better equipped center.

This policy seems to be generally accepted, but unfortunately it is quite often not followed. We must not forget that financial and other more "subjective" factors can be of importance. However, the fetus prefers early intrauterine rather than late neonatal emergency transport.

When?

Poor intrauterine conditions are dangerous for the fetus but so is poor adaptation to extrauterine life. For every growth-retarded fetus there is an optimal delivery date.

I shall not discuss the particular problems associated with high maternal risk. It is evident that eclampsia, heavy vaginal hemorrhage, or other critical conditions for the mother must lead to immediate delivery, as a life-saving procedure. Fortunately, we see few such situations providing we practice adequate prophylactic obstetrics. Of course, these conditions vary considerably from one country to the other.

It is difficult to cover all the different pathological conditions leading to elective delivery of an IUGR baby at given time. I shall try to be pragmatic.

IUGR: Fetal Pathology

Very early and severe IUGR must be discussed first and separate from other conditions. If growth retardation starts during the second trimester of pregnancy, one should think of major congenital defects. We try in these cases to get a fetal karyotype from amniotic fluid cell culture or direct placental biopsy. We look for major defects of the central nervous system (microcephaly, early hydrocephalus), Potter's syndrome, and other severe malformations. In some rare cases, intrauterine passive euthanasia can or must be discussed. This question is of course very complex and depends on medical, legal, and ethical practice. But if there is a minimal chance of long-term survival, we have to do all we can to deliver the baby in optimal condition.

Fetal pathology leading to IUGR, compatible with (eventual) favorable outcome, is frequently related to cardiovascular diseases or malformations, lower urinary tract, and gastro-intestinal disorders and fetal infections. In our material, 5 out of 11 fetuses infected with human immunodeficiency virus were growth-retarded; the same can happen with toxoplasmosis, cytomegalovirus, and other infections.

In general, the obstetrician has to ask the following questions:

Can the fetal pathology leading to IUGR be treated *in utero*?

If not (which is the usual situation), is the extrauterine prognosis better than the intrauterine one? If the answer to this question is yes, then delivery should be arranged. If the answer is no, then optimal maternal conditions for intrauterine survival of the fetus must be created. Monitoring of vital signs in the fetus and a team approach involving obstetrician, pediatrician, pediatric surgeon, etc., are essential aspects of management. Determination of the optimal delivery date is the product of team work.

IUGR: Placental Pathology

With improved biometry and echographic analysis of the placenta, we realize that this organ is quite frequently in sub-optimal anatomic condition (small placentas, excluded cotyledons, abnormal lie, retroplacental hematomas, etc.). Functional assessment of the placenta is interesting for research and theoretical considerations, but routine clinical use of the different indices of placental function is not very useful (hormones, enzymes, dehydroepiandrosterone sulfate loading tests, etc.). They tell us that the "growth climate" is not favorable and therefore the obstetrician must be particularly alert. But decision-making based on these variables is difficult.

The most important technique for monitoring fetal health is based on the analysis of fetal heart rate (FHR). The use of stress tests and the evaluation of fetal movements, fetal breathing, and other vital signs are helpful. We have also to consider the quantity and quality of the amniotic fluid, especially those variables relating to lung maturity. Most of these observations tell us that the fetus is in danger but FHR patterns give the best clue for the optimal timing of delivery.

IUGR: Mother

Understanding maternal pathology means thinking of medical *and* social conditions. The outcome of previous pregnancies can be the clue to a current problem. It is important not to forget that occupation, nutritional habits, smoking, alcohol, drugs, and all aspects of everyday life may be relevant and should be known.

The more specific illnesses leading to IUGR are often out of reach of any treatment. Thus, cardiovascular disorders, pre-existing hypertensive disease, malformation of the genital tract, etc., can rarely be improved. The patient needs to be under constant supervision, since any direct influence on fetal well-being is difficult. We have to create the optimal conditions for maternal health and utero-placental blood flow. Physical activity should be minimal. A high-protein diet with vitamins, trace elements, etc. may be helpful but we should not be too optimistic about this. If uteroplacental insufficiency has already led to severe IUGR, we can offer whatever nutrients we like on the maternal side, but the fetus cannot be reached. Intrauterine alimentation is an interesting field of research, but does not yet have a practical use. The basic premise must be to provide optimal conditions for the mother and very close supervision of fetal well-being, with the hope that fetal maturation will continue until we can deliver the fetus.

Intrauterine growth retardation of around 1 to 2 weeks is compatible with normal obstetric practice, but if there is more pronounced retardation, very careful attention to fetal progress is required. If growth achievement is more than 3 to 4 weeks delayed, this is usually incompatible with favorable fetal outcome, unless the fetus is delivered. Placental respiratory function has to be assessed regularly and the fetus must be delivered as soon as any signs of hypoxia appear. After 36 weeks, any fetus with severe IUGR should be delivered, even if there is no immediate danger.

How?

Cesarean Section or Vaginal Delivery?

From the start of fetal viability at ± 25 weeks to the end of the 32nd week of gestation, cesarean section is indicated in most IUGR cases. Oligo-hydramnios, and poor development and maturation of the lower uterine segment and cervix are negative factors for vaginal delivery. The fetus has minimal reserves for his energy metabolism and placental oxygen transport reserve is poor. Therefore, vaginal delivery is dangerous.

The technique of cesarean section needs to be adapted to this special situation. The typical transverse incision of the lower uterine segment is often insufficient. A corporeal (classical) incision with or without a transverse one is necessary. It is bad surgical practice to extract a severely retarded fetus through a small incision.

It may be possible to avoid cesarean section in the following situations:

1. Where there is very bad fetal prognosis and good prognosis for the mother and for future pregnancies. Imminent intrauterine death with very poor neonatal

prognosis may lead to the acceptance of vaginal delivery ("passive" euthanasia).

2. If there are very favorable local conditions (multiparous mother, very soft cervix, etc.); in this situation vaginal delivery without major mechanical impact on the fetus can be anticipated.

3. From the 33rd week onwards vaginal delivery is possible but cesarean section frequent. I shall not discuss the different indications in detail, because they are basically the same as for any other obstetric situation.

Of course, breech presentation means cesarean section for any infant with severe IUGR.

Induction of Labor

Induction of labor is frequently necessary. We do not believe that the use of prostaglandins is the best way to do this. Intracervical prostaglandin gel application seems relatively safe, but we have nevertheless observed some rapid, traumatic deliveries in normal term babies, usually after some hours of ineffective and uncoordinated labor. We might occasionally use very small quantities of prostaglandins to mature rigid cervical tissue before we induce labor with oxytocin.

Currently, tocolysis by oxytocin perfusion in the presence of a surgical team, ready to work at any time in cases of hypoxia, seems to be the safest way to induce labor. Artificial rupture of membranes should be done only if labor is well under way and the mechanical indices are favorable.

At this point we should remember that intrauterine monitoring, especially the application of scalp electrodes and fetal blood sampling, can be dangerous. The fetus is susceptible to bacterial and viral diseases which may be introduced in this way, causing harm. The fetal scalp is also very thin and trauma is possible. Heart rate monitoring by modern multifocal Doppler technique is usually sufficient. Non-invasive monitoring of Po_2 and Pco_2 is now possible, and blood flow monitoring using pulsed Doppler techniques will help us further in the future. The mother must also be monitored throughout labor, with attention to hydration, administration of glucose, control of electrolytes, etc.

The delivery of the baby should be as atraumatic as possible. A large and carefully performed episiotomy is important to reduce mechanical resistance of the pelvic floor. Forceps delivery, if necessary, is better than the application of a suction device. Once again, vaginal breech delivery in IUGR is dangerous and should not be attempted.

Minimal Neonatal Assistance for IUGR Infants

After birth the following are essential:

1. Adequate attention to the thermal environment.

2. Adequate and prompt resuscitation, including aspiration of meconium via laryn-
   goscope.
3. Determination of blood gases and acid-base status in cord blood samples.
4. The presence of a pediatrician.

Analgesia and Anesthesia

If general anesthesia is required, the obstetrician should insist on last-minute induction. Careful preparation for cesarean section or forceps delivery is required, ensuring that disinfection, catheterization, etc., are performed before induction of
anesthesia. Only when everything is ready should narcosis be induced and the fetus
delivered in the shortest possible time.

We disapprove of the use of systemic anaesthetic drugs in IUGR deliveries.
Given in an effective dosage to the mother, the fetus may be equally affected and its
unstable homeostasis disturbed. Growth-retarded infants are struggling for intrauterine survival by adapting their energy control. Preferential perfusion of vital organs
is maintained by reducing the perfusion of less important territories (subcutaneous
and muscle tissue, etc.). Systemic analgesia can interfere with this adaptation and
lead to intrauterine shock: shunts are opened, and acidotic tissue is washed out leading to severe acidemia with loss of blood pressure and cardiovascular and cerebral
failure. We therefore recommend anesthesia with only very limited or no side effects. Regional anesthesia by epidural block can be used. We obtain sufficient analgesia or anesthesia in about 95% of cases, and mechanical resistance (pelvic floor)
is reduced. The most important negative effect can be the fall of maternal blood
pressure. This can be overcome by the use of epinephrine and sufficient fluid
support.

CONCLUSION

Every IUGR infant must be treated as a unique problem and delivered in the optimal way. This depends not only on good medical care, but also on a full understanding of the particular human situation. It must not be forgotten, even if this is not the
subject of my contribution, that the prevention of IUGR should be the principal goal
of every obstetric team.

Real prevention means the suppression of the pathology leading to IUGR. We
know that this is extremely difficult. In many countries, poor intrauterine growth is
due mostly to poor maternal conditions, including economic and social deprivation
and other negative factors. It is therefore a political problem, which is beyond the
reach of any medical symposium. Nevertheless, I think it is important to stress that
only by improving maternal health can we make a major worldwide improvement in
the quality of intrauterine life and extrauterine survival. The same is true of intrauterine infections. Prevention is possible but difficult.

If the other basic causes of slow uterine growth (placental insufficiency, malformations of the uterus, maternal heart disease, etc.) cannot be cured, we can at least prevent major fetal damage by good medical care.

REFERENCES

1. Baumgarten K, van Assche A. Intrauterine growth retardation. *Europ J Obstet Gynecol Reprod Biol* 1983;15:367–83.
2. Bhargava SK, Sachdev HPS, Ghosh S. Distribution of live births and early neonatal mortality in relation to gestation and intrauterine growth. *Ind J Med Res* 1985;82:95–7.
3. Bolte A, Schlensker KH, Breuker KH, Wolff F. Geburtshilfe bei schwerer fetaler Wachstumsretardierung. *Geburtshilfe Frauenheilkd* 1983;43(Suppl.1):93–8.
4. Brustman LE, Langer O, Anyaegbunam A. The heightened significance of prolonged bradycardia associated with intrauterine growth retardation. *Am J Perinatol* 1985;2:288–91.
5. Chew FT, Drew JH, Oats JN, Riley SF, Beischer NA. Nonstressed antepartum cardiotocography in patients undergoing elective cesarean section—Fetal outcome. *Am J Obstet Gynecol* 1985;151:318–21.
6. Chiswick ML. Intrauterine growth retardation. *Br Med J* 1985;291:845–8.
7. Heinonen K, Matilainen R, Koski H, Launiala K. Intrauterine growth retardation (IUGR) in preterm infants. *J Perinat Med* 1985;13:171–8.
8. Huisjes HJ, Baarsma R, Hadders-Algra M, Touwen BCL. Follow-up of growth-retarded children born by elective cesarean section before 33 weeks. *Gynecol Obstet Invest* 1985;19:169–73.
9. Krause W, Michels W, Wagner U. Retardierungsproblematik im Rahmen der "Frühgeburtlichkeit." *Geburtshilfe Frauenheilkd* 1985;45:864–8.
10. Nicolaides KH, Rodeck CH, Soothill PW, Campbell S. Ultrasound-guided sampling of umbilical cord and placental blood to assess fetal well-being. *Lancet* 1986;ii:1065–7.
11. Saling E. Versuch einer neuen kompensatorischen Versorgung des hypotrophen Feten. *Geburtshilfe Frauenheilkd* 1987;47:90–2.
12. Seeds JW. Impaired fetal growth: ultrasonic evaluation and clinical management. *Obstet Gynecol* 1984;64(Suppl.3):577–84.
13. Simpson GF, Creasy RK. Obstetric management of the growth retarded baby. *Clin Obstet Gynecol* 1984;11:481–97.
14. Schmidt W, Boos R, Hendrik HJ, Schmidt R. Pathologischer Placentasitz nach der 20. Schwangerschaftswoche-Bedeutung für den Schwangerschafts- und Geburtsverlauf. *Geburtshilfe Frauenheilkd* 1986;46:206–12.
15. Taylor DJ. Low birthweight and neurodevelopmental handicap. *Clin Obstet Gynecol* 1984;11:525–43.
16. Thoulon JM. Le retard de croissance intra-utérin idiopathique. *Rev Fr Gynecol Obstet* 1984;79:263–7.
17. Vasa R, Vidyasagar D, Winegar A, Peterson P, Spellacy WN. Perinatal factors influencing the outcome of 501- to 100-gm newborns. *Clin Perinatol* 1986;13:267–84.
18. Worthington D, Davis LE, Grausz JP, Sobocinski K. Factors influencing survival and morbidity with very low birth weight delivery. *Obstet Gynecol* 1983;62:550–5.

DISCUSSION

Dr. Seeds: I want to mention one additional technique that we use occasionally in cases of intrauterine growth retardation with suspected fetal compromise and an undilated cervix: fetal cord blood sampling. There is some advantage in determining fetal umbilical blood gases and base deficit. It has on many occasions helped us in the diagnosis of the compromised fetus and over the decision to deliver.

Dr. Bossart: When you say cord blood sampling, do you mean intrauterine cord blood sampling?

Dr. Seeds: Yes. Ultrasound-guided percutaneous umbilical cord sampling.

Dr. Bossart: This is a beautiful technique. However, I don't think we can yet say "go ahead and do intrauterine fetal blood sampling in the umbilical vein" as a general approach. Do you think this technique will ever come into general use?

Dr. Seeds: I hope it does not come into general use since there are obviously considerable dangers involved with it. However, it should be something that is available in referral centers.

Dr. Bossart: Dr. Seeds, I would appreciate your comments about the unrestricted availability of ultrasound in industrialized countries like yours or mine. Ultrasound examinations can easily be performed and ultrasound is said to be innocuous, at least in the short term, in contrast to X-rays and other techniques. But it is also available to any physician, even without adequate knowledge or experience. I wonder whether in any community there should be one specialist in ultrasound for, say, 10 obstetricians. Or whether it should be available to all of them?

Dr. Seeds: In the United States, ultrasound is available to anyone with the money to buy the machine. There is no legal restriction on availability of machines, there is no legal requirement for training. What we have seen over the last five years in our particular area is a dramatic improvement in referrals, an improvement in attitudes about referrals, and an improvement in communication, all based on ultrasound training and ultrasound availability. What we see now is much greater willingness by the private physician to refer the complicated patient. Certainly, the ideal to achieve would be what you say: isolated specialists who do superb work with everyone else referring to them. In fact, five years ago, these isolated specialists existed, but the referrals did not occur. The private physician held on to patients for too long, until too late. So for reasons that I did not expect, it has ended up empirically being a good thing, although theoretically there are certainly the many dangers that you spoke of. Of course, we have also a problem with the malpractice and litigation in the United States.

Dr. Marini: There are two kinds of ultrasound: sophisticated equipment that should be available in referral centers, and simple machines that every obstetrician should be able to use. I fully agree with Dr. Seeds that due to the spread of this technique more women are now referred before delivery. I would like to ask Dr. Bossart what he recommends in order to accelerate lung maturation, when a premature infant with intrauterine growth retardation and evidence of lung immaturity has to be taken out of the uterus: steroids or glucocorticoids, thyroid hormones, or other agents?

Dr. Bossart: In cases of growth retardation in very early gestation, I don't think that we have to worry about surfactant (apart from the fact that we are not always able to obtain enough liquor to do the surfactant determination) because the baby is going to die in the next 48 hr if we don't take it out. We have no experience with thyroid hormones. Our pediatric colleagues can now instill surfactant into the newborn's trachea right after delivery.

Dr. Marini: We recently reviewed our cases of IUGR during the last two years. The major problem in our series is maternal hypertension/preeclampsia. I agree with you that there is no way to improve fetal nutrition by giving nutrients to the mother, because the circulation to the placenta is already impaired. The only alternative would thus be to identify mothers at risk of preeclampsia before irreversible damage has been caused to the placental circulation, and then to expand plasma volume, improve the microcirculation, and so on, in order to minimize the extent of IUGR. I would appreciate your comments on this, or on the Dutch experience with the "angiotensin test" for screening of primigravidae at risk of preeclampsia and providing treatment with low doses of aspirin.

Dr. Bossart: I agree with you that any intervention should ideally occur before harm has been caused to the placenta. However, I don't have any experience with the detection of pre-eclampsia as they did in the Netherlands.

Dr. Cédard: I agree with Dr. Marini that IUGR in Western Europe is usually due to maternal pathology. But I think that, at least in Paris, this may vary quite a lot from hospital to hospital depending on the socio-economic background of the patients, and the quality of the follow-up of the pregnancy. Some hospitals, for example, have a large proportion of immigrants among their patients; these mothers are not so well-followed during pregnancy, and indeed present with toxemia. In our hospital, where the follow-up is of high quality, indications for the determination of fetal maturity have more or less disappeared. Thus, the indications for preterm delivery are not necessarily the same in different hospitals. I just want to add that, at least in our experience, obstetricians and pediatricians prefer to have IUGR babies outside the uterus, in order to be able to take care of them.

Dr. Bossart: I don't think that obstetricians should just take babies out. I believe in fetal pediatrics. We have been able to treat heart block, ascites, and some other conditions *in utero*. I think there is a future for intrauterine therapy. However, we need to be aware that at a particular moment intrauterine life becomes more hazardous than extrauterine life. And we need to get this moment right, by considering all the available information. I agree that this is quite complicated in reality.

Dr. Pearse: You made a very provocative suggestion that there was an indication sometimes to leave a baby with a flat cardiotocograph trace *in utero*. Could you expand on it?

Dr. Bossart: My question is the following: When we have an absolutely non-reactive, flat, silent intrauterine trace, should we take the baby out under all circumstances even if we think that he will not survive for more than a few hours, or are we allowed in such circumstances to accept intrauterine death without intervening. This is never a simple decision; it may be more easy in extreme situations.

Dr. Seeds: I don't have the answer, but if I may express an opinion, we should always give the baby the benefit of the doubt.

Dr. Chessex: This sort of decision is extremely complex and should depend on quite a large number of factors, including, for example, the situation of the mother, the available facilities for taking care of the newborn, and so on.

Dr. Segre: Do you inform the mother of the situation and does she participate in the decision to leave the baby in the uterus in such circumstances?

Dr. Bossart: That is a very difficult question. This situation fortunately presents very seldom. Of course, when we hesitate to perform a cesarean section for a baby which will die a few minutes later, we discuss that with patients, if they are capable of understanding the problem. Another problem now is the viable fetus (30 to 32 weeks) with malformations. When the parents know that the baby has a major problem, they sometimes start asking us to get rid of it. We think that we have no right ethically to let the baby die if there is anything that can be done, for example, an operation. Let's turn to the neonates. Our pediatric colleagues quite often give 1 or 2 days of assisted ventilation and then, after considering the whole problem, turn off the machine. I think you would do that too.

Dr. Pearse: Yes, we may withdraw therapy in a severely sick newborn, not because he is severely sick, but because we have almost definite evidence that the child is going to be severely handicapped. Those are the grounds upon which we might discontinue ventilation.

Dr. Marini: The situation is quite different in Italy. This is a legal problem in our country. We are not allowed to withdraw any kind of therapy once we have started it. The neonatologist who starts resuscitating a neonate in the delivery room, and puts him on a ventilator, has to go on with the ventilatory support. The first decision is very important. This should clearly indicate that neonatologists need to have a very close working relationship with obstetricians; we need to know precisely before delivery what kind of malformation a baby has, so as to avoid starting resuscitation when the prognosis is desperate.

Dr. Pearse: I don't agree that once we have started we have to go on. I think we should start treatment. I don't think it would be ethical to withdraw therapy unless we have all the available evidence at our disposal. We must wait until we have all the facts before we make a decision. But if everything points to a hopeless prognosis, then I think we are quite justified in withdrawing therapy, even though we have started ventilating the baby from birth.

Dr. Bossart: I agree with you. That is what we do.

Dr. Priolosi: What is your attitude in the case of a twin pregnancy, when you have evidence that one twin is severely growth-retarded and the other one is growing well?

Dr. Bossart: From our ultrasound examination, we know now that twin pregnancy is much more frequent than we thought 10 years ago. Very often one twin dies, sometimes both. In cases of twin pregnancy, we monitor the growth and well-being of both, though of course we cannot look at hormonal levels, unless we could obtain blood samples from the two cords individually. If the weaker fetus has problems after, say, the 30th week, we may take them both out of the uterus. We should concentrate on the smallest one and not on the strongest. Of course, there is no general rule in managing these pregnancies.

Dr. Kuletharn: I agree with you that regional anesthesia is the best type of anesthesia during labor, but not everybody has the facility available. You said that the baby is not able to react to the stress of labor when the mother receives morphine, and we all know that these babies get a flat trace. But are you suggesting that deceleration patterns arise because the baby is not able to react anymore?

Dr. Bossart: Chronically stressed fetuses are particularly sensitive to narcotics, which paralyze neurovegetative regulatory centers. When morphine derivatives are injected into the mother, you can observe this side effect in the fetus about 20 to 30 min later. We should therefore avoid these substances in growth-retarded infants who have very labile homeostasis and, rather than systemic drugs, use drugs with a well-controlled local action.

Dr. Kuletharn: What is the effect of morphine in a normal fetus?

Dr. Bossart: From a clinical point of view, morphine slows down the reaction of the fetus towards stress.

Dr. Toubas: We studied the effects of morphine in the fetal sheep, e.g., on fetal breathing movements. We expected the breathing movements to disappear. But to our great surprise, and for an unknown reason, we generated very intense breathing activity for periods of about one hr, as well as very slight hypoxia. Morphine induced changes in the electrocortical activity of the fetus, characterized by permanent high frequency and low voltage. So although morphine did not cause severe hypoxia, it definitely does something to the fetus. Similar observations have been made during experimentation on baboons, which are closer to the human species: Fetal breathing movements first stop, but then continuous breathing movements of very high amplitude are observed. This could be due to a withdrawal phenomenon; others regard it as a sort of fetal gasping.

Dr. Bogg: In our institution, we follow intrauterine growth retardation by serial Doppler velocimetry and by the Manning score (1). Reduction of the diastolic flow in the umbilical artery and the fetal aorta are warning signs, but we cannot predict how many days will separate the disparition of end-diastolic flow in these arteries from a documented fetal distress. For the past 6 months we have been measuring the cerebral resistance index

$$cR = \frac{S - D}{S}$$

according to Pourcelot (2) at the bifurcation of internal carotid artery as described by Wladimiroff (3). We observed 15 cases in which there was an increase in diastolic flow in the cerebral arteries. This is a sign of preferential blood supply to the brain, whereas vasoconstriction occurs in other parts of the fetal body. We also observed severe acidosis in these 15 infants. Thus, alterations of the Doppler spectrum in the brain seem to be a useful and predictive parameter of impending fetal death. Have you any experience in this field?

Dr. Bossart: There are still quite a lot of technical problems with the Doppler technique. I don't have any experience with it. Prof. Calame, who is neonatologist in Lausanne, and his group used it to look at cerebral blood flow (but not *in utero*).

Dr. Seeds: Doing Doppler flow studies, looking at flow with velocity profiles, is one issue and there are still many technical variables that impinge on the accuracy of flow measurements. But if you are looking at patterns of increased or decreased flow, then the pattern is clearly going to be valid, even though there might be technical variability in the absolute determination of flow rate in ml per minute. It takes some practice to be able to perform Doppler flow studies on the internal carotid artery of a fetus *in utero*, and it is a very exciting technique. It may be limited in availability right now, but I would like to ask Dr. Bogg if there were no other clinical or ultrasonic signs of distress in these 15 babies.

Dr. Bogg: In all cases we noted ultrasonic signs of fetal growth retardation and oligohydramnios, as well as a decrease of diastolic flow in umbilical arteries. The increase in diastolic flow at the level of cerebral arteries preceded severe alterations of the fetal heart rate in 60% of cases.

Dr. Bossart: You said that all the newborns were acidotic. How profound was the acidosis?

Dr. Bogg: In all 15 cases a high cerebral telediastolic flow was associated with fetal distress (mean Apgar score at 5 min was 3.8 and mean umbilical artery pH was 7.10). Until today, we have only been able to rely on cardiotocography in order to decide at what moment the fetal extraction is to take place. We feel that, using Doppler ultrasound measurement of brain blood flow, it might be possible to decide the extraction a bit earlier, in the pre-acidotic phase, before severe alterations of cardiac rhythm occur. In order to confirm this hypothesis, we are conducting a prospective study using fetal blood samples.

Dr. Marini: Prof. Battaglia, in collaboration with G. Pardi and his group in our institution, was able to demonstrate a rather good relationship between impairment of diastolic blood flow, measured by ultrasound, and biochemical changes in the fetus, by fetal sampling. Evaluation of diastolic flow by ultrasound thus seems to be a very promising, and not invasive technique for estimating fetal well-being. There is also another group in Italy, directed by Prof. Romanini from the Catholic University in Rome, who have given a calcium antagonist to mothers of fetuses with abnormal diastolic blood flow and they have sometimes observed an improvement in diastolic blood flow. This seems to indicate that intrauterine growth retardation due to maternal hypertension can sometimes be treated in this way.

Dr. Dias-Correa: Dr. Bossart, did the patients in whom you performed a classical cesarean section present any problem in subsequent gestations? For instance, does the risk of uterine rupture not increase after a classical incision? Is there an increased risk of placental insufficiency?

Dr. Bossart: It has always been said that the risk of rupture is higher after classical than after lower segmental section, although I don't think this has ever been demonstrated. However, it is likely that an incision of the myometrium causes more complications than an incision of the lower segment. But, if you decide to perform a cesarean section for a severely growth-retarded infant because you don't want to submit the baby to a stressful vaginal delivery, why then extract it through a small segmental incision? Classical section is certainly indicated for the extraction of a severely growth-retarded fetus, at least between 27 and 30 to 32 weeks. Otherwise we always perform lower transverse segmental section.

Dr. Dias-Correa: Don't you think that it is dangerous to induce labor with oxytocin in cases of placental insufficiency (as is the rule in IUGR)?

Dr. Bossart: We never use prostaglandins to induce labor in cases of IUGR, because we don't know yet how to monitor these drugs. We use oxytocin only in favorable local circumstances, and of course we monitor the situation very strictly. We don't use oxytocin, for instance, when the cervix is rigid, posterior, and 3 cm long, but we might use it in a multipara under favorable circumstances. However, I agree with you that it can be dangerous.

REFERENCES

1. Manning FA, Baskett TF, Morrison I, Lange I. Fetal biophysical profile scoring: a prospective study in 1184 high-risk patients. *Am J Obstet Gynecol* 1984;140:289–94.
2. Pourcelot L. Applications cliniques de l'examen Doppler transcutané: vélocimétrie ultrasonore Doppler. Séminaire INSERM 1974;34:213–40.
3. Wladimiroff JW, Tonge HM, Stewart PA. Döppler ultrasound assessment of cerebral blood flow in the human fetus. *Br J Obstet Gynaecol* 1986;93:471–5.

Intrauterine Growth Retardation, edited by
Jacques Senterre. Nestlé Nutrition Workshop
Series, Vol. 18. Nestec Ltd., Vevey/Raven Press,
Ltd., New York © 1989.

Morbidity and Mortality in Intrauterine Growth Retardation

Pedro Rosso

Department of Pediatrics, School of Medicine, Pontifical Catholic University of Chile, Santiago, Chile

Nearly three decades ago it became apparent that a significant number of low birthweight newborns classified as premature were born at term. The small size of these infants could only be explained by retarded prenatal growth (1,2). The recognition of fetal growth retardation as a new syndrome was soon followed by studies demonstrating that mortality rates were much higher in these infants than in normally grown newborns of similar gestational age, although lower than in premature infants. It was also found that infants suffering from fetal growth retardation were more susceptible to certain types of neonatal complication (3,4). This information greatly stimulated research in the area, thus contributing to the progress of high-risk obstetrics and neonatal care.

In spite of considerable advances in recent years, key aspects of the problem of intrauterine growth retardation (IUGR) remain undefined. Retarded fetal growth occurs under many different conditions. Affected infants may have severe congenital anomalies and infections; some of them may have suffered the effects of prenatal drug or alcohol abuse; in other cases gestation has been complicated by various diseases; and finally, there are cases where growth retardation seems to be the only abnormal finding. Presumably, morbidity and mortality risks are greatly influenced by these various circumstances, but this aspect of the problem remains to be clarified.

The study of perinatal death involves an understanding of its association with cultural, behavioral, and social factors, as well as the more specific biologic and medical aspects of the health of the mother and her infant. Most studies on the relationship between IUGR and perinatal mortality have ignored these factors, apparently because they are considered to be common to both, implying that growth retardation per se leads to higher mortality.

Growth-retarded neonates without congenital anomalies or infections are generally considered as one group. The majority of studies on IUGR and neonatal and long-term morbidity have been devoted to these infants. However, clinical evidence indicates that they are not a homogeneous group and different types have been recognized, based on their anthropometric characteristics. Some of these types seem to be more susceptible to perinatal complications than others. Postnatal growth and subsequent development is also apparently related to the particular type of intrauterine growth retardation, suggesting the need to revise some of the current concepts. These are the main issues addressed by the present chapter.

DEFINITION OF INTRAUTERINE GROWTH RETARDATION IN MORTALITY STUDIES

Weight-specific perinatal mortality curves from different countries have a similar shape; only the actual rates differ. Mortality is very high at the lowest birthweight but falls sharply as birthweight increases; it is at its lowest within the range of the most frequent birthweights but rises again for the heaviest birthweights. Such a curve can be displayed and modeled by plotting the ratio of deaths to survivors in a logarithmic scale (5). Transformed in this way, perinatal risk may be considered as the sum of three components: one component independent of birthweight; one which decreases linearly with birthweight; and one which increases linearly with birthweight. The latter two have slopes of equal magnitude. This type of weight-specific perinatal mortality curve maintains similar characteristics when applied to specific causes of death such as congenital malformations or birth injuries, indicating that the shape of the curve is determined by weight-specific susceptibility to certain problems rather than by the cumulative effect of diseases specific to either low or high birthweight (Fig. 1). Based on these considerations, it seems highly predictable that growth-retarded neonates would have greater mortality rates because of their lower birthweight, but their causes of morbidity and mortality would be similar to those affecting other neonates.

One of the main problems faced by large-scale epidemiological studies of morbidity and mortality in IUGR is the clinical definition of this syndrome. Two approaches have been used: (a) defining as growth-retarded all low birthweight infants born at term; (b) (more recently) defining normal and abnormal ranges for birthweight at various gestational ages. Both approaches have advantages and disadvantages.

Several research workers have defined fetal growth retardation as low birthweight

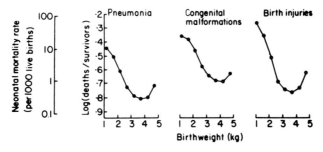

FIG. 1. Birthweight-specific neonatal mortality curves for three specific causes of death in United States whites, 1960. (From ref. 5.)

($<$2,500 g) after week 37 of gestation (3,6,7). This criterion is relatively easy to apply and, as an additional advantage, it allows comparisons between markedly different populations. Unfortunately, as pointed out by Keirse (8), by considering only term infants, this approach excludes growth-retarded infants born before term, who constitute a significant percentage of the total.

Another problem is the use of 2,500 g as a single cut-off point for infants born within a range of gestational ages. Since mean birthweight is lower at week 37 of gestation than at week 40, the same cut-off point applied to this range of gestational ages will identify as growth-retarded considerably more infants at week 37. Moreover, a newborn weighing less than 2,500 g is more severely growth-retarded at week 40 than at week 37 and therefore more susceptible to the complications associated with retarded prenatal growth.

In the more precise approach, defining birthweight for gestational age (9,10), newborns are considered to be growth-retarded if their birthweight falls below a predefined cut-off point of "normality." In studies of this type, mortality rates would vary depending both on the fetal growth standard applied and on the cut-off point selected.

Intrauterine Growth Standards

Over the last two decades, numerous intrauterine growth curves have been published (11–22). Their influence on neonatal care has been considerable; however, these curves have promoted the use of body weight as the main criterion to assess adequacy of size at birth, thus contributing to current uncertainties regarding normal and abnormal fetal growth. Newborn infants of similar gestational age, race, sex, and body length can vary by as much as 1,100 g in their birthweights (23). Such wide variations can only reflect marked differences in fetal fat deposition, skeletal muscle mass, and the size of various organs. In turn, this implies different prenatal growth rates and circumstances. Some of these infants may have suffered severe growth retardation in the last weeks of pregnancy, which might, for example, have reduced birthweight from an expected 3,800 g to 3,100 g instead. Since this reduced birthweight still falls within the normal range of weight for age, the infant is considered "normal." Obviously, these unrecognized cases of fetal growth retardation are not included in morbidity and mortality statistics.

The fetal growth curves in the various intrauterine growth standards are of similar shape but differ with respect to the range of normal values. Since the 10th percentile of these standards is usually taken as the cut-off point for normal growth (see below), the use of different growth standards will result in great differences in the number of infants classified as "small-for-gestational-age" (Table 1).

The different ranges of birthweight values in the available intrauterine growth standards seem to reflect different characteristics of the study populations which are known to influence birthweight, such as race, average maternal height, and living conditions. They also reflect diversity in selection criteria; factors associated with

TABLE 1. *Comparison of 10th percentile values for birthweight at week 40 of gestation in different prenatal growth standards (both sexes)*

Author	10th percentile (g)	Location
Lubchenco et al. (11)	2,630	(Denver, Colorado, U.S.A.)
Thomson et al. (12)	2,840	(Aberdeen, Scotland)
Brenner et al. (18)	2,750	(North Carolina, U.S.A.)
Naeye & Dixon (19)[a]	2,776	(Various U.S. cities)
Williams et al. (21)	2,848	(California, U.S.A.)
Blidner et al. (22)	2,985	(Ontario, Canada)

[a]Blacks and whites combined.

abnormal fetal growth in both mothers and infants will determine higher or lower average values for various indices of fetal growth. For example, the growth standard of Lubchenco et al. (11), widely used throughout the world, includes women living at high altitudes and, most probably, a proportion of smokers, since the negative effect of smoking on birthweight was not known when this study was conducted. Most earlier standards incorporated all births, though Meredith (15) included singleton live births. Some standards included only infants of "certain" gestational age, while others have included infants of approximate and uncertain gestational age. A review of six intrauterine growth curves from the United States (24) revealed some of the potential sources of discrepancy. Five excluded multiple births, two excluded major anomalies, two excluded toxemia, and one excluded up to 30 growth-retarding factors. Four of the standards made allowance for ethnicity, two corrected for sex of the infant, one allowed for parity, one for maternal weight, and none for maternal height.

Ideally, fetal growth standards should include only infants who were fully able to express their genetic growth potential. However, it is impossible to determine prenatal growth potential, so the only alternative is to exclude those neonates with maternal and fetal factors known to affect fetal growth. This can only be achieved in a prospective study similar to that conducted by Miller and Merritt (20). Not surprisingly, these authors report higher birthweight and other anthropometric values than all previous growth studies.

Normal Growth and Fetal Growth Retardation

Different cut-off points of "normality" have been used in the past to identify "normal" and "growth-retarded" infants. These include two standard deviations below mean values, and the 10th, 5th, and 3rd percentiles. As previously mentioned, each of these cut-off points will result in significant differences in the number of neonates presumed to be growth-retarded. Lower cut-off points, e.g., the 3rd percentile or 2 SD below the mean, will lead to a smaller number of infants being considered growth-retarded in comparison with, say, the 10th percentile cut-off point. In addition, the proportion of infants with severe growth retardation will be higher when a lower cut-off point is selected, and therefore morbidity and mortality rates in these infants will also appear higher.

The use of birthweight as the only criterion for detecting fetal growth retardation leads to additional problems. As discussed above, regardless of the cut-off point selected, a number of growth-retarded neonates with birthweights above the cut-off value will be considered "normal." On the other hand, a group of normal infants whose birthweights are below the cut-off point will be classified as growth-retarded. It is likely that the morbidity and mortality risk in these normally small infants is lower than in growth-retarded infants of the same weight. It therefore seems more accurate to refer to them as "small-for-gestational-age" or "small-for-dates" rather than as suffering from intrauterine growth retardation.

The analysis of birthweight variability explains why a number of small-for-gestational-age infants are normal and not growth-retarded. Birthweight is the expression of genetic influences interacting with maternal and environmental factors. Individually, these factors contribute to only a fraction of the normal birthweight variability but their combination may lead to significant effects. Thus, a female infant born to a short (less than 155 cm), primiparous mother is likely to have a birthweight considerably below mean values for that population. Clearly, this infant is small but not growth-retarded. However, it could be argued that while the influence of female sex is purely genetic, maternal height and parity are maternal constraints on fetal growth. Therefore, while it would be correct to take into account the infant's sex in assessing the adequacy of fetal growth, it would be incorrect to include other factors which have a restraining influence. Furthermore, in a developing country, reduced maternal stature may reflect growth stunting due to undernutrition during childhood, and thus be a pathologic condition. This remains an unresolved issue. Currently, only one intrauterine growth standard includes correction factors for sex, parity, and maternal height (12). This standard, however, also includes corrections for maternal weight at mid-gestation which seems erroneous since low weight gain during pregnancy reflects maternal undernutrition.

Available studies on perinatal mortality in IUGR can hardly be compared because of the different definitions of fetal growth retardation applied. Considering the lack of an accurate method of identifying growth-retarded neonates, the mortality data should be considered as only a partial, and probably biased, picture of reality.

MORTALITY ASSOCIATED WITH INTRAUTERINE GROWTH RETARDATION

Compared with the numerous studies on mortality of low birthweight infants, there are relatively few reports on mortality of growth-retarded infants.

One of the earliest and best known studies in this field is the analysis by Butler and Bonham (3) of the British Perinatal Mortality Survey of 1958. In this survey, social, biologic, and clinical data on mother, pregnancy, labor, and newborn were obtained in 17,400 singleton and twin births. Gestational age, based on date of the last menstrual period, was considered "known" in 89% of the cases. Birthweights at each completed week of gestation were expressed either as percentiles or as standard deviations below or above the mean birthweight. The results showed that intrapartum and first-week mortality was extremely high when mean birthweight was more than 2 SD below the mean. The lowest perinatal mortality was observed in infants whose birthweights were between zero and 1 SD above the mean. Low birthweight infants with gestational age over 36 weeks were considered "small-for-dates." Mortality in these infants was eight times higher than in their heavier peers (Table 2). The main causes of death were asphyxia, pulmonary infection, and massive pulmonary hemorrhage.

Other studies conducted in various populations have confirmed the higher neonatal and perinatal mortality risk of small-for-dates infants compared with normal size infants of similar gestational age (9,25–27). Furthermore, some of the studies indicate a strong correlation between the severity of growth retardation and perinatal mortality in infants weighing less than 2,500 g at weeks 40–41 of gestation compared with infants in the 3,000–3,499 g birthweight category (28) (Table 3). Similar striking differences are demonstrated in the contour plots of perinatal mortality for gestational age and birthweight of various populations (9,29,30). In addition, the contour plots confirm the conclusions of previous studies that the association of perinatal mortality with birthweight is stronger than with fetal age, and this also holds true for small-for-dates infants (21).

Few studies on perinatal mortality and intrauterine growth retardation have provided data on specific cause of death. In a study conducted by Van den Berg and Yerushalmy (4) in a United States population, growth retardation was identified as birthweight in the lowest quartiles of weight for gestation observed for the entire population. The infants, who were presumably most growth-retarded, had a mean birthweight of 2,254 g at 40 weeks of gestation. Neonatal mortality rate in this

TABLE 2. *Percentage distribution and mortality ratio of major birthweight groups by gestational age*

Birthweight (g)	Gestational age (weeks)		
	38–39	40–41	42–43
≤ 2,500			
Percent	22.2	13.0	2.8
Mortality ratio	333	321	500
> 2,500			
Percent	28.2	45.2	11.2
Mortality ratio	40	36	61

Adapted from ref. 3.

TABLE 3. *Perinatal mortality by gestational age and birthweight,*
based on 93,156 births

Birthweight (g)	Gestational age (weeks)		
	38–39	40–41	42–43
2,000–2,499	22.9	58.6	52.6
2,500–2,999	8.6	7.7	13.1
3,000–3,499	2.5	2.5	5.1
3,500–3,999	1.4	1.5	2.0

Adapted from ref. 28.

group was 43.5 per 1,000 live births. Asphyxia and respiratory problems were the most common causes of death (approximately 38%), followed by congenital malformations, birth injury, "immaturity," and miscellaneous causes.

A study by Usher and McLean (26) in a Canadian population provides one of the most detailed information on causes of death in small-for-gestational age infants published so far. In this study "small-for-dates" was defined as birthweight below 2 SD of mean values for a given gestational age. These infants were compared with appropriate-for-gestational-age infants (birthweight over 2 SD). Perinatal mortality was increased 12-fold in small-for-dates compared with normal sized infants. "Obscure" causes of death were the most common, followed by congenital malformations, asphyxia, infection, and respiratory distress, in decreasing order. The "obscure" causes group, which included 56% of the total, showed no major lesions at necropsy.

The largest and most recently published study on mortality and morbidity in infants with intrauterine growth retardation was conducted in several urban and rural areas in the United States (10). Data on all births and infant deaths were provided by local and state Vital Statistics Units. All infants whose birthweights were in the lowest quartile for gestational age were considered small-for-dates, and all other infants were considered to be appropriate-weight-for-gestation. The data indicate that small-for-dates and appropriate-for-dates infants of similar weight differ in the nature of their risk of adverse outcome at 1 year of age. In each group, the total proportion of infants who either died before 1 year of age or were handicapped at 1 year of age was similar, but appropriate-for-dates infants were at greater risk of neonatal death while the small-for-dates infants were at greater risk of problems presenting later during the first year of life. The differences in mortality were present only in the infants weighing 2,500 g or less, indicating the presence of factors independent of birthweight. These were presumably linked to maturity. In the weight groups over 2,500 g, neonatal and postneonatal mortality was similar in small-for-dates and appropriate-for-gestational-age infants (Table 4).

Over the last two decades, significant progress in both high-risk obstetrics and the management of critically ill newborns has greatly decreased mortality rates in various birthweight-gestational age categories. A comparison of neonatal mortality risk

TABLE 4. *Neonatal, postneonatal, and total infant mortality in live-born singletons, by birthweight and weight for gestation*

Birthweight (g)	Weight for gestation	Mortality		Total during first year
		Neonatal	Postneonatal	
< 1,501	SGA	463.5	56.1	519.6
	AGA	533.1	78.1	611.2
1,501–2,000	SGA	76.7	19.5	96.2
	AGA	116.3	19.6[a]	135.9
2,001–2,500	SGA	15.2	10.4	25.6
	AGA	39.3	7.7[a]	47.0
2,501–3,000	SGA	4.6	5.2	9.8
	AGA	6.0	5.4	11.4
3,001–3,500	SGA	2.3	3.1	5.4
	AGA	2.4	3.1	6.5
3,501–4,000		1.7	2.6	4.3
≥ 4,001		2.2	2.7	4.9

Adapted from ref. 10.
SGA, small-for-gestational-age; AGA, appropriate-for-gestational-age.
[a]Number of cases used to calculate death was less than 10.

in the same clinical center for the years 1958–1969 and 1974–1980 (25,31) showed the most important difference in predicted neonatal mortality to be a shift towards the lower (birthweight) gestational age categories. For example, a 50% mortality group, which encompassed 1,000 g at 30 weeks of gestation in the most recent data, now includes 750 g at 26 weeks of gestation. The lowest risk group, which encompassed a small subgroup at 3,250 g at 40 weeks of gestation, has expanded to include a large group of infants with birthweights ranging from 2,500 g at 34 weeks gestation. In both studies the small-for-dates infants had the highest mortality risk at any gestational age; however, the differences were proportionally smaller in the 1974–1980 period.

MORBIDITY ASSOCIATED WITH INTRAUTERINE GROWTH RETARDATION

Numerous studies have consistently shown that fetal growth retardation is associated with the following neonatal complications: asphyxia, hypoglycemia, hyperviscosity, and hypothermia (32) (Table 5). These studies have only included those infants without severe congenital malformations or infections, thus the type of growth retardation presumably caused by an "inadequate supply line" (33) including reduced uterine blood flow.

In the absence of congenital malformations, infections, and/or other maternal problems known to retard fetal growth, a small size at birth is generally considered to be the consequence of a reduced utero-placental blood flow. This idea is well-

TABLE 5. *Perinatal complications in small-for-gestational-age infants with normal and low ponderal index (PI)*

Complications	Normal PI (21)	Low PI (23)
Asphyxia	2/21	7/23
Hypoglycemia	0/21	4/23
Hyperviscosity	1/21	7/23
Hypothermia	1/21	6/23

Adapted from ref. 50.
Intergroup differences are all statistically significant.

supported by measurements of placental blood flow in women carrying growth-retarded fetuses (34,35) and by observations in animal models (36). Indirect support is also provided by observations of spontaneous fetal heart rate decelerations during antepartum non-stress testing in growth-retarded neonates (37).

Asphyxia

A chronic reduction in uterine blood flow and therefore of intervillous space blood flow results in persistently low Po_2 and, in addition, limits glucose availability to the fetus, causing a reduction in fetal glycogen stores. The combination of these two factors produces an extremely high risk of intrapartum hypoxia and asphyxia for the growth-retarded infants. Numerous studies have shown an increased percentage of abnormal fetal heart rate patterns and fetal acidosis during the course of labor and delivery in growth-retarded neonates (38–42). If the use of intermittent positive pressure ventilation for more than 1 min after delivery is taken as a sign of intrapartum asphyxia, this complication would be 5 to 10 times more common in growth-retarded neonates than in their fully grown peers (43).

Fortunately, the management of asphyxia in these infants does not present particular difficulties and the long-term sequelae associated with birth asphyxia of equivalent severity is apparently similar in small-for-dates and normal-sized infants (44).

Despite a higher frequency of intrapartum asphyxia, small-for-gestational-age infants do not seem to suffer a proportionally increased risk of meconium aspiration (45). This finding appears paradoxical since meconium aspiration pneumonia is most frequently seen in newborns who have suffered intrapartum asphyxia and passed meconium *in utero*.

Massive Pulmonary Hemorrhage

Massive pulmonary hemorrhage was believed to be a typical complication of growth-retarded neonates. In the 1958 British Perinatal Mortality (46) survey, massive pulmonary hemorrhage was found to be 10 times more common in low birthweight term infants than in large infants. However, such an association was not apparent in the 1970 survey (47). This fall in incidence is likely to reflect progress in neonatal care during the intervening years, especially the reduction in the number of cases of severe birth asphyxia and hypothermia, and a more cautious use of intravenous base, all factors believed to contribute to pulmonary hemorrhage (48).

Hypoglycemia

Both preterm and full-term small-for-gestational-age infants are more likely to develop hypoglycemia than their normal sized peers. In the early 1970s the incidence of hypoglycemia in infants below the 10th percentile of weight for gestational age was reported to be approximately 10 times higher than in larger infants (49). More recent studies have reported a lower incidence of hypoglycemia, a fact attributed to early feeding (50).

The tendency of growth-retarded neonates to develop hypoglycemia is believed to reflect an imbalance between a high glucose consumption rate and a reduced glucose production rate (51). The reasons for the increased glucose consumption are unknown, but several factors might be involved. In some growth-retarded infants, the size of the brain is relatively well-preserved in comparison with that of the liver and other organs. Since the brain is the main glucose-consuming organ of the body, those infants with a selectively large brain would have proportionally greater glucose demands. Moreover, their brain:liver weight ratio is considerably greater than normal. Thus the liver should produce considerably more glucose per gram of tissue in order to maintain a normal balance. Red cells are also important glucose consumers. As discussed below, growth-retarded fetuses frequently have a relative increase in red cell mass. Finally, hypothermia, also a common problem in growth-retarded neonates, leads to increased glucose utilization.

The reduced glucose production rate of growth-retarded neonates apparently reflects a reduced hepatic glycogen content (52) and a reduced activity of glycolytic and gluconeogenetic enzymes. The size of fetal glycogen stores depends on glucose availability and insulin levels. In the growth-retarded fetus both factors are reduced due to the reduction in placental blood flow.

Amino acids normally used as substrate during gluconeogenesis are utilized more slowly by small-for-dates infants (53), suggesting a reduced gluconeogenetic capacity. Other studies have shown an inverse relationship between blood glucose and both alanine and lactate levels in small-for-dates neonates, lending further support for the possibility of impaired gluconeogenesis (54). A delay in the synthesis of key gluconeogenetic enzymes has been suggested as an explanation for this (55). Hydrocortisone administration in these infants increases alanine utilization (56), a finding compatible with the possibility of enzyme induction.

Hyperviscosity

Small-for-dates infants born at term have an increased hematocrit and red cell volume (57,58) and, as a consequence, may develop hyperviscosity (59). Hyperviscosity affects 18% of all small-for-dates neonates (60). This is a considerably higher incidence than the 5% reported in fully grown neonates (61).

The increased red cell mass of small-for-dates infants has been attributed to various factors, including chronic hypoxia (62), *in utero* placental-fetal transfusion caused by hypoxia and acute fetal distress, with intact umbilical circulation (63,64), and to postnatal placental transfusion due to late clamping of the umbilical cord (65). All these explanations remain speculative. Meberg (66) investigated the possibility that chronic fetal hypoxia could stimulate erythropoietin production (which, in turn, would stimulate red cell production), and found no significant differences in cord blood erythropoietin levels between small-for-dates and normal-sized infants.

Hypothermia

Small-for-dates infants are highly susceptible to the development of hypothermia because they have a reduced capacity to retain and generate body heat.

Body insulation is greatly dependent on the quantity of subcutaneous fat, which is reduced in small-for-dates infants. In addition, they tend to lose more radiant heat than larger infants because of a greater surface area/bodyweight ratio.

Neonates generate heat by non-shivering thermogenesis through the exothermic metabolism of fatty acids in brown adipose tissue (67). The quantity of brown adipose tissue is markedly reduced in small-for-dates infants, especially in those that appear to be severely growth-retarded (68). Consequently, the contribution of brown adipose tissue to non-shivering thermogenesis is considerably smaller in the growth-retarded infant. The presence of hypoglycemia may further reduce the efficiency of this mechanism (69,70).

When small-for-dates neonates are exposed to environmental temperatures below 33°C, they increase their oxygen consumption, but this response is not sufficient to maintain their core temperature for more than 20 min (71). This limited response is consistent with reduced brown adipose tissue.

MORBIDITY IN DIFFERENT TYPES OF FETAL GROWTH RETARDATION

Types of Fetal Growth Retardation

A review of the fetal effects of intrauterine growth retardation in various animal models, as well as the limited available data on organ weight in small-for-gestational-age infants, led Rosso and Winick (72) to propose a classification of fetal growth retardation based on the etiology of the problem and its clinical characteristics. Two clinical types of growth retardation were considered in this classification: Type I, where the infants appeared proportionally growth-retarded; and Type II, where the infants were disproportionally growth-retarded, with head circumference spared relative to other body segments. Post-mature infants, of the type described by Clifford (73), who usually have a normal head circumference, were also included in the Type II category.

The anthropometric differences between Type I and Type II fetal growth retardation were attributed to the combined effects of the causal factor and the gestational age at which growth retardation began (72). Thus Type I (proportionate growth retardation) was believed to reflect an early onset (before week 30 of gestation), while Type II represented a later onset (after week 30 of gestation). Clinical observations by Urrusti et al. (74), based on intrauterine growth curves extrapolated from small-for-gestational-age infants with normal and low weight:length ratios, supported the "timing" hypothesis put forward by Rosso and Winick (72). A more conclusive set of data was presented by Campbell (75) who, using ultrasound measurements of fetal biparietal diameter (BPD), observed two major patterns of growth retardation. One, described as "low growth profile," was characterized by early onset, as indicated by BPD values below the normal range before week 25 of gestation. The second type of pattern, described as "late flattening," corresponds to a fall-off from the normal curve from approximately week 32 of gestation.

The "timing" hypothesis to explain the major clinical groups of growth-retarded neonates was further elaborated by Villar and Belizan (76). These authors proposed that, independent of causal factors, Type I growth retardation resulted from reduced nutrient availability for the fetus dating from the first trimester and continuing throughout the remainder of the gestational period. Type II growth retardation would reflect growth retardation starting between weeks 27 and 30. In addition, they proposed a Type III category to include infants whose growth was negatively affected in the last 2 to 3 weeks of gestation, when prenatal organ and skeletal growth is nearly completed.

Numerous recent anthropometric studies on small-for-dates infants without congenital malformations have confirmed the existence of different types of growth retardation, but general agreement has not been reached concerning the anthropometric characteristics of each type.

The distinction between the two major types of fetal growth retardation is usually based on ponderal index, a measure introduced by Rohrer in 1921 (77). This index is calculated as weight (g) $\times$ 100, divided by (length)^3 (cm), and shows how heavy an infant is for a given length. Using this index, Walther and Ramaekers (50) found that 23 out of 46 consecutive term infants with a birthweight below the 3rd percentile had a ponderal index below the 3rd percentile and 21 had a ponderal index above the 10th percentile for gestational age. These data confirm previous observation by Ounsted and Ounsted (78) that 30% to 50% of small-for-gestational-age infants have a reduced weight for length.

The use of the ponderal index to classify growth-retarded neonates offers practical advantages but it may help to confuse the problem by not considering "skeletal growth" which could be more a reliable index of the severity and time course of growth retardation (23). "Skeletal growth," as reflected by body length and head circumference, might be a better index of the impact of growth retardation in various organs, including the brain. Its degree of compromise could have prognostic value for subsequent growth and development. In contrast, ponderal index and other indices which reflect body fat and muscle mass, including skinfold thickness and mid-arm circumference, may have a better prognostic value for short-term complications. The degree of brain sparing could be quantified by comparisons of the head circumference:body length ratio rather than the head circumference:body weight ratio.

Theoretically, various combinations of compromised skeletal growth and soft tissue growth could result from the combined effect of time of onset and severity of fetal growth retardation, but in general they will all fall within the major classifications of fetal growth retardation recognized so far (79). Type I would have severely compromised skeletal growth but a normal ponderal index. Type II, or late onset IUGR, would have moderately compromised skeletal growth and a reduced ponderal index. In addition, most of these infants would have an increased head circumference:body length ratio. Type III, or term onset IUGR, would have a normal skeletal size and a low ponderal index; the head circumference:body length ratio will probably be normal.

The importance of timing rather than of causal factors as the major determinant of the anthropometric characteristics of small-for-dates infants is illustrated by a study by Crane and Kopta (80). These authors studied 33 small-for-dates infants to test the hypothesis that "asymmetric" growth retardation is caused by "utero-placental insufficiency" while "symmetric" growth retardation is caused by other factors. In 21 cases assigned to the "asymmetric" group the presence of "utero-placental insufficiency" was established by abnormal estriol patterns, low human placental lactogen levels, antepartum meconium, an abnormal contraction stress test and/or late deceleration in labor, and abnormal histologic features of the placenta. The rest of the infants (13 cases) were assigned to the "symmetric" group, based on the existence of factors considered to predispose to this type of growth retardation including maternal smoking, drug addiction, congenital anomalies, chemotherapy treatment, and others. In addition, these cases did not suffer fetal distress during labor and ultrasonography demonstrated a "reduced growth potential" pattern.

The results showed no differences between the two groups with respect to birthweight, body length, head circumference, and ponderal index. The authors concluded that none of these variables was useful in distinguishing infants with "asymmetric" and "symmetric" growth retardation, and emphasized the fact that the reduced growth in head circumference was similar in both groups.

The study by Crane and Kopta (80) clearly demonstrates that different causal factors may determine similar types of growth retardation, thus supporting the idea that in most cases, timing and possibly severity of the growth retardation is more important than a specific causal factor. However, since certain causal factors are likely to affect the course of pregnancy at a particular time, it is conceivable that they may be strongly associated with one of the clinical types of growth retardation, for example, preeclampsia and Type II neonatal growth retardation.

Timing of Growth Retardation and Morbidity

The susceptibility of infants with various types of growth retardation to neonatal complications remains a poorly explored field. At present, the study by Walther and

Ramaekers (50) continues to be the most relevant one. These authors studied 46 consecutively born term infants whose weight was ≤2 SD below mean values for gestational age, correcting for sex, birth order, and maternal height. All were Caucasian and singletons, and none had congenital anomalies or intrauterine infections. Based on their ponderal index the infants were divided into two groups, those whose ponderal index was above the 10th percentile (23 infants) and those whose ponderal index was below the 3rd percentile (21 infants). Two infants whose ponderal index was between these limits were excluded from the study. The data showed that infants with a low ponderal index were more prone to develop asphyxia, hypoglycemia, hypothermia, and hyperviscosity than those with a normal ponderal index (Table 5). The authors concluded that the identification of proportionately and disproportionately growth-retarded neonates is clinically useful, since the risk of neonatal complications is markedly influenced by the type of growth retardation.

If the assumption is correct that in small-for-gestational-age babies a normal ponderal index reflects a longer period of intrauterine growth retardation, the study by Walther and Ramaekers (50) would indicate that infants with proportionate fetal growth retardations are better adapted to intrapartum stress and to the early post-natal environment.

PATHOPHYSIOLOGY AND MORBIDITY OF INTRAUTERINE GROWTH RETARDATION

In Type I fetal growth retardation, utero-placental blood flow will not expand normally from the early states of gestation. Both the fetus and the placenta will grow more slowly, but proportionately, to the reduced amount of oxygen and nutrients supplied by the maternal circulation. In this type of growth retardation critical fetal demands will be met by the supply line throughout pregnancy, so fetal homeostasis will remain within normal limits. The marked growth retardation of these infants will reflect a proportionate reduction in cell number of all the organs and tissues, including the skeleton. As suggested by various follow-up studies, including those in twins of unequal size, their post-natal recovery of the growth deficit is never complete, so affected infants reach adult size considerably below their genetic potential (81–83).

In Type II and Type III growth retardation utero-placental blood flow will be normal during the first 25 to 30 weeks of gestation and then, for unknown reasons, it will continue to expand at a slower than normal rate. Thus, a fetus who up to that time was growing normally begins to receive less than the required amount of nutrients. The rather abrupt change will elicit various adaptive responses and ultimately growth retardation will occur. In this situation, one of the main factors influencing fetal homeostasis will be reduced glucose availability caused by the relative reduction in placental blood flow. Observations in the fasting pregnant sheep illustrate the fetal adaptive mechanisms to reduced maternal glucose levels and reduced utero-placental blood flow. In this model, maternal blood glucose level falls after 5 days of fasting and uterine blood flow decreases by approximately 25% (84). Uterine up-take of oxygen, glucose, and essential amino acids decreases by nearly 50%, al-though total amino acid uptake remains constant (84,85). The fetus becomes hypoglycemic and insulin release is decreased (86). Since fetal glucose utilization is insulin-dependent (87), fetal glucose utilization decreases markedly. In the fetal lamb this is reflected by a reduction in the glucose/oxygen quotient from 0.70–0.80 in the fed state to 0.30–0.40 after 5 days of fasting (85). This change indicates that other metabolic substrates are utilized instead of glucose to maintain fetal oxidative metabolism. An 80% increase in urea production rates suggests that amino acids may be providing the additional energy substrate (85).

The sheep model of prolonged fasting is not comparable to the human situation in terms of the drop in maternal glucose levels. However, it seems logical to assume that reduced utero-placental blood flow determines a decrease in daily placental transfer of glucose.

The combined effects of reduced glucose and oxygen supply will result in cate-cholamine secretion and redistribution of fetal cardiac output. Brain blood flow will be relatively preserved compared with other organs such as liver, kidney, and mus-cle, thus contributing to the disproportionate growth of these organs. In addition, the reduced glucose availability and low insulin secretion will drastically reduce he-patic triglyceride synthesis and fat deposition. This would explain the progressive relative thinning of the growth-retarded fetus compared with the normally growing fetus. The reduced fat deposition would make these infants more susceptible to hy-poglycemia, while chronic hypoxia and the resulting enhanced erythropoiesis would be factors contributing to polycythemia and hyperviscosity.

Growth retardation in Type II infants is generally less severe than in those suffer-ing Type I fetal growth retardation. The less severe compromise of skeletal growth is apparently one of the factors which explains the better rate of postnatal growth and improved likelihood of complete recovery in these infants (88). Studies on early post-natal malnutrition in rats suggest that the capacity of a growing organism to re-cuperate from a period of arrested growth is related to the magnitude of the deficit in cell number (89). Furthermore, complete recovery is only possible when cell number has been preserved but cell size is reduced.

Human fetal growth occurs mainly by cell division. Cell enlargement, which be-gins approximately at week 25 of gestation, is only a minor component of the pro-cess (90). Therefore, the capacity of a growth-retarded neonate to recover from this initial deficit would largely depend on the magnitude of the relative reduction in cell number. From this point of view, some of the Type II, or disproportionately growth-retarded infants, may also have a reduced expectancy of achieving their full growth potential if prenatal growth was severely affected.

REFERENCES

1. Douglas JWB. Some factors associated with prematurity. *J Obstet Gynaecol Br Cwlth* 1950;57:143–70.

2. Scott KE, Usher R. Fetal malnutrition: its incidence, causes and effects. *Am J Obstet Gynecol* 1966;94:951–63.
3. Butler NR, Bonham DG. *Perinatal mortality*. Edinburgh, London: Churchill Livingstone, 1963.
4. Van den Berg B, Yerushalmy J. The relationship of intrauterine growth of infants of low birthweight to mortality, morbidity and congenital anomalies. *J Pediatr* 1966;69:531–45.
5. Wilcox AJ, Russell IT. Birthweight and perinatal mortality: II. On weight-specific mortality. *Int J Epidemiol* 1983;12:319–25.
6. Fedrick J, Adelstein P. Factors associated with low birth weight of infants delivered at term. *Br J Obstet Gynecol* 1978;85:1–7.
7. Kaltreider DF, Kohl S. Epidemiology of preterm delivery. *Clin Obstet Gynecol* 1980;23:17–31.
8. Keirse MJNC. Epidemiology and aetiology of the growth retarded baby. *Clin Obstet Gynecol* 1984;11:415–36.
9. Goldstein H, Peckham C. Birthweight, gestation, neonatal mortality and child development. In: Roberts DF, Thomson AM, eds. *The biology of human fetal growth*, London: Taylor and Francis, 1976;81–103.
10. Starfield B, Shapiro S, McCormick M, Bross D. Mortality and morbidity in infants with intrauterine growth retardation. *J Pediatr* 1982;101:978–83.
11. Lubchenco L, Hansman C, Dressler M, Boyd E. Intrauterine growth as estimated from liveborn birthweight data at 24 to 42 weeks of gestation. *Pediatrics* 1963;32:793–800.
12. Thomson AM, Billewicz WZ, Hytten FE. The assessment of fetal growth. *J Obstet Gynaecol Br Cwlth* 1968;75:903–16.
13. Usher R, McLean F. Intrauterine growth of infants at sea level: standards obtained from measurements of infants born between 25 and 44 weeks of gestation. *J Pediatr* 1969;74:901–10.
14. Sterky G. Swedish standard curves for intrauterine growth. *Pediatrics* 1970;46:7–8.
15. Meredith H. Body weight at birth of viable human infants: a worldwide comparative treatise. *Human Biol* 1970;42:217–64.
16. Tanner JM, Thomson AM. Standards for birthweight at gestation periods from 32 to 42 weeks, allowing for maternal height and weight. *Arch Dis Child* 1970;45:566–9.
17. Wong KS, Scott KE. Fetal growth at sea level. *Biol Neonate* 1972;20:175–88.
18. Brenner WE, Edelman DA, Hendricks CH. A standard of fetal growth for the United States of America. *Am J Obstet Gynecol* 1976;126:555–64.
19. Naeye RL, Dixon JB. Distortions in fetal growth standards. *Pediatr Res* 1978;12:987–91.
20. Miller HC, Merritt TA. *Fetal growth in humans*. Chicago, London: Year Book Medical Publishers, 1979;31–56.
21. Williams RL, Creasy RK, Cunningham GC, et al. Fetal growth and perinatal viability in California. *Obstet Gynecol* 1982;59:624–32.
22. Blidner IN, McClemont S, Anderson GD, Sinclair J. Size at birth: standards for an urban Canadian population. *Can Med Assoc J* 1984;130:133–40.
23. Miller HC, Hassanein K. Diagnosis of impaired fetal growth in newborn infants. *Pediatrics* 1971;48:511–22.
24. Miller HC. Intrauterine growth retardation. An unmet challenge. *Am J Dis Child* 1981;135:944–8.
25. Lubchenco LO, Searls DT, Brazie JV. Neonatal mortality rate: relationship to birthweight and gestational age. *J Pediatr* 1972;81:814–82.
26. Usher RH, McLean FH. Normal fetal growth. In: Davis JA, Dobbling J, eds. *Scientific foundations of paediatrics*. London: Heinemann, 1974;69–80.
27. Friedman E, Neff R. *Pregnancy hypertension: A systematic evaluation of clinical diagnosis criteria*. Acton (Mass., U.S.A.): Publishing Sciences Group, 1977.
28. Bakketeig LS, Hoffman HJ, Titmuss Oakley AR. Perinatal mortality. In: Bracken MB, ed. *Perinatal epidemiology*. New York, Oxford: Oxford University Press, 1984;99–151.
29. Hoffman HJ, Lundin FE, Bakketeig LS, Harley EE. Classification of births by weight and gestational age for future studies of prematurity. In: Reed DM, Stanley FJ, eds. *The epidemiology of prematurity*. Baltimore, Munich: Urban and Schwarzenberg, 1977;297–325.
30. Goldstein H. Factors related to birthweight and perinatal mortality. *Br Med Bull* 1981;37:259–64.
31. Koops BL, Morgan LJ, Battaglia FC. Neonatal mortality risk in relation to birthweight and gestational age: update. *J Pediatr* 1982;101:969–77.
32. Lin C, Evans MI. *Intrauterine growth retardation. Pathophysiology and clinical management*. New York: McGraw-Hill, 1984;315–51.
33. Gruenwald P. The supply line of the fetus: definitions relating to fetal growth. In: Gruenwald P, ed.

The placenta and its maternal supply line. Effects of insufficiency on the fetus. Baltimore: University Park Press, 1975;1–17.

34. Chatfield WR, Rogers TGH, Brownlee BEW, Rippon PE. Placental scanning with computer-linked gamma camera to detect impaired placental blood flow and intrauterine growth retardation. *Br Med J* 1975;i:120–3.

35. Lunell NO, Sarby B, Lewander R, Nylund L. Comparison of uteroplacental blood flow in normal and in intrauterine growth-retarded pregnancy. Measurements with Indium 113 and a computer-linked gammacamera. *Gynecol Obstet Invest* 1979;10:106–18.

36. Robertson WB, Brosens IA, Dixon HG. Maternal blood supply in fetal growth retardation. In: Van Assche FA, Robertson WB, eds. *Fetal growth retardation.* Edinburgh: Churchill Livingstone, 1981;126–38.

37. Pazos R, Vuolo K, Aladjem S, Luek J, Anderson C. Association of spontaneous fetal heart rate decelerations during antepartum nonstress testing and intrauterine growth retardation. *Am J Obstet Gynecol* 1982;144:574–7.

38. Low JA, Pancham SR, Worthington D. Fetal heart deceleration patterns in relation to asphyxia and weight for gestational age percentile of the fetus. *Obstet Gynecol* 1976;47:14–9.

39. Tejani N, Mann LI. Diagnosis and management of the small-for-gestational age fetus. *Clin Obstet Gynecol* 1977;20:943–55.

40. Cetrulo CL, Freeman R. Bioelectric evaluation in intrauterine growth retardation. *Clin Obstet Gynecol* 1977;20:979–86.

41. Hutchins CJ. Delivery of the growth-retarded infant. *Obstet Gynecol* 1980;56:683–90.

42. Lin CC, Moawad AH, Rosenow PJ et al. Acid base characteristics of fetuses with intrauterine growth retardation during labor and delivery. *Am J Obstet Gynecol* 1980;137:553–9.

43. McDonald HM, Mulligan JC, Allen AC, Taylor P. Neonatal asphyxia. I. Relationship of obstetric and neonatal complications in neonatal mortality in 405 consecutive deliveries. *J Pediatr* 1980;96:898–902.

44. Mulligan JC, Painter MJ, O'Donoghue PA, et al. Neonatal asphyxia. II. Neonatal mortality and long-term sequelae. *J Pediatr* 1980;96:903–7.

45. Gregory GA, Gooding CA, Phibbs RH, Tooley WH. Meconium aspiration in infants—a prospective study. *J Pediatr* 1974;85:848–52.

46. Fedrich J, Butler NR. Certain causes of neonatal deaths. IV. Massive pulmonary haemorrhage. *Biol Neonate* 1971;18:243–62.

47. Chamberlain R, Chamberlain GVP, Howlett B, Claireaux A. *British births 1970.* London: William Heinemann, 1975;236–56.

48. Jones RAK, Robertson NRC. Problems of the small-for-dates baby. *Clin Obstet Gynecol* 1984;11:499–524.

49. Lubchenco LO, Bard H. Incidence of hypoglycemia in newborn infants classified by birthweight and gestational age. *Pediatrics* 1971;47:831–8.

50. Walther FJ, Ramaekers LHJ. Neonatal morbidity of SGA infants in relation to their nutritional status at birth. *Acta Pediatr Scand* 1982;71:437–40.

51. Salle B, Ruitton-Uglienco A. Glucose disappearance rate, insulin response and growth hormone response in the small for gestational age and premature infant of very low birthweight. *Biol Neonate* 1976;29:1–17.

52. Shelley HJ, Neligan GA. Neonatal hypoglycemia. *Br Med Bull* 1966;22:34–9.

53. Williams PR, Fiser RH, Sperling MA. Effects of alanine feeding on blood glucose, plasma glucogen and insulin concentrations in small for gestational age infants. *N Engl J Med* 1975;292:612–4.

54. Haymond MW, Karl ILE, Pagliara AS. Increased gluconeogenic substrates in the small-for-gestational age infant. *N Engl J Med* 1974;291:332–8.

55. Marsac C, Sandubray JM, Mancion A, Leroux JP. Development of glyconeogenic enzymes in the liver of human newborns. *Biol Neonate* 1976;28:317–25.

56. Sann L, Ruitkon A, Mathieu M. Effect of intravenous hydrocortisone administration on glucose homeostasis in small for gestational age infants. *Acta Paediatr Scand* 1979;68:113–8.

57. Usher R, Lind J. Blood volume of the newborn premature infant. *Acta Paediatr Scand* 1965;54:419–31.

58. Cassady G. Plasma volume studies in low birthweight infants. *Pediatrics* 1966;38:1020–7.

59. Gross GP, Hathaway WE, McGaughey HR. Hyperviscosity in the neonate. *J Pediatr* 1973;82:1004–12.

60. Hakanson DO, Oh W. Hyperviscosity in the small-for-gestational age infant. *Biol Neonate* 1980;37:109–12.

61. Wirth FH, Goldberg KE, Lubchenco LP. Neonatal hyperviscosity. Incidence and effect of partial plasma transfusion. *Pediatr Res* 1975;19:372 (abstr).
62. Humbert JR, Abelson H, Hathaway WE, Battaglia FC. Polycythemia in small for gestational age infants. *J Pediatr* 1969;75:812–9.
63. Michael AF, Mauer AM. Maternal-fetal transfusion as a cause of plethora in the neonatal period. *Pediatrics* 1961;28:488–96.
64. Oh W, Omori K, Emmanouilides GC, Pheeps DL. Placenta to lamb fetus transfusion in utero during acute hypoxia. *Am J Obstet Gynecol* 1975;122:316–22.
65. Usher RH, Stephad M, Lind J. The blood volume of the newborn infant and placental transfusion. *Acta Pediatr Scand* 1963;52:497–512.
66. Meberg A. Haemoglobin concentration and erythropoietin levels in appropriate and small for gestational age infants. *Scand J Haematol* 1980;24:162–8.
67. Hey EN. The care of babies in incubators. *Recent Adv Pediatr* 1971;4:1711–6.
68. Aherne W, Hull D. Brown adipose tissue and heat production in the newborn infant. *J Path Bact* 1966;911:223–34.
69. Hey EN, Katz G. Temporary loss of metabolic response to cold stress in infants of low birthweight. *Arch Dis Child* 1969;44:323–30.
70. Bhakoo ON, Scopes JW. Minimal rates of oxygen consumption in small dates babies during the first week of life. *Arch Dis Child* 1974;49:583–5.
71. Hey EN. The relation between environmental temperature and oxygen consumption in the newborn baby. *J Physiol* 1969;200:589–603.
72. Rosso P, Winick M. Intrauterine growth retardation. A new systematic approach based on the clinical and biochemical characteristics of this condition. *J Perinat Med* 1974;2:147–60.
73. Clifford SH. Postmaturity with placental dysfunction. *J Pediatr* 1954;44:1–13.
74. Urrusti J, Yoshida P, Velasco L, et al. Human fetal growth retardation: I. Clinical features of sample with intrauterine growth retardation. *Pediatrics* 1972;50:547–58.
75. Campbell S. Physical methods of assessing size at birth. In: *Size at birth*. Ciba Foundation Symp. 27 (new series). Amsterdam: Elsevier, 1974;275–93.
76. Villar J, Belizan JM. The timing factor in the pathophysiology of the intrauterine growth retardation syndrome. *Obstet Gynecol Survey* 1982;37:499–506.
77. Rohrer R. Der Index der Körperfülle als Mass des Ernährungszustandes. *Munch Med Wochensch* 1921;68:580–8.
78. Ounsted M, Ounsted C. *On fetal growth rate*. Clinics in Dev Med no. 46. Spastics International Medical Publications. London: William Heinemann Medical Books, 1973;78–93.
79. Miller HC. Fetal growth and neonatal mortality. *Pediatrics* 1972;49:392–9.
80. Crane JP, Kopta MM. Comparative newborn anthropometric data in symmetric versus asymmetric intrauterine growth retardation. *Am J Obstet Gynecol* 1980;138:518–22.
81. Beck GJ, van den Berg BJ. The relationship of the rate of intrauterine growth of low-birth-weight infants to later growth. *J Pediatr* 1975;86:504–11.
82. Low JA, Galbraith RS, Muir D, Killen H et al. Intrauterine growth retardation: a preliminary report of long-term morbidity. *Am J Obstet Gynecol* 1978;130:534–45.
83. Fujikura T, Froehlich LA. Mental and motor development in monozygotic co-twins with dissimilar birth weights. *Pediatrics* 1974;53:884–9.
84. Morris FH, Rosenfeld CR, Crandell SS, Adcock EW. Effect of fasting on uterine blood flow and substrate uptake in the sheep. *J Nutr* 1980;110:2433–43.
85. Lemons JA, Schreiner RL. Amino acid metabolism in the ovine fetus. *Am J Physiol* 1983;244:E459–66.
86. Bassett JM, Madill D. The influence of maternal nutrition on plasma hormones and metabolite concentrations of fetal lambs. *J Endocrinol* 1974;61:465–77.
87. Simmons MA, Battaglia FC, Meschia G. *In vivo* effect of insulin on fetal glucose utilization and transplacental glucose transport. *Pediatr Res* 1978;12:90–2.
88. Davies DP, Platts P, Pritchard JM, Wilkinson PW. Nutritional status of light-for-date infants at birth and its influence on early postnatal growth. *Arch Dis Child* 1979;54:703–6.
89. Winick M, Noble A. Cellular response in rats during malnutrition at various ages. *J Nutr* 1966;89:300–6.
90. Widdowson EM, Crabb DE, Milner RDG. Cellular development of some human organs before birth. *Arch Dis Child* 1972;47:652–5.

DISCUSSION

Dr. Canosa: Dr. Rosso presented an important part of the intrauterine growth retardation (IUGR) story, which is the early morbidity and mortality, but perhaps the long-term morbidity and mortality is even more important. How long should follow-up studies go on, and what kind of variables should be examined in a morbidity follow-up?

Dr. Rosso: I don't want to preempt later discussion, but I will say that I share the views of others that there are still many unanswered questions about the long-term consequences of IUGR in terms of physical growth and mental capacity. The reason these questions are so hard to answer is that it is virtually impossible to set up a study in which you can adequately account for the effects of perinatal pathology and the variations in postnatal environment, especially during the early years. If you look at the results of studies in developed countries there does seem to be a lasting impact, reflected both in terms of physical growth and intellectual capacity, but mental capacity is only seriously affected when there has been very early or severe IUGR.

Dr. Hay: I'd like to ask Dr. Rosso about the treatment of hyperviscosity. There seems to be a great deal of variation in the way people treat this condition. Some people do nothing, others perform exchange transfusions at a certain hematocrit (Hct) value, others according to the baby's condition, and so on. There also seems to be uncertainty about the outcome.

Dr. Rosso: I am not involved in clinical management so I don't feel confident to discuss this. Perhaps there are others better equipped.

Dr. Toubas: We must be careful about definition. Are you defining hyperviscosity in terms of Hct or in terms of viscosity measurement?

Dr. Hay: I was defining it as a Hct greater than 65%. In most studies this value is 2 SD above the mean, and at this level there is a direct linear correlation with viscosity.

Dr. Toubas: Some people do an exchange transfusion if the Hct is 65% or over; others will wait until it reaches 70% unless the baby has symptoms.

Dr. Bracci: We have made many determinations of erythrocyte filtration rate and our impression is blood abnormalities due to asphyxia, such as low pH, may cause hyperviscosity independently from high Hct, at least in some cases.

Dr. Chessex: There are two main contributors to hyperviscosity—the plasma and the red cells. In asphyxia there is an increase in fibrinogen which causes increased plasma viscosity. One must distinguish this form of hyperviscosity from that due to a high Hct. I do not know whether this has been looked at carefully in small-for-gestational-age (SGA) infants.

Dr. Bracci: I think it is very difficult to distinguish between factors related to the red cells and factors related to plasma, and I do not know of any studies which have examined this in SGA infants. The characteristics of fetal erythrocytes can affect blood viscosity independently of plasma factors, and the extent to which they do this may also be influenced by asphyxia.

Dr. Priolisi: Returning to the question of intervention when there is a high Hct, it is of relevance to consider that the interplay between pulmonary artery resistance and systemic resistance is affected by Hct. At Hct above 65%–70%, the ratio pulmonary artery resistance/systemic resistance becomes >1. This can produce disturbances of the lung function which are a good clinical indicator for intervening to lower the Hct by doing plasma exchange.

Dr. Wharton: My impression is that in developed countries the problems of immediate management of SGA babies have receded. The cause for concern is much more related to the long-term outlook. I suppose the reason for the improvement in short-term prognosis is primarily better obstetrics, with many fewer cases of severe asphyxia and massive meconium aspiration. Hypoglycemia simply should not occur on a well-run neonatal unit, since we are so well aware of it as a problem. So far as hyperviscosity is concerned, I recall that some years ago we used to do exchange transfusions quite often for this reason, but more recently people have questioned the value of *in vitro* viscosity measurements and whether they bear much relationship to true viscosity *in vivo* in view of the laminar flow of blood within the vessels. We have now stopped intervening except on very rare occasions and I do not think this has made any difference to mortality or morbidity. On the other hand, we certainly had some morbidity when we were doing plasma exchanges for hyperviscosity, such as necrotizing enterocolitis, for example.

Dr. Senterre: I do not treat babies just because they have a Hct above 65%. I look for clinical signs and only do plasma exchanges if there are respiratory difficulties, cardiac difficulties, or hypoglycemia (which can be caused by polycythemia) in babies with more than 6 million erythrocytes per mm^3 or Hct of 75% or more.

Dr. Toubas: We have been discussing acute medical problems, but we need to remind ourselves all the time that these babies, who were in a poor environment *in utero,* are being released into a poor environment after birth. What happens to these babies at 1 year of age? What is the infant mortality? How many are victims of sudden infant death syndrome? We physicians must pinpoint the problems and try to ensure that our respective governments are aware of them.

Intrauterine Growth Retardation, edited by
Jacques Senterre. Nestlé Nutrition Workshop
Series, Vol. 18. Nestec Ltd., Vevey/Raven Press,
Ltd., New York © 1989.

Causes of Low Birthweight in Developing Countries

Brian Wharton

Sorrento Maternity Hospital, Wake Green Road, Birmingham, B13 9HE, United Kingdom

Low birthweight was originally defined as 2,500 g or below, but more recently it has been revised to less than 2,500 g. It is a simple definition requiring only an accurate measurement of weight. It does not infer that all light babies will require special care but, like all babies whatever their weight, special attention will be necessary to provide adequate warmth, food, and love—and if they come to medical attention—to prevent cross-infection from one baby to another.

It is of course also necessary to characterize the baby's weight in relation to other features as well, particularly his gestational age, and then to compare this with some external reference data (or standard) of weight for gestational age. There are varied and strongly held views on whether local or international reference data should be used and whether they should be based on the total or on only a selected "normal healthy" population; we have discussed this in detail previously (1). Even after these allowances other adjustments must be made: Some intrinsic biological law results in boys being heavier than girls (this is intriguing in its own right, but it would be unreasonable to expect girls on average to be as heavy as boys); first born children are lighter than subsequent births wherever birthweight has been studied; and so on. There is probably no end to the adjustments and allowances one can make. Crude as it is, therefore, "birthweight," lone and unadorned, summarizes an amalgam of biological and pathological factors which have affected the child's growth.

In this chapter I have drawn on published work from many developing countries, and for those who wish to pursue particular points in further detail, I have tried to give at least a passing reference to many of the papers concerned with the causes of low birthweight in developing countries which have been published in English since 1983. Rather than give a mere literature review, however, I have also drawn on our own experience at Sorrento Maternity Hospital in Birmingham, England, which has for many years looked after many mothers and their babies from the Indian subcontinent, particularly from Pakistan. A number of recent papers have also drawn lessons from ethnic differences in birthweight (2–10). Elsewhere in this volume, Canosa describes the problems as actually seen in India and Bangladesh.

143

THE SORRENTO EXPERIENCE

Immigration from the Indian subcontinent to Britain began during the Second World War and gathered pace thereafter. People came from particular areas such as Gujarat and the Punjab and tended to settle in local communities. Immigration of Asian British subjects from East Africa also occurred and this was enhanced by the expulsion of Asian people from Uganda in 1974. The East African Asians had probably enjoyed a higher standard of living than those from India and Pakistan. Last to arrive were people from Bangladesh who had often been living in conditions of extreme privation.

As immigration declines and the newcomers acclimatize to their new environment the opportunity to study and learn from them will similarly decline and so it is useful to have this opportunity to summarize our experience to date. Table 1 shows the changes which have occurred in the weight of Pakistani babies born at Sorrento and the changes in some of the major factors known to affect birthweight, i.e., gestational age, parity, and the height of the mother. Table 2 shows a multiple regression analysis of these factors as they affect birthweight, first in a single year (1983) (i.e., a static or "one point in time" analysis), and second as an explanation of the change occurring in the decade 1968–1978. Many multivariate analyses of birth-

TABLE 1. *Details of Pakistani babies and their mothers at Sorrento Maternity Hospital, Birmingham, England*

	1968[a]	1978[a]	1983[b]
n	152	228	260
Birthweight (kg)			
Mean	3,022	3,161	3,204
Percent < 2500 g	9	7	—
Gestational age (weeks)			
Mean	38.2	38.5	39.12
Percent < 37 weeks	13	10	5
Previous births			
Mean	2.1	2.5	2.2
Percent none	32	19	22
Percent 1–4	55	61	58
Percent > 4	14	20	20
Maternal height (cm)			
Mean	152.8	153.3	153.7
Percent < 150 cm	37	24	
Mean time elapsed since previous birth (years)	1.9	2.2	
Percent teenage mothers	11	8	

[a]Data from ref. 42.
[b]Data from ref. 17.

TABLE 2. *Influence of various factors on birthweight of Pakistani babies born at Sorrento, Birmingham, England*

	Factor				
	Gestation	Sex (M vs. F)	Parity (subsequent vs. first pregnancy)	Maternal height	Unexplained by the factors considered
Births in 1983[a]	+ 150 g/week	+ 124 g	+ 134 g	+ 12 g/cm	78%
Change 1968–1978[b]	+ 0.3 week		+ 0.4 birth	+ 0.5 cm	
Effect of change on birthweight[b]	+ 23 g		+ 34 g	+ 16 g	47%

[a]Data from ref. 17.
[b]Data from ref. 42.

weight have been published. Recent ones from developing countries include those by Lun et al. (11) and Bantje (12). Perhaps the outstanding conclusion from such analyses, including ours, is that so much of the variance in birthweight remains "unexplained" after taking all of these factors into account. Presumably it is in this unexplained sector where there is progress to be made. It is interesting that in a static analysis, i.e., that for 1983, our mathematical approach cannot account for 78% of the spread in birthweight, but when analyzing change, i.e., from 1968–1978, the unexplained proportion has fallen to 47%. I am wary of over-interpreting this but perhaps a continued analysis of secular change in birthweight is likely to be more fruitful in identifying the crucial factors in the determination of birthweight.

Having discussed the "parameters" of birthweight using an essentially mathematical analysis, this chapter now turns to a developmental approach, following the fetus from before conception to birth.

BEFORE CONCEPTION

Maternal Height

Shorter mothers tend to have lighter babies. In our own studies of Pakistani mothers in Birmingham an extra centimeter of maternal height was associated with an extra 12 g of baby weight (± 2 SEM, range 4–20 g).

Clearly then, the health of the mother during her own girlhood is an important factor in the epidemiology of low birthweight. Anything that improves growth in childhood will make some contribution to improved fetal growth in the next generation, but it is more important that the particular pregnancy is healthy.

In 10 years, although the height of our Pakistani mothers in Birmingham had increased by only 0.5 cm, this had made an estimated 16 g contribution to the observed increased birthweight of 139 g seen during that time. This accounts for 12% of the total increase, hardly dramatic but at least an encouragement for steady endeavor. The effect of maternal stature on birthweight in Thailand has been recently reported (13).

Fertility Behavior

There are various behavioral aspects of fertility which appear to affect intrauterine growth, including age of the mother, birth interval, and parity.

Teenage mothers tend to have lighter babies. In many parts of the world, teenage pregnancy, although accepted with reluctance, is not regarded as ideal. Consequently, mothers are more likely to be unsupported and to live in poorer socioeconomic circumstances. This is true for example in Nairobi, where 14% of babies born to teenage mothers were of low birthweight and 24% were preterm compared with 7% and 7%, respectively, in non-teenage mothers (14). Other recent studies on the development and nutritional aspects of pregnancy in teenagers are those by Frisancho et al. (15,16). However, in some parts of the world early teenage marriage and pregnancy are common and quite accepted. It is not known whether these girls carry on growing throughout their pregnancy, or what effect pregnancies during the growing period have on ultimate adult stature.

Short birth intervals, particularly of less than 12 months, are associated with an increased risk of low birthweight. Effective contraception is therefore part of a strategy of reducing the prevalence of low birthweight; as breast feeding has receded in some countries, so birth intervals have got less. Again the exact mechanisms are not understood. It is tempting to suggest there has been insufficient time to recover from the nutritional stress of pregnancy, but is this true? After all, at birth the mother has some energy stored as fat to help her through lactation. If lactation is very short because another pregnancy occurs, is this nutritionally more demanding for the mother?

In all societies studied, parity has an effect on birthweight; second babies are heavier than first babies but thereafter the difference is small. We found the difference in weight between the first and subsequently born infants to be 120 g (± 2 SE, range 5–240 g). Presumably the policy towards smaller families in China could lead to a reduction in mean birthweight if there were no other concurrent changes.

CONCEPTION AND EARLY PREGNANCY

Genes

Clearly genes affect intrauterine growth. Many of the major chromosome and specific gene disorders are associated with definite reductions in birthweight, but often the deficiency of growth apparent at birth is small compared to that in later life (e.g., Turner's syndrome).

We are not concerned with these major abnormalities here. While sometimes devastating in their effect on the individual, their effect on the mean birthweight of the population is small. Some "genetic" factors might however have a population effect; parental consanguinity is one such factor. Some studies have shown that consanguinity impairs intrauterine growth while others have not. Table 3 summarizes the results of our own and previous studies on this subject. Our own conclusions were that consanguinity does result in an increase in the number of poorly grown babies (17% of the babies of first cousin parents were below the 10th percentile of weight for gestational age) but overall the effect on mean birthweight of the population is quite small—less than 100 g (17). The mechanism whereby consanguinity results in an increased prevalence of poorly grown babies is not clear. Although the evidence is inconclusive, consanguinity seems to be associated with a higher prevalence of congenital malformations and this may mean that whatever causes the congenital malformation in early pregnancy also begins to retard growth at the same time.

Many mothers in the developing world are Moslem and consanguinous marriages, particularly of first cousins, are preferred.

Another genetic factor is the tendency to have multiple ovulation and therefore multiple births. This is particularly common in Nigeria (18,19). More general reviews of the various factors affecting birthweight in Nigeria were summarized in 1985 by Ransome-Kuti (20) and since then there have been several further analyses (21–24).

LATER PREGNANCY

Gestational Age

In all analyses, gestational age is the most important factor affecting birthweight. In our study of Pakistani mothers, an extra week of gestation was associated with an increase in birthweight of 150 g (± 2 SEM, range 110–190). This was 20 g more than the difference due to parity and 30 g more than that due to sex. It was the equivalent of an extra 12.5 cm in maternal height.

Although the prevalence of low birthweight in different environments has received considerable attention, the prevalence of preterm birth has received much less, perhaps because the determination of gestational age is more difficult.

Gestational age is less easily assessed in developing societies, and so many of the lessons which may be relevant to the developing world have to be drawn from developed industrial societies. In Birmingham we found part of the secular increase in the weight of Pakistani babies was due to a slight lengthening of gestational age (2 days) and a slight fall in the number of preterm births (from 13% to 10%). Small as these changes are they contributed 23 g to the overall increase in birthweight of 139 g.

Perhaps more attention should be paid to gestational age. Possibly even small increases would have a measurable effect on birthweight.

TABLE 3. *Comparison of studies of effect of parental consanguinity on fetal growth*

| Study | Country (population studied) | Numbers | | | Birthweight (g) | | | | Weight for gestational age, parity, sex, and maternal height (% < 10th percentile) | Other factors affecting birthweight allowed for in statistical analysis | Other body measurements |
		Total	Consanguineous	Unrelated	Mean consanguineous	Mean unrelated	Difference (consanguineous-unrelated)	Significance of difference			
Siben (43)	India (Tamil Nadu)	322	UN 126 C1 52 C2 61 13	196	UN 2,731 C1 2,650 2,794	2,834	−103	p < 0.01		Gestational age—term babies only included	Length, head circumference, skinfold thickness
Morton (44)	Japan	75,180	C1 2,928 C2 2,144	70,088	C1 3,046	3,074	−28			Gestational age, parity, city	
Schork (45)	Japan	2,314	230	2,084	3,099	3,091	+8	NS		Parity, sex, maternal age, paternal age, month of birth	Head circumference, chest girth

Reference	Population	N	Subgroup	n (consanguineous)	n (controls)	Birth weight, consanguineous (g)	Birth weight, controls (g)	Difference (g)	Significance	Variables controlled	Variables measured
Rao (46)	India (Tamil Nadu)	14,243	Rural: UN, C1, C2	3,889 (1,308, 1,991, 590)	4,449	2,740	2,772	−32	NS		Length, head circumference, chest girth
			Urban: UN, C1, C2	1,654 (371, 989, 294)	4,251	2,883	2,867	+16	NS		
Slatis (47)	United States (white)	108		63	45	3,247	3,352	−105	NS	Sex, socioeconomic state	
Paddaiah (48)	India (Andhra Pradesh)	1,823		1,821	3,002	2,820	2,880	−60	$p < 0.001$		Length, head circumference, chest girth, calf girth
Honeyman (17)	United Kingdom (Pakistani Moslems)	260	C1, C2	122, 62	76	C1 3,178, C2 3,192	3,258	−80, −66	NS, NS	Gestational age, sex, parity, maternal height	Length, head circumference, skinfold thickness; C1 (17)*, C2 (6), Unrelated (5)

*$p < 0.05$.
NS = Not significant.
C1 = first cousins; C2 = more distant than first cousin. UN = uncle/niece.
From ref. 17.

Since preparing this table Khoury et al. (49) have published their study of consanguinity in the Amish. They also found an increased prevalence of intrauterine growth retardation, but their method of presenting their results makes it difficult to summarize them in this table.

Anemia

It may be that anemia has not received sufficient attention as an indicator of poor intrauterine growth. The situation is complex, however. In normal pregnancy the hemoglobin falls, and this is partly but not wholly explained by hemodilution. We and many others have observed that this "normal" fall in hemoglobin does not occur in European mothers who produce a poorly grown baby (25, and see also Marini in this volume). However, a low hemoglobin may also be a marker of poor maternal reserves. A large study in Indonesia showed that primiparous mothers of low birthweight babies had a hemoglobin level 0.3 g below those having babies weighing 3.0–3.499 kg and this difference increased with increasing parity up to a difference of 0.6 g at parity 5 or more (26). There have been other recent studies on this subject (e.g., 27). Reduced hemoglobin is not necessarily evidence of a specific deficiency—only an intervention study with iron supplements could determine that. It is more likely to be just one component of the mothers' poor environment.

Hypertension

It is well-established that maternal hypertension, whether it is the pregnancy-specific variety developing after the 20th week (i.e., preeclampsia) or due to some pre existing problem, is associated with poor intrauterine growth and an increased perinatal mortality. In the British Perinatal Mortality Survey of 1958, severe preeclampsia (i.e., diastolic pressure above 110 mm Hg, or above 90 with proteinuria) was associated with a reduction in mean birthweight of 225 g (28).

The prevalence of preeclampsia in different communities varies. The reason for this is not clear, although two of our colleagues contributing to this volume have suggested a relationship between calcium intake and pregnancy hypertension (29). In Birmingham we found that fewer of our primiparous Asian mothers (25%) had hypertension when compared with our European mothers (46%) and with the UK national average (34%) (30). Interestingly, this difference was not apparent in the multiparae (20%, 24%, and 24%, respectively).

Smoking

Again, it is well-established that smoking in later pregnancy is associated with poor intrauterine growth. There has been considerable discussion as to whether smoking itself is the true cause or whether it is merely a marker for poorer socioeconomic circumstances, poorer diet, and perhaps a higher alcohol intake. However, one study of a health education intervention did result in increased birthweight (31). Maternal smoking is uncommon in most rural areas of the developing world but it is becoming increasingly frequent in urban areas. I have not been able to trace studies concerned with the effects of smoking on birthweight specifically in developing countries, though Verma et al. (32) have described the effect of tobacco chewing on fetal outcome in India. I suspect, to use a vernacular phrase, that this would be "one more nail in the coffin," but this may not necessarily be the case. Perhaps, in developing countries, major influences such as nutrition act as the limiting factors, and so other environmental influences have little effect.

Malaria

The association of malaria with perinatal pathology is well established (33), but just as with smoking it has not been made absolutely clear whether the relationship between maternal malaria and low birthweight is causal or merely an association. More affluent mothers would tend to avoid malaria and these mothers could have larger babies for other reasons. Perhaps the best evidence of a direct cause and effect association is the experience in the Solomon Islands (34) where an anti-mosquito campaign, though relying on a historical control technique, was quickly followed by a substantial reduction in the number of low birthweight babies.

We are certainly not winning the battle against malaria at present, and the result of this is that more low birthweight babies are likely to be born. Robyn, elsewhere in this volume, discusses malaria in more detail.

Energy Balance

A report of the discussion on maternal supplementation appears later in the volume. I have therefore reviewed supplementation in more detail there.

I would in this chapter, however, like to develop in more detail the concept of energy balance in mid-pregnancy. During the second trimester a substantial amount of the mother's weight gain is due to an increase in her own fat stores—not only is her fetus growing, she is growing too. In later pregnancy most of the weight gain is due to the rapidly growing fetus and placenta. The mother herself has stopped growing, her fat stores are no longer increasing; in fact they decrease a little.

We noted that Asian mothers who went on to have poorly grown babies had put on little fat in the second trimester (35); indeed, their triceps skinfold thickness hardly increased at all. The increment in triceps skinfold also indicates which mothers will benefit from nutritional supplementation (36,37). In a larger and more recent study (38) we have confirmed the value of triceps skinfold increments during the second trimester in predicting intrauterine growth (See Table 4).

We consider that the increment in skinfold thickness represents the state of energy balance, i.e., intake minus output over a 10-week period at a crucial time in mid-pregnancy, when the mother is laying down stores in anticipation of later fetal demands. Nutrition in pregnancy is concerned with the input side of the balance. There is little point in increasing the input if there is not a potential negative balance and, indeed, there is some evidence of an adverse effect.

The output side of the balance is concerned with energy expenditure, and in recent years this has received increasing attention. It seems that many women in de-

TABLE 4. *Birthweight, birthweight percentile,[a] and placental weight in mothers who accumulate fat inadequately (triceps skinfold increment ≤ 20 μm/week) and in mothers who accumulate fat adequately (triceps skinfold increment > 20 μm/week) during the second trimester of pregnancy. From Viegas et al. (38). Results are means (SD).*

Measurement	Babies born to mothers who accumulate fat inadequately n = 35	Babies born to mothers who accumulate fat adequately n = 46	p
Crude birthweight (kg)	2.96 (0.33)	3.14 (0.42)	< 0.05
Gestational age (weeks)	39.2 (1.2)	38.9 (1.1)	NS
Thomson SD score[a]	− 0.685 (0.66)	− 0.255 (0.80)	< 0.02
Sorrento SD score[a]	− 0.411 (0.79)	0.198 (0.81)	< 0.005
Other baby anthropometry Head circumference (cm)	33.8 (1.2)	34.6 (1.2)	< 0.005
Length (cm)	49.8 (1.9)	50.3 (2.1)	NS
Triceps skinfold (mm)	3.62 (0.63)	3.80 (0.76)	NS
Biceps skinfold (mm)	3.33 (0.62)	3.93 (0.76)	NS
Suprailiac skinfold (mm)	3.17 (0.75)	3.93 (0.85)	NS
Mid upper arm muscle circumference (cm)	8.83 (0.59)	9.13 (0.72)	< 0.05
Placental weight (g)	551 (98)	616 (112)	< 0.01

p values indicate significance of difference between the two groups. NS: *p* > 0.09.
[a]Birthweight percentile for gestational age, sex, parity, and maternal height according to data from refs. 36, 37, and 50.

veloping countries carry on doing strenuous work throughout their pregnancies (39). There have also been a number of accidental "experiments" suggesting that work in later pregnancy is deleterious, e.g., flooding in Tanzania led to less work in the fields, a strike in Bombay led to less work in the cotton mills, and in both instances, birthweight was improved (40,41).

CONCLUSIONS

Low birthweight is commoner in developing countries than in the remainder of the world. There is a tendency to relate this difference solely to differences in maternal nutrition. Undernutrition makes a contribution to the problem, and I have no doubt it makes a considerable contribution. Nevertheless, it is not realistic to brood over nutrition alone without due consideration for other genetic and environmental characteristics of the developing world, such as parity, birth interval, consanguinity, smoking, malaria, hypertension, anemia, and so on.

The ills of geographical pathology are not susceptible to isolated nutritional explanation.

ACKNOWLEDGMENTS

It is a pleasure to acknowledge the help of colleagues who joined me in the various studies quoted above. Dr. J. G. Bissenden and Mr. O. A. Viegas were Mary Crosse Research Fellows at Sorrento Maternity Hospital. I am grateful to all of them and Mrs. Shirley Kane for valued secretarial assistance.

REFERENCES

1. Wharton BA, Dunn PM. Perinatal growth. The quest for an international standard for reference. *Acta Paediatr Scand* 1985; suppl 319:1–123.
2. Bhan A, Viegas OA, Huang HS, Ratnam SS. Neonatal anthropometry in relation to ethnic distribution of birthweight in Singapore. *J Trop Pediatr* 1985;31:124–8.
3. Chetcuti P, Sinha SH, Levene MI. Birth size in Indian ethnic subgroups born in Britain. *Arch Dis Child* 1985;60:868–70.
4. Condie RG, Terry PB. Ethnic differences in birthweight-related parameters with particular reference to possible maternal nutritional risk factors. *Postgrad Med J* 1983;59:655–6.
5. DaVanzo J, Habicht JP, Butz WP. Assessing socioeconomic correlates of birthweight in peninsular Malaysia: ethnic differences and changes over time. *Soc Sci Med* 1984;18:387–404.
6. Hughes K, Tan NR, Lun KC. Ethnic group differences in low birthweight of live singletons in Singapore, 1981–83. *J Epidemiol Community Health* 1986;40:262–6.
7. Kurji KH, Edouard L. Ethnic differences in pregancy outcome. *Public Health* 1984;98:205–8.
8. McFadyen IR, Campbell Brown M, Abraham R, North WR, Haines AP. Factors affecting birthweight in Hindus, Moslems and Europeans. *Br J Obstet Gynaecol* 1984;91:968–72.
9. Shiono PH, Klebanoff MA, Graubard BI, Berendes HW, Rhoads GG. Birthweight among women of different ethnic groups. *JAMA* 1986;255:48–52.
10. Yadav H. Birth weight distribution, mean birth weights, and low birthweights among various ethnic groups in Malaysian newborns. *Singapore Med J* 1983;24:145–9.
11. Lun KC, Tan NR, Hughes K. Multivariate analysis of Singapore birth weights. *Asia Oceania J Obstet Gynaecol* 1985;11:189–97.
12. Bantje H. A multiple regression analysis of variables influencing birthweight. *Trop Geogr Med* 1986;38:123–30.
13. Nondasuta A, Chaturachinda K, Watthana Kasetr S. Birthweight in relation to maternal height and weight. *J Med Assoc Thai* 1986;69:243–7.
14. Bwibo NO. Birthweights of infants of teenage mothers in Nairobi. *Acta Paediatr Scand* 1985;Suppl 319:89–94.
15. Frisancho AR, Matos J, Bollettino LA. Influence of growth status and placental function on birth weight of infants born to young still-growing teenagers. *Am J Clin Nutr* 1984;40:801–7.
16. Frisancho AR, Matos J, Leonard WR, Yaroch LA. Developmental and nutritional determinants of pregnancy outcome among teenagers. *Am J Phys Anthropol* 1985;66:247–61.
17. Honeyman MM, Bahl L, Marshall T, Wharton BA. Consanguinity and fetal growth in Pakistani Moslems. *Arch Dis Child* 1987;62:231–5.
18. Fakeye OO. Twin birthweight in Nigeria and the effect of sex-pair and parity. *Trop Geogr Med* 1986;38:265–70.
19. Oni GA. Twins and their birth sizes in a Nigerian community. *East Afr Med J* 1983;60:492–7.

20. Ransome-Kuti O. Intra-uterine growth, birthweights and maturity of the African newborn. *Acta Paediatr Scand* 1985;Suppl 319:95–102.
21. Dawodu AH, Laditan AA. Low birthweight in an urban community in Nigeria. *Ann Trop Paediatr* 1985;5:61–6.
22. Ogbeide O, Alakija W. Birthweights of babies in Benin, Bendel State of Nigeria. *J Trop Pediatr* 1985;31:139–42.
23. Oni GA, Ariganjoye O. A study of some of the predisposing factors to low birthweight in a Nigerian community. *East Afr Med J* 1986;63:121–30.
24. Oshuhor PC, Ibrahim M. Birthweights in Katsina, Northern Nigeria. *J Trop Pediatr* 1986; 32:200–2.
25. Bissenden JG, Scott PH, Hallum J, Mansfield HN, Scott P, Wharton BA. Racial variations in tests of fetoplacental function. *Br J Obstet Gynaecol* 1981;88:109–14.
26. Kessel E, Sastrawinata S, Mumford SD. Correlates of fetal growth and survival. *Acta Paediatr Scand* 1985;Suppl 319:120–7.
27. Kuizon MD, Cheong RL, Ancheta LP, Desnacido JA, Macapinlac MP, Baens JS. Effect of anaemia and other maternal characteristics on birthweight. *Hum Nutr Clin Nutr* 1985;39:419–26.
28. Butler NR, Alberman ED. Perinatal problems: the second report of the 1958 British perinatal mortality survey. Edinburgh: Churchill Livingstone, 1969.
29. Belizan JM, Villar J. The relationship between calcium intake and oedema, proteinuria and hypertension gestosis: an hypothesis. *Am J Clin Nutr* 1980;32:2202–10.
30. Wharton BA, Smalley C, Millns C, Nirmal J, Bissenden JG, Scott PH. The Asian mother and her baby at Sorrento. In: Wharton BA, ed. *Topics in perinatal medicine*. Tunbridge Wells: Pitman Medical, 1980;141–51.
31. Sexton M, Hebel JR. A clinical trial of change in maternal smoking and its effect on birth weight. *JAMA* 1984;251:911–5.
32. Verma RC, Chansoriya M, Kaul KK. Effect of tobacco chewing by mothers on fetal outcome. *Indian Pediatr* 1983;34:507–14.
33. McGregor IA, Wilson ME, Billewicz WZ. Malaria infection of the placenta in The Gambia, West Africa; its incidence and relationship to stillbirth, birthweight and placental weight. *Trans R Soc Trop Med Hyg* 1983;77:232–44.
34. MacGregor JD, Avery JG. Malaria transmission and fetal growth. *Br Med J* 1974;3:433–6.
35. Bissenden JG, Scott PH, Hallum J, Mansfield HN, Scott P, Wharton BA. Anthropometric and biochemical changes during pregnancy in Asian and European mothers having well grown babies. *Br J Obstet Gynaecol* 1981;88:992–7.
36. Viegas OAC, Scott PH, Cole TJ, Mansfield HN, Wharton P, Wharton BA. Dietary protein energy supplementation of pregnant Asian mothers at Sorrento, Birmingham. I. Unselective during second and third trimesters. *Br Med J* 1982;285:589–92.
37. Viegas OAC, Scott PH, Cole TJ, Eaton P, Needham PG, Wharton BA. Dietary protein energy supplementation of pregnant Asian mothers at Sorrento, Birmingham. II. Selective during the third trimester only. *Br Med J* 1982;285:592–5.
38. Viegas OAC, Cole TJ, Wharton BA. Impaired fat deposition in pregnancy: an indicator for nutritional intervention. *Am J Clin Nutr* 1987;45:23–8.
39. Jimenez MH, Newton N. Activity and work during pregnancy and the postpartum period: a cross-cultural study of 202 societies. *Am J Obstet Gynecol* 1979;135:171–6.
40. Bantje H. Seasonal variations in birthweight distribution in Ikwiriri village, Tanzania. *J Trop Paediatr* 1983;29:50–4.
41. Balfour MI, Talpade SK. The maternity conditions of women mill workers in India. *Indian Medical Gazette* 1930;65:241–249, quoted by Ashworth A, Feachem RG. *Bull Wld Hlth Org* 1985;63:165–84.
42. Clarson CL, Barker MJ, Marshall T, Wharton BA. Secular change in birthweight of Asian babies born in Birmingham. *Arch Dis Child* 1982;57:867–71.
43. Sibert JR, Jadhav M, Inbaraj SG. Fetal growth and parental consanguinity. *Arch Dis Child* 1979;54:317–9.
44. Morton NE. Empirical risks in consanguinous marriages: birth weight, gestational time and measurements of infants. *Am J Hum Genet* 1958;10:344–9.
45. Schork MA. The effects of inbreeding on growth. *Am J Hum Genet* 1964;16:292–9.
46. Rao PSS, Inbaraj SG. Inbreeding effects on fetal growth and development. *J Med Genet* 1980;17:27–33.

47. Slatis HM, Hoene RE. The effect of consanguinity on the distribution of continuously variable characteristics. *Am J Hum Genet* 1961;13:28–31.
48. Paddaiah G, Reddy GG. Effect of consanguinity on anthropometric measurements in the newborn. *Ind J Pediatr* 1980;47:133–6.
49. Khoury MJ, Cohen BH, Diamond EL, Chase GA, McKusick VA. Inbreeding and reproductive mortality in the old order Amish. III. Direct and indirect affects of inbreeding. *Am J Epidemiol* 1987;125:473–83.
50. Thomson AM, Billewicz WZ, Hytten FE. The assessment of fetal growth. *J Obstet Gynaecol Br Cwlth* 1968;75:903–16.

Intrauterine Growth Retardation, edited by
Jacques Senterre. Nestlé Nutrition Workshop
Series, Vol. 18. Nestec Ltd., Vevey/Raven Press,
Ltd., New York © 1989.

Anthropometry in Brazilian Newborn Infants: Studies of Association with Some Maternal Factors

Fernando José de Nóbrega, Fábio Ancona Lopez, and
Conceição A.M. Segre

Department of Pediatrics, Escola Paulista de Medicina, 01235 Perdizes, São Paulo, Brazil

This paper describes a study coordinated by Professor Fernando José de Nóbrega and produced by a working team on undernutrition from the Brazilian Society of Pediatrics (1). A population of 101,126 live newborn infants was investigated. These infants were born during the period of 1 year (1978 through 1979) in maternity hospitals of all the state capitals of Brazil. The data used in this study were collected by medical or auxiliary personnel who were coordinated locally. Standardized data collection forms were used to relay the information to the central coordinators.

MATERNAL FACTORS

The authors studied the relationship between anthropometry of the newborn (weight, length, head circumference) and the following eight maternal variables: socioeconomic level, age, birth order, smoking habits, weight before pregnancy, height, adequacy of weight/height, and prenatal care. The socioeconomic level was defined according to a score made up from the father's occupation, education, and marital status. These criteria provided a classification into groups corresponding to high (1), medium (2), and low (3) social class. The adequacy of weight/height was obtained from the ratio between pre-gestational weight and the ideal weight for height according to Jelliffe (2). Prenatal care was considered to be effective if the mothers attended at least three antenatal clinics during the pregnancy.

NEWBORN DATA

Birthweight in grams was measured in the first 3 hr of life, using a baby scale which was checked for accuracy before the measurement was done. Length and head circumference (in cm) were determined in the first 24 hr of life.

157

STATISTICAL ANALYSIS

The association between each one of the maternal variables and anthropometric measures of the newborn was tested with the use of the χ^2 statistics. For the study of contrasts between proportions the Goodman statistics were calculated.

RESULTS

Table 1 shows the birthweight data according to socioeconomic level. Analysis using the Goodman (g) statistics test showed that there was no significant difference between socioeconomic levels 1 and 2 in the numbers of infants with birthweights <2,500 g and between 2,501 g and 3,000 g, but significantly more infants in these weight categories were born to women in the lowest social class group. The opposite was true for birthweights over 3,000 g.

If birthweights below 3,000 g are considered inadequate (i,e., low birthweight <2,500 g, and insufficient birthweight 2,501–3,000 g), then the number of infants of inadequate birthweight in this population was 34.6%.

Table 2 shows the distribution of birthweight according to maternal weight, which is divided into six bands. As maternal weight increased, there was a significant decrease in the number of infants with birthweights <2,500 g and between 2,501 and 3,000 g, and an increase in infants weighing >3,000 g.

Tables 3 and 4 show the distribution of birthweight according to maternal height and adequacy of weight/height, which are again divided into bands. The same pattern was repeated, with fewer infants <3,000 g as height and weight/height increased. The results obtained for birthweight were the same as for length and head circumference measurements.

TABLE 1. *Distribution of birthweight according to socioeconomic level (SEL)*

| | Birthweight (g) | | | | | | Total | |
| | ≤ 2,500 | | 2,501–3,000 | | > 3,000 | | | |
SEL	n	%	n	%	n	%	n	%
1	131	4.6	637	22.2	2,102	73.2	2,870	3.4
2	457	5.2	1,848	21.1	6,463	73.7	8,768	10.3
3	6,459	8.8	19,780	27.0	46,917	64.2	73,156	86.3
Total	7,047	8.3	22,265	26.3	55,482	65.4	84,794	100.0

Association test: calc χ^2 = 435.52; crit χ^2 = 9.49.
Contrasts study:
  ≤ 2,500 = {(prop SEL 1) = (prop SEL 2)} < {(prop SEL 3)}.
  2,501–3,000 = {(prop SEL 1) = (prop SEL 2)} < {(prop SEL 3)}.
  > 3,000 = {(prop SEL 1) = (prop SEL 2)} > {(prop SEL 3)}.
prop, proportion.

TABLE 2. *Distribution of birthweight according to maternal weight*

Maternal weight (kg)	≤ 2,500		2,501–3,000		> 3,000		Total	
	n	%	n	%	n	%	n	%
< 45	1,114	13.1	3,075	36.3	4,316	50.7	8,505	11.6
45–49	1,560	9.9	4,814	30.6	9,370	59.5	15,744	21.4
50–54	1,466	7.8	4,885	29.9	12,519	66.4	18,870	25.7
55–59	856	6.1	3,306	23.6	9,822	70.3	13,984	19.0
60–69	653	5.1	2,375	18.7	9,693	76.2	12,721	17.3
≥ 70	151	4.1	546	14.7	3,010	81.2	3,707	5.0
Total	5,800	7.8	19,001	25.9	48,730	66.3	73,531	100.0

Association test: calc χ^2 = 2,328.60; crit χ^2 = 18.307.
Contrasts study:
≤ 2,500g = (< 45) >(45–49) > (50–54) > (55–59) > (60–69) > (≥ 70) // (60–69) = (≥ 70).
2,501–3,000g = (<45) > (45–49) > (50–54) > (55–59) > (60–69) > (≥ 70).
> 3,000g = (< 45) < (45–49) < (50–54) < (55–59) < (60–69) < (≥ 70).

TABLE 3. *Distribution of birthweight according to maternal height*

Maternal height (cm)	≤ 2,500		2,501–3,000		> 3,000		Total	
	n	%	n	%	n	%	n	%
< 145	215	17.7	539	34.4	815	51.9	1,569	2.1
145–149	680	13.1	1,679	32.5	2,813	54.4	5,172	6.8
150–154	1,748	9.8	5,430	30.4	10,700	59.9	17,878	23.7
155–159	1,732	8.3	5,661	27.1	13,497	64.6	20,890	27.6
160–169	1,726	6.4	6,136	22.8	19,025	70.9	26,887	35.6
≥ 170	168	5.4	576	18.5	2,364	76.1	3,108	4.1
Total	6,269	8.3	20,021	26.5	49,214	65.3	75,504	100.0

Association test: calc χ^2 = 1,214.21; crit χ^2 = 18.307.
Contrasts study:
≤ 2,500 = (< 145) > (145–149) > (150–154) > (155–159) > (160–169) > (≥ 170) // (160–169) = (≥ 170).
2,501–3,000 = (<145) = (145–149) = (150–154) > (155–159) > (160–169) > (≥ 170).
> 3,000 = (< 145) = (145–149) < (150–154) < (155–159) < (160–169) < (≥ 170).

TABLE 4. *Distribution of birthweight according to the maternal adequacy of weight/height (W/H, % of standard values)*

| Maternal W/H adequacy (%) | Birthweight (g) | | | | | | Total | |
| | ≤ 2,500 | | 2,501–3,000 | | > 3,000 | | | |
	n	%	n	%	n	%	n	%
70 ⊣ 80	431	9.9	1,249	8.6	1,958	5.2	3,638	6.4
80 ⊣ 90	1,247	28.6	3,838	26.6	7,970	21.1	13,055	23.2
90 ⊣ 100	1,371	31.5	4,561	31.6	11,564	30.6	17,496	30.9
100 ⊣ 110	778	17.9	2,867	19.9	8,673	22.9	12,318	21.9
> 110	525	12.0	1,880	13.0	7,588	20.0	9,993	17.6
Total	4,352	7.7	14,395	25.5	37,753	66.8	56,500	100.0

Cases without information about socioeconomic level omitted.
Association test: calc χ^2 = 945.23; crit χ^2 = 15.507.
Contrasts study:
  ≤ 2,500 = (70 ⊣ 80) > (80 ⊣ 90) > (90 ⊣ 100) > (100 ⊣ 110) > (> 110).
  2,501–3,000 = (70 ⊣ 80) > (80 ⊣ 90) > (90 ⊣ 100) > (100 ⊣ 110) > (> 110).
  > 3,000 = (70 ⊣ 80) < (80 ⊣ 90) < (90 ⊣ 100) < (100 ⊣ 110) < (> 110).

Table 5 shows the distribution of birthweight according to the level of prenatal care. It was found that 82% of this population attended three or more prenatal visits. Mothers of infants weighing <3,000 g were more likely to have had inadequate prenatal care than mothers of infants weighing >3,000 g.

Tables 6–10 show the distribution of birthweight in relation to the combined effects of prenatal care and socioeconomic level. It was found that in the high and medium socioeconomic levels, there were no birthweight differences related to the

TABLE 5. *Distribution of birthweight according to prenatal care*

| Prenatal care | Birthweight (g) | | | | | | Total | |
| | ≤ 2,500 | | 2,501–3,000 | | > 3,000 | | | |
	n	%	n	%	n	%	n	%
Yes	5,011	7.5	17,080	25.6	44,734	66.9	66,825	81.8
No	1,807	12.2	4,401	29.6	8,652	58.2	14,860	18.2
Total	6,818	8.3	21,481	26.3	53,386	65.4	81,685	100.0

Association test: calc χ^2 = 533.96; crit χ^2 = 5.99.
Contrasts study:
  ≤ 2,500 = (prop yes) < (prop no).
  2,501–3,000 = (prop yes) < (prop no).
  > 3,000 = (prop yes) > (prop no).
prop, proportion.

TABLE 6. *Distribution of birthweight according to socioeconomic level (SEL) in mothers* *without prenatal care*

	Birthweight (g)							
	≤ 2,500		2,501–3,000		> 3,000		Total	
SEL	n	%	n	%	n	%	n	%
1	2	9.1	4	18.2	16	72.7	22	0.1
2	20	8.5	55	23.3	161	68.2	236	1.6
3	1,785	12.2	4,342	29.7	8,475	58.1	14,602	98.3
Total	1,807	12.2	4,401	29.6	8,652	58.2	14,860	100.0

Association test: calc χ^2 = 12.0; crit χ^2 = 9.49.
Contrasts study:
  ≤ 2,500 = without contrast.
  2,501–3000 = without contrast.
  > 3,000 = (prop SEL 2) > (prop SEL 3).
prop, proportion.

TABLE 7. *Distribution of birthweight according to socioeconomic level in mothers* with *prenatal care*

	Birthweight (g)							
	≤ 2,500		2,501–3,000		> 3,000		Total	
SEL	n	%	n	%	n	%	n	%
1	86	4.7	397	21.8	1,336	73.5	1,819	2.7
2	421	5.0	1,732	21.0	6,130	74.0	8,283	12.4
3	4,504	7.9	14,951	26.4	37,268	65.7	56,723	84.9
Total	5,011	7.5	17,080	25.5	44,734	67.0	66,825	100.0

Association test: calc χ^2 = 278.27; crit χ^2 = 9.49.
Contrasts study:
  ≤ 2,500 = { (prop SEL 1) = (prop SEL 2) } < (prop SEL 3).
  2,501–3,000 = { (prop SEL 1) = (prop SEL 2) } < (prop SEL 3).
  > 3,000 = { (prop SEL 1) = (prop SEL 2) } > (prop SEL 3).
prop, proportion.

TABLE 8. *Distribution of birthweight according to presence or absence of prenatal care in socioeconomic level 1*

	Birthweight (g)						Total	
	≤ 2,500		2,501–3,000		> 3,000			
Prenatal care	n	%	n	%	n	%	n	%
Yes	86	4.7	397	21.8	1,336	73.5	1,819	98.8
No	2	9.1	4	18.2	16	72.7	22	1.2
Total	88	4.8	401	21.8	1,352	73.4	1,841	100.0

Association test: calc χ^2 = 1.0; crit χ^2 = 5.99.
Contrasts study: without contrast.

TABLE 9. *Distribution of birthweight according to presence or absence of prenatal care in socioeconomic level 2*

	Birthweight (g)						Total	
	≤ 2,500		2,501–3,000		> 3,000			
Prenatal care	n	%	n	%	n	%	n	%
Yes	421	5.1	1,732	20.9	6,130	74.0	8,283	97.2
No	20	8.5	55	23.3	161	68.2	236	2.8
Total	441	5.2	1,787	21.0	6,291	73.8	8,519	100.0

Association test: calc χ^2 = 6.77; crit χ^2 = 5.99.
Contrasts study: without contrast.

TABLE 10. *Distribution of birthweight according to presence or absence of prenatal care in socioeconomic level 3*

	Birthweight (g)						Total	
	≤ 2,500		2,501–3,000		> 3,000			
Prenatal care	n	%	n	%	n	%	n	%
Yes	4,504	7.9	14,951	26.4	37,268	65.7	56,723	79.5
No	1,785	12.2	4,342	29.7	8,475	58.1	14,602	20.5
Total	6,289	8.8	19,293	27.1	45,743	64.1	71,325	100.0

Association test: calc χ^2 = 396.98; crit χ^2 = 5.99.
Contrasts study:
  ≤ 2,500 = (prop presence of prenatal care) < (prop absence of prenatal care).
  2,501–3,000 = (prop presence of prenatal care) < (prop absence of prenatal care).
  > 3,000 = (prop presence of prenatal care) > (prop absence of prenatal care).
prop, proportion.

presence or absence of adequate prenatal care. In the lowest socioeconomic group, however, it was shown that a greater number of mothers of infants <3,000 g did not attend antenatal care, while the opposite was observed for babies weighing >3,000 g. It became clear that for this low socioeconomic group prenatal care was an important factor in obtaining favorable conditions for fetal growth.

Tables 11–13 show the distribution of birthweight according to maternal smoking habits and socioeconomic level. Analysis of the influence of smoking showed that in the low birthweight and inadequate birthweight categories there was a greater number of smoking mothers than non-smoking mothers. The opposite was true for

TABLE 11. *Distribution of birthweight according to maternal smoking habit*

Maternal smoking	Birthweight (g)							
	≤ 2,500		2,501–3,000		> 3,000		Total	
	n	%	n	%	n	%	n	%
Yes	3,063	11.1	8,505	30.9	15,922	58.0	27,490	34.2
No	3,653	6.9	12,649	23.9	36,579	69.2	52,881	65.8
Total	6,716	8.4	21,154	26.3	52,501	65.3	80,371	100.0

Association test: calc χ^2 = 1,077.24; crit χ^2 = 5.99.
Contrasts study:
  ≤ 2,500 = (prop yes) > (prop no).
  2,501–3,000 = (prop yes) > (prop no).
  > 3,000 = (prop yes) < (prop no).
prop, proportion.

TABLE 12. *Distribution of birthweight in smoking mothers according to socioeconomic level (SEL)*

SEL	Birthweight (g)							
	≤ 2,500		2,501–3,000		> 3,000		Total	
	n	%	n	%	n	%	n	%
1	28	5.5	125	24.4	359	70.1	512	1.9
2	190	7.7	621	25.1	1,664	67.2	2,475	9.0
3	2,845	11.6	7,759	31.7	13,899	56.7	24,503	89.1
Total	3,063	11.1	8,505	31.0	15,922	57.9	27,490	100.0

Association test: calc χ^2 = 141.14; crit χ^2 = 9.79.
Contrasts study:
  ≤ 2,500 = { (prop SEL 1) = (prop SEL 2) } < { (prop SEL 3) }.
  2,501–3,000 = { (prop SEL 1) = (prop SEL 2) } < (prop SEL 3).
  > 3,000 = { (prop SEL 1) = (prop SEL 2) } > (prop SEL 3).
prop, proportion.

TABLE 13. *Distribution of birthweight in nonsmoking mothers according to socioeconomic level (SEL)*

SEL	Birthweight (g)						Total	
	≤ 2,500		2,501–3,000		> 3,000			
	n	%	n	%	n	%	n	%
1	55	4.4	253	20.3	936	75.3	1,244	2.3
2	249	4.2	1,165	19.5	4,545	76.3	5,459	11.3
3	3,349	7.3	11,231	24.6	31,098	68.1	45,678	86.4
Total	3,653	7.0	12,649	24.1	36,579	69.9	52,881	100.0

Association test: calc χ^2 = 207.93; crit χ^2 = 9.49.
Contrasts study:
  ≤ 2,500 = { (prop SEL 1) = (prop SEL 2) } < (prop SEL 3).
  2,501–3,000 = { (prop SEL 1 = prop SEL 2) } < (prop SEL 3).
  > 3,000 = { (prop SEL 1) = (prop SEL 2) } > (prop SEL 3).
prop, proportion.

infants weighing >3,000 g. However, when these results were analyzed according to socioeconomic level it was shown that smoking habit did not appear to influence birthweight in the higher socioeconomic group. This suggests that the influences of smoking habits are somehow compensated for in higher social groups, perhaps by factors related to better economic conditions.

CONCLUSIONS

The findings of this study show that the main factors related to intrauterine growth in Brazil are:

1. Low socioeconomic conditions found in 86% of the population. The chronic effects of social deprivation can limit maternal weight and height, and hence affect birth size in the next generation.
2. Lack of prenatal care, affecting 18% of the population, particularly those of low social class (98% of the pregnant women in this particular group).
3. Smoking habits, particularly in the lowest socioeconomic group.

REFERENCES

1. Nóbrega FJ. Antropometria, patologias e malformações congênitas do recém-nascido brasileiro e estudos de associação com algumas variáveis maternas (Anthropometry, pathology and congenital malformations in Brazilian newborn infants. Studies of association with some maternal factors). *Jornal de Pediatria*, 1985; suppl 59.
2. Jelliffe DB. *Assessment of the nutritional status of the community. WHO* Monograph no. 53. Geneva: WHO, 1968.
3. Curi PR, Morais RV. Associação, homogeneidade e contrastes entre proporções em tabelas contendo distribuições multino-miais (Association, homogeneity and contrasts between proportions on tables with multinomial distributions). *Ciência e Cultura* 1981;33:712–22.

Intrauterine Growth Retardation, edited by
Jacques Senterre. Nestlé Nutrition Workshop
Series, Vol. 18. Nestec Ltd., Vevey/Raven Press,
Ltd., New York © 1989.

Intrauterine Growth Retardation in Africa

C. Robyn, M. S. Keita, and S. Meuris

*Human Reproduction Unit, Université Libre de Bruxelles, Hôpital Saint-Pierre,
1000 Brussels, Belgium*

In 1979, some 21 million low birthweight babies ($<$2,500 g) were born in the world. This represents about 17% of all births in that year (1). In those countries where the proportion of low birthweight is the highest and where action is needed, data on birthweight are scarce or even non-existent. The relative influences of genetic factors and environmental factors (socioeconomic, cultural, health) are still poorly elucidated.

Morbidity and neonatal mortality are higher in low birthweight babies than in those of normal weight, and among survivors, there is a higher incidence of neurological handicaps and mental retardation. Infections occur more frequently and are more severe and longer lasting after intrauterine growth retardation (2). In countries with high rates of low birthweight, there is an urgent need to promote measures aimed at reducing the environmental causes of intrauterine growth retardation, such as maternal diseases, chronic undernutrition, and poor socioeconomic conditions. However, effects and side effects of specific preventive interventions such as food supplements, chemoprophylaxis of malaria, etc., have not been thoroughly investigated so far. Therefore, no consensus can exist on health and social programs to be initiated. A prerequisite for any further progress is that birthweight should be more systematically measured.

EPIDEMIOLOGY

Low birthweight ($<$2,500 g) is a public health concern in Africa. It is, however, difficult to obtain an accurate evaluation of the incidence of low birthweight babies in this part of the world, since only a rather small number of babies born in Africa are weighed. Most data on birthweight available in Africa are from hospitals (3), but the majority of mothers are not delivered in hospital. In Nigeria, for example, most deliveries take place at home assisted by elder multiparous women, traditional birth attendants, or by herbalists; or in church dispensaries or private maternity homes (3). In Lagos, 46% of babies are born in hospitals while in the Kainji Lake area this figure falls to 2.6% (4). Average birthweights often tend to increase from teaching hospitals, through non-teaching hospitals and health centers, to homes. For exam-

TABLE 1. *Mean birthweight, rates of low birthweight, and rates of low birthweight for gestational age > 37 weeks in Africa*

Country	Region or city	Year	Number	Mean weight (g)	Percent < 2500 g or < 37 weeks	Percent < 2500 g and > 37 weeks
Western Africa						
Guinea-Bissau		1977	3,239	3,229	8.0	
Ivory Coast	Abidjan	1975	7,154	2,950	14.1	
Nigeria	Ibadan	1968–72	10,839	2,920	19.2	60
	Ibadan	1973–74	1,290	3,053	24.9	43
	Ibadan	1968–72	20,651	2,940	15.3	60
	Igbo-Ora	1971–75	4,334	—	11.0	
	Katsina	1975–76	1,460	3,030	15.8	
	Lagos	1966	9,104	3,230	13.1	
	Benin	1970–71	4,821	3,033	10.8	
Senegal	Dakar	1959	8,409	3,115	9.9	
Eastern Africa						
Ethiopia	Addis Ababa	1964–68	8,469	3,132	8.8	
	Addis Ababa	1971	3,144	3,139		
Kenya	Nairobi	1971	3,160	3,345	13.6	34
	Nairobi	1974	3,700		18.9	34
	Nairobi	1975	1,595		17.5	
	Nairobi	1971	14,326	3,143		
Rwanda		1971	7,929	2,890	17.0	
Tanzania	Dar es Salaam	1964	8,139	2,950	11.0	
	Dar es Salaam	1973	2,070	3,117		
	Dar es Salaam	1975–76	16,532	2,991	15.2	
	Dar es Salaam	1976–77	2,828	2,906	22.3	
	Moshi	1960–63	2,166	3,040	10.1	
	Moshi	1971–72	1,251	3,151	2.0	
	Tanga	1955–60	3,355	2,970		
	Tanga	1966	1,000		11.2	56
	Nzega	1955–60	2,007	2,900		
Zambia	Kitwe	1971–72	2,401		14.2	
Middle Africa						
Central African Republic		1973	19,496	2,873	23.0	
Chad		1965	3,000	3,114	10.5	
Gabon		1970–72	7,032	2,979	13.0	
Cameroun		1971–73	8,071	3,119		
Zaire	Lubumbashi	1969	5,206	3,163	12.6	
	Rutshuru	1983	1,121	2,850	16.6	
	Kabare	1983	1,224	2,940	13.6	
	Bagira	1983	806	3,020	6.7	
Southern Africa						
South Africa	Capetown	1964–65	4,657	3,050	14.9	42
	Capetown	1964–65	2,045	3,300	8.2	38
	Johannesburg	1971–72	1,800	883	19.5	73

Data from ref. 1 and ref. 6 for series of more than 1,000 deliveries.

ple, mean birthweight in Oluyoro Hospital, a mission hospital in Ibadan (Nigeria), is significantly higher than that of babies born in the University College Hospital (UCH) (5). This can be expected, since the University Hospital delivers more women with abnormal obstetric cases. There are fewer low birthweight babies in urban areas (6.7%) than in rural areas (13.5%–19.6%), as seen in Kivu (Table 1) (6). Data collected in only one hospital or only one health center are therefore rarely representative of the region where the hospital is located, and even less of the entire country.

Another difficulty is that in most cases the date of the last menstrual period is not available. This makes it difficult to differentiate between preterm deliveries and cases of intrauterine growth retardation (IUGR). As the date of the last menstrual period is generally not known, the maturity of the newborn has been evaluated in recent studies with reference to a scale of maturity (7). Unknown menstrual period is associated with high rates of low birthweight and with low socio-economic and socio-demographic status: these characteristics are themselves associated with a high rate of preterm deliveries (8). Thus, deleting the group of women with unknown last menstrual period may bias epidemiological studies on low birthweight and the consequences of such a choice must be carefully checked.

In Africa, the rates of low birthweight (<2,500 g) vary greatly from one study to another, sometimes within the same country (Table 1). They range between 8% and 25%. The average value estimated in 1980 for the continent was 15% (1). Average values estimated for Northern (13%), Western (17%), Eastern (14%), Middle (15%), and Southern (15%) Africa were fairly uniform (1). The mean birthweight in Africa is about 3,000 g, in comparison with 3,100 g in Latin America, and 3,200 g in Europe and Northern America (1).

ETIOLOGY

Olowe reported on the relation between birthweight and gestational age (from 26 weeks) in 436 newborn African infants delivered by healthy Nigerian mothers from middle to high socio-economic social classes, living at sea level and taking prophylactic antimalarial drugs, iron, and folic acid routinely throughout pregnancy (9). The growth curve based on these data is identical to the curves reported for newborns delivered by healthy mothers in industrialized countries (10,11).

The proportion of low birthweight babies with gestational age of >37 weeks is less frequently recorded. It appears to range from 34% to 74% of low birthweight babies in Africa. In a group of 250 low birthweight babies from Baragwanath Hospital (Johannesburg, South Africa) Stein and Ellis (12) observed that 73% were small-for-gestational age. Toxaemia (9%) was not a very important factor. "When the incidence of low birthweight is higher than 10%, it is almost exclusively due to the increase of intrauterine growth retardated low birthweight infants, while prematurity remains almost unchanged" (13).

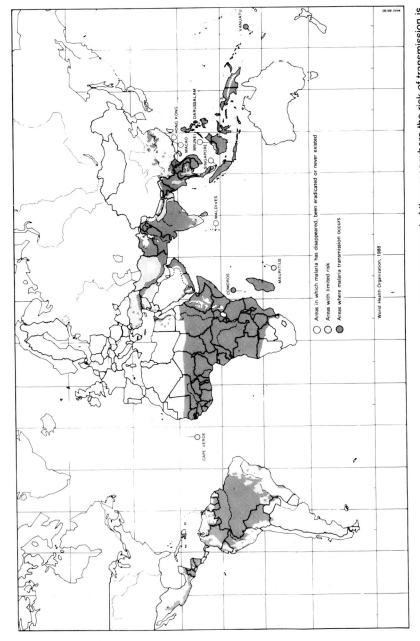

FIG. 1. Geographic distribution of the areas where malaria transmission occurs and of the areas where the risk of transmission is limited: world situation in 1986. (From ref. 14.)

MALARIA

Malaria remains one of the last plagues of mankind. Half of the world population is confronted with Plasmodium. Extensive successes have been obtained by anti-malarial campaigns based on eradication of the anopheline vectors and on the reduction of the human source of Plasmodium by chemoprophylaxis (14). However, a new expansion of the disease has been observed in Asia, South America, and to a lesser extent, in Africa. This derives from the selection of strains of anopheline vectors resistant to insecticides and strains of *Plasmodium falciparum* resistant to quinine derivatives (14).

The malaria areas are located between the tropics of Cancer and Capricorn where almost half of the world population lives. Africa is the continent where the malarial endemic is of the greatest concern: Some 39 million people live in hypoendemic areas, about 115 million in mesoendemic zones, and 231 million in areas where malaria is hyperendemic to holoendemic (Fig. 1). About 1 million children die every year as a direct consequence of the disease. As children and pregnant women represent the high-risk groups for malaria, this results in an excess of low birthweight babies and of neonatal and infantile morbidity and mortality (15).

In epidemic conditions, in a population with a rather low level of immunization, such as that reported from Ceylon in 1934–35 (16), Saigon (17), and Malaysia (18), malaria is highly virulent, leading to frequent maternal death, high rates of abortion, stillbirth, and premature deliveries. In these conditions, *in utero* infection of the fetus and congenital malaria are frequent, too. Where malaria is endemic and where adult women have acquired protective immunity through repeated prior infections, it is agreed that during pregnancy women show an increased prevalence and density of malaria. But the effects of the disease on pregnancy are less apparent and not yet completely understood. This situation prevails in most parts of tropical Africa. Clark (19) and Blacklock and Gordon (20) were the first to report that placental malaria is a common feature at parturition in endemic conditions, and that it is asymptomatic in most cases. This has since been largely confirmed throughout tropical Africa, with incidences of placental malaria varying from 15% to 85%, and usually higher than those of peripheral parasitemia found in the same women (21).

PARASITEMIA AND PLACENTAL INFECTION

Placental infections are sometimes substantially heavier than suggested by the density of parasites in peripheral blood: the placenta may contain a large number of infected red blood cells (up to 65%) while the peripheral blood is free from parasites (21). Erythrocytes infected by *Plasmodium falciparum*, which in Africa is the most common cause of pregnancy malaria, are sequestered in the human placenta (22). Erythrocytes containing *Plasmodium falciparum* develop electron-dense excrescences at the cell surface, called knobs (23). These knobs adhere to endothelial cells and form focal junctions with the endothelial cell membrane. This phenomenon is likely to contribute to the observed sequestration of mature erythrocytic forms of *Plasmodium falciparum* in the deep organs (24).

Placental malaria occurs more frequently (27%) in residents of rural communities than in those of urban ones (12%). Furthermore, in some areas there are seasonal variations in the prevalence of the parasitemia. It is highest in the 3 months following the end of the rainy season and lowest in the second half of the dry season (25).

It has been suggested that the higher prevalence of malaria during gestation is due to a decrease in the immune response of pregnant women. However, there have been several observations which do not support this idea. For example, the specific tetanus antibody response (IgG) in pregnant women is comparable to that in non-pregnant healthy adults. No apparent influence of gestational age on the immune response to the absorbed tetanus toxoid has been observed during pregnancy (26). Field studies in an area of stable malaria showed that mean serum levels of IgG and IgA were depressed during pregnancy, the lowest levels being observed during the last weeks of gestation (27). However, although protective antibodies against malaria are of the IgG type, assays of specific malarial antibodies in relation to pregnancy have failed to yield consistent results, and most authors have not found any significant difference in anti-malarial antibody titers between pregnant and non-pregnant women when aparasitemic, even in primigravidas (25,28,29). In Gambia, during the wet season of August, the prevalence and the density of parasitemia and also the specific antibody levels increase in pregnant women, just as in other adults and in children (28). This also favors the concept that the immune response to malaria is not impaired during pregnancy. Furthermore, the extreme rarity of congenital malaria in newborns throughout regions in which the disease is highly endemic seems to argue against any serious breakdown of anti-malarial immunity during pregnancy. Malarial antibodies are readily demonstrable in sera from Gambian newborns. They are responsible for the "relative freedom that the infant born in highly endemic areas appears to enjoy over the early weeks of life" (25). Finally, the increased prevalence and severity of malarial infection takes place early in pregnancy, with progressive recovery to non-pregnant levels close to delivery (21). This development bears no relationship to changes in immunoglobulin concentrations, since IgG declines progressively to reach the lowest levels at the time of delivery or even during the postpartum period (30).

An alternative explanation would be that a pregnancy-specific factor enhances the virulence of the Plasmodium. The trophoblastic origin of such a factor and its local production would explain the high density of parasites seen in the intervillous spaces: The idea of the pregnant uterus acting as a haven of safety for the parasite is not new, since Clark (19) proposed it in one of his earliest papers describing placental malaria. Studies conducted in areas of perennial transmission revealed that the prevalence of parasitemia increases rather early in pregnancy, with a calculated peak at around day 100 of gestation (21). Thereafter the prevalence of infection pro-

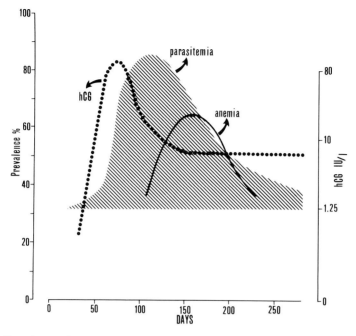

FIG. 2. Prevalence of malaria infection (parasitemia) and hemolytic anemia associated with splenomegaly in primigravidas, together with the development of human chorionic gonado-trophin (hCG) in urine during pregnancy. Day 1 = first day of last menstrual period. (From ref. 21.)

gressively declines and at the end of pregnancy it is only slightly higher than the level seen in non-pregnant women. The curve published by Brabin (21) runs parallel to that of the blood concentration of human chorionic gonadotrophin (hCG) during early pregnancy (Fig. 2).

The concept of pregnancy-induced immunosuppression also does not satisfactorily explain why primigravidas are much more susceptible than multigravidas to malarial infection during pregnancy, the prevalence of both parasitemia and placental infection being twice as high (21). Densities of infections are also higher in primigravidas (28). The significance of such differences is not known. However, the lower prevalence of parasitemia during pregnancy in multigravidas may simply be the consequence of the development of the age-dependent immunity against the parasite. In Africa, at the time of their first pregnancy, almost all women are below 20 and may not have yet acquired the optimal immune protection. If one considers the first pregnancy as a challenge due to an increased virulence of the infection under the influence of some specific pregnancy factors, then the difference in prevalence between primigravidas and multigravidas can be interpreted as the result of the higher degree of immunity developed in response to malarial infection in the first pregnancy (21).

PLACENTAL LESIONS

Galbraith et al. (31) and Walter et al. (32) produced a detailed histological and ultrastructural study of placentas from mothers infected with malaria. They developed
techniques for the recognition of hemozoin, the brown malarial pigment, and parasites in the placenta. Thickening of the trophoblastic basement membrane is seen in
all infected placentas. Monocytes containing phagocytosed pigment are found in the
intervillous spaces. In heavily infected placentas, monocytes form aggregates or
pseudo-inflammatory masses in the intervillous spaces, together with fibrin and par-
asitized erythrocytes. In these cases, malarial pigment is also observed in the cyto-
plasm of the trophoblast. This is associated with focal syncytial necrosis and
cytotrophoblastic proliferation. The ultimate stage of villous necrosis is the formation of clumps of fibrinoid. In most placentas, a few deposits of pigment are apparent within the Hofbauer cells and within the stroma of scattered healthy villi. Even
in placentas with dense parasitemia in the intervillous spaces, no plasmodias are
seen in the placental tissue (32). Parasites are seldom found in cord blood, as congenital malaria is exceptional in areas of endemic malaria (33,34).

In practice in regions where malaria is endemic, malarial pigment and thickening
of the basal membrane of the trophoblast are often seen in the absence of peripheral
and placental parasitemia. Infected maternal erythrocytes were found in only some
40% of the placentas with malarial lesions (32). Conversely, parasitemia in maternal peripheral blood at the time of delivery is not necessarily associated with malarial lesions of the placenta: Only some 50% of parturient women with peripheral
parasitemia had typical lesions in the placenta (32). Similar observations were reported by Watkinson and Rushton (35) in a study on the outcome of pregnancy in
West African mothers. In 9 out of the 12 women with parasitemia but unpigmented
placentas, however, malarial parasitemia had been last detected before 20 weeks of
gestation. Thus when infection takes place early in pregnancy, the pigment may be
"cleared" from the placenta, at least in some cases. The fact that the peak of
monthly incidence (October–November) of placental pigmentation was synchro-
nous with the peak incidence of parasitemia provides further evidence that pigmentation is associated with a relatively recent infection. According to Watkinson and
Rushton (35), microscopic examination of biopsy specimens, even full-thickness
slices of the placenta, may not always detect focal placental lesions. This could help
to explain some of the discrepancies between the rate of placental lesions and the
prevalence of parasitemia.

BIRTHWEIGHT

It has been consistently reported that the birthweights of infants born of mothers
with infected placentas were lower than those of infants born from non-infected
mothers: The differences in weights vary from 55 g to 310 g (34–46) (Table 2).
There is a slight excess of female births (n = 150) over males (n = 120) in the series

TABLE 2. *Influence of placental malaria on birthweights in Africa (1952–1983): Positive mothers are mothers with placental malaria*

Ref.	n	Placental malaria (%)	Mothers positive for placental malaria		Mothers negative for placental malaria		Difference in weight
			Mean birthweight (g)	< 2500 g (%)	Mean birthweight (g)	< 2500 g (%)	
Bruce-Chwatt (36)	310	23.5	2,903	20.5	3,048	11.0	145
Archibald (37)	463	14.7	2,722	29.4	2,892	16.5	170
Archibald (38)	440	14.1	2,776	21.0	3,076	8.2	298
Cannon (39)	392	33.2	2,610	36.9	2,920	12.2	310
Spitz (40)	576	23.6	—	41.2	—	27.0	89
McLaren and Ward (41)	400	21.5	3,037	14.0	3,092	7.3	55
Jelliffe (42)	570	16.1	2,085	19.6	3,063	10.0	263
Jilly (43)	50	43.7	2,855	—	3,033	—	178
Kortmann (44)	413	34.1	2,945	—	3,020	—	75
Reinhardt et al. (45)	198	33.7	2,960	—	3,080	—	120
Walter et al. (46)	115	34.7[a]	2,770	—	2,920	—	220
Watkinson and Rushton (35)	65	41.5[a]	2,580	—	3,150	—	570[b]

[a]Placentas with malarial lesions.
[b]Difference calculated only for first-born babies.

of babies with infected placentas reported by McLaren and Ward (41) and by Jelliffe (42): The sex ratio (male/male + female) was 0.44 when it is classically over 0.50 at birth. It should be remembered that during the last trimester of pregnancy, the tro-phoblast of female fetuses produces more hCG than that of males (47). In areas of endemic malaria, there is no clear association between placental malaria and still-birth or maternal death (34).

Chandra (48) has reported impaired T-cell function in infants who are small for their gestational age, a feature widely accepted as evidence of fetal malnutrition. This impaired T-cell function persists during the first months and even years of life and may adversely influence the infant's prospects for survival. To date, no studies have determined whether infants with low birthweight resulting from placental ma-laria show similar immunologic defects.

Reduction in birthweight associated with placental infection is greater in primi-gravidas, with mean reported values of 321 g (42) and 636 g (49). In some studies, it is even statistically significant only in first born infants (34). Dense placental in-fection is also more frequent in primigravidas. Birthweight deficits tend to be the greatest in association with the highest parasite density and this is particularly true for first born children (34). In order to understand the relation between placental malaria *(Plasmodium falciparum)* and impaired fetal growth, McGregor and Avery (50) investigated the consequences on birthweight of a malaria eradication campaign initiated in the British Solomon Islands. The main antimalarial measure employed was spraying DDT in order to kill as many adult female anopheline mosquitoes transmitting malaria as possible. Birthweights rose substantially within a few months after starting the antimalarial operations. The average increase between 1969 and 1971 was 165 g for all babies and 252 g for the first born babies. The rate of low birthweight babies (<2,500 g) declined from 21% to 12% for all newborns and from 41% to 21% for first borns. During this period, the consumption of antimalarial drugs did not increase.

Taking biopsy specimens from 65 placentas in a region where *Plasmodium falciparum* malaria is endemic and where pregnant women traditionally receive only curative treatment for parasitemias and no chemoprophylaxis, Watkinson and Rushton (35) reported a 40% rate of pigmented placentas, i.e., with macrophages containing phagocytosed malarial pigment in the intervillous spaces. Parasitemias had been diagnosed antenatally in only 18% of these women despite frequent antenatal follow-up. Primigravidas had the highest incidence (67%) of pigmented placenta and of parasitemia. Mean birthweight of babies with pigmented placentas was lower than that of babies with non-pigmented placentas: The difference was the greatest for first born babies (570 g). All babies weighing less than 2,500 g at birth had pigmented placentas. The mean gestational age and the rate of preterm babies were the same whether the placenta was pigmented or not. The presence of malarial pigment did not influence the weight of the placenta (35).

In the same group of mothers, Watkinson et al. (51) also reported lower plasma estradiol levels in those who delivered babies with pigmented placentas. This was significant from the 32nd week of pregnancy. The plasma progesterone levels also tended to be lower. More recently, similar results have been obtained for estriol (52) and for human placental lactogen (53). All these endocrine changes seen during late pregnancy in mothers with pigmented placentas indicate that malarial infection causes damage to the trophoblast. These are likely to be responsible for intrauterine growth retardation. However, peripheral parasitemia is not a good marker of the morbidity of the fetoplacental unit. "As pigmented placentas were related to low birthweights and weights for gestational age whereas non-pigmented placentas, even in women with early parasitemias, were not, it may be only the later parasitemia and later placental infection that cause major morbidity for the feto-placental unit" (35).

Since, in the Gambian study, less than half of the women with pigmented placentas had parasitemia detected and treated during pregnancy, many of the malarial episodes must have caused either trivial symptoms or no symptoms at all. Neither the easily accessible daily clinic nor regular antenatal clinics ensured diagnosis and adequate protection against the morbidity of placental infection (35). Thus in regions of Africa where malaria is endemic, curative treatment for parasitemia is ineffective in preventing placental lesions and fetal growth retardation.

Since malarial lesions of the placenta cannot be predicted by detection of peripheral parasitemia, all pregnant women in endemic malarial areas should be given antimalarial chemoprophylaxis. This should start early and at least during the second trimester of pregnancy: the crucial period for protection of the feto-placental unit is, according to Watkinson and Rushton (35), the last trimester of pregnancy. The limited number of studies that have been undertaken so far show that chemoprophylaxis of malaria produces a fall in malaria antibody levels in protected populations and that the magnitude of the fall is related to the efficiency of the control program. It is unlikely, however, that pregnant women with established immunity to malaria will lose this immunity as a result of taking chemoprophylaxis for only a few months during pregnancy, although the situation may be different in children (54). Therefore, effective antimalarial measures result in reduced rates of parasitemia, anemia, fetal and maternal morbidity, and intrauterine growth retardation.

UNDERNUTRITION

Data on the influence of maternal malnutrition on birthweight came from observations made in Europe during the Second World War. The siege of Leningrad (55) and the Dutch situation in 1944–45 (56) are usually quoted as examples of a significant decrease of birthweight, by 500 g and 250 g, respectively, resulting from acute starvation. It was also reported that birthweight was reduced more when the restriction took place during the last trimester of pregnancy: The mean birthweight of infants born 9 weeks after the end of the starvation period was higher than that of infants born at the end of this period (56). In Ethiopia, the absence of further intrauterine growth of the fetus observed between the 36th and 40th week of gestation is considered to be the consequence of poor nutrition of the mother (57). However, altitude might also be a factor since the population investigated lives 2,500 m above sea level (58). A diet deficiency in all nutrients during the third trimester of pregnancy in healthy young non-privileged primigravidas results in the delivery of babies 470 g lighter than those delivered from similar women of the privileged group (59). In some regions of Africa, such as Ethiopia and Kenya, pregnant women purposely reduce their diet for fear of having big babies and difficult deliveries (60).

Seasonal variations in food supply influence the birthweight as well. The lowest mean birthweights were recorded in Ethiopia during the pre-harvest season when staple foods were scarce and prices at a maximum and when this period coincided with pregnancies in the third trimester (58). In Nigeria the mean birthweight of babies born from primiparas during the months of May–August, which corresponded to the rainy season, was significantly lower than for the other months of the year. However, this period of May–August is also a period of high malaria parasitemia in addition to food shortage (61).

The growth rate of the fetus is not only influenced by the energy supply to the mother but also by her energy consumption. Indeed, heavy physical labor during pregnancy affects the birthweight when mothers have energy intakes below WHO/FAO-recommended standards (62). In this study, the low energy and protein intakes were not entirely due to limited family income. Full-term infants of mothers engaged in heavy physical labor had a mean birthweight (3,060 g) significantly lower (3,270 g) than that of infants born from less physically active mothers on a similar low energy diet. Physically active mothers gained less body weight during pregnancy (3.3 kg) than the less active mothers (5.9 kg). Thus, in a situation of borderline energy balance, such as in chronic undernutrition, the mother still continues to gain weight during pregnancy, even if weight gain is reduced to a minimum and even if this results in a significant although limited decrease in birthweight.

Change in third trimester skinfold measurements is a good predictor of birthweight. Changes in skinfold thickness reflect changes in maternal fat stores (63). In well-nourished women, 3 kg of fat are stored before the 30th week of gestation (64). Part of this is supplied to the fetus during the last trimester, when fetal growth rate is at its highest. Fat storage correlates with an increase in triceps skinfold thickness during the first two trimesters of pregnancy, and a progressive decrease of the skinfold during the last 3 months (63). Deficit in energy intake both limits the normal increase of skinfold thickness during pregnancy and reduces birthweight. In Ethiopia, women with very thin triceps skinfold in early gestation gave birth to infants weighing less than 2.9 kg. Women with large triceps skinfold and whose skinfold decreases during the third trimester produce heavy neonates (>3.2 kg).

ANEMIA

In many tropical areas, anemia is caused or aggravated by parasitic diseases, mainly malaria and intestinal parasites such as the hookworm (>2,000 eggs per g of feces). During pregnancy the hemoglobin iron of the mother increases by 500 mg. The total iron needed during the whole of pregnancy is about 1,000 mg. The daily requirements are six times greater during the last trimester than in non-pregnant women. In normal conditions, half the total requirement of iron comes from the iron stores. Abortions, premature births, low birthweight, and postpartum hemorrhage are associated with low hemoglobin levels during pregnancy (65). Anemia is more frequent in mothers giving birth to low birthweight babies. In Togo (66), 24% of such mothers are anemic in contrast to 10% in the group of mothers delivering babies weighing more than 2,500 g Kessel et al. (67) reported that the duration of pregnancy is independent of the anemia status. Thus, anemia is an important correlate of intrauterine growth retardation.

Anemia related to malaria in pregnancy is common. It is usually hemolytic. There is however no direct association between the hemoglobin level and the prevalence of parasitemia during pregnancy. In children, the peak incidence of anemia and splenomegaly follows the period of acute malarial infection. In pregnancy, patients with hemolytic anemia and splenomegaly are observed between the 16th and 24th week, coinciding with the peak of acute infection (21) (Fig. 2). Immunological factors seem to play an important role in the etiology of anemia associated with malaria: A reduction in red blood cell life span persists for several weeks after the acute infection (68). Secondary megaloblastic anemia may occur, but later in pregnancy. This may have important consequences for the child. The peak of the prevalence of anemia before the 24th week of pregnancy is not suppressed by the sole administration of antimalarials at this time. Indeed, antimalarials given after 20 to 28 pregnancy weeks do not correct established anemia unless folic acid is given as well. However, chemoprophylaxis initiated from early pregnancy was successful in preventing pregnant women developing hemolytic anemia.

Iron is essential for the development of *Plasmodium falciparum*. It seems that in erythrocytes, parasites do not take iron from hemoglobin. There is no metabolism of the iron-containing moiety of hemoglobin. No parasite enzymes that degrade hemin have been identified. Hemin is even toxic to parasite carbohydrate metabolism. How then is it that iron is sequestered in infected red cells as hemozoin, the characteristic malarial pigment? The answer is that *Plasmodium falciparum* synthesizes a transferrin receptor and localizes it at the surface of the infected erythrocyte, allowing iron transfer to the parasite: Red cells lose their own transferrin receptor during erythrocyte maturation (68).

High frequencies of α-thalassemia and of sickle cell disease are the result of natural selection by malaria (69). However, in areas of high transmission, antimalarial immunity acquired by adult women is sufficient for the sickle cell trait to confer no advantage. The situation is different for children: Individuals with the sickle cell gene are more resistant to attacks of severe malaria. Parasite invasion of red cells and parasite growth within these cells are decreased when they contain sickle hemoglobin, but only under low oxygen tension as in deep tissues (70). Peak prevalence of parasitemia occurs before 24 weeks of gestation in women with the sickle cell trait as in women without the gene (71). Its amplitude is the same for the two types of pregnant women. Sickle cell anemia is seldom encountered during pregnancy in Africa, since most homozygous subjects do not reach adulthood as a result of the high mortality due to malnutrition and associated infectious diseases (72). The presence of the sickle cell trait, encountered in 20 to 25% of people from West Africa, is largely an asymptomatic condition and is not of great hazard in pregnancy for either mother or child (73). However, urinary tract infections and hematuria are more frequent in pregnant women with the trait. In the West Indies, the mean birthweight of babies born from women with the sickle cell trait was found significantly lower than that of a matched population without the trait (74). A similar observation has been made by Hoff et al. (75) in a population of black pregnant women in Alabama (USA). Mean femur lengths were found to be reduced at each gestational period when compared with similar measurements in women with normal hemoglobin (74).

TEENAGERS

In the Nairobi Birth Survey, conducted from June to August 1981, teenage mothers, aged 19 and below, were 19% of the total group. The rate of low birthweight among teenagers was 18% (76). In a large series of deliveries in Nigeria, the incidence of low birthweight rate among the Hausa was 27% in mothers aged less than 15, 26% in mothers aged 15 to 19, 20% in those aged 20 to 24, and 18% in the 25 to 29 year age group (77).

The mean birthweight increases with parity up to the third (78), fourth (77), or fifth (44) pregnancy and with maternal age up until 34 to 36 years (57,77).

TWINS

The high rate of twins in some populations of Africa sometimes contributes importantly to the high rates of low birthweight babies. Among the Yorubas in Nigeria and in Ethiopians, twins represent about 5% of all births (57,79,80). In Togo, among 888 newborn babies with low birthweight (<2,500 g) investigated by Bégué et al. (81), 165 were twins (18.2%). Babies from multiple pregnancies represented 22% of all low birthweight infants in Hausa, Northern Nigeria (77) and 25% in Yoruba, Western Nigeria (5,82). In a group of 250 low birthweight babies, Stein and Ellis (12) found 26% were twins. This represented 32% of the babies who were small for their gestational age.

REFERENCES

1. World Health Organization, Division of Family Health. The incidence of low birthweight. A critical review of available information. *World Health Stat Q* 1980;33:197–224.
2. Xanthou M. Immunologic deficiencies in small-for-date neonates. *Acta Paediatr Scand* 1985;319:143–9.
3. Ransome-Kuti O. Intra-uterine growth, birthweights and maturity in the African newborn. *Acta Paediatr Scand* 1985;Suppl. 319:95–102.
4. Morley D, Knox G. The birthweights of Yoruba babies. *J Obstet Gynecol* 1960;67:975–80.
5. Effiong CE, Laditan AAO, Aimakhu VE, Ayeni O. Birthweight of Nigerian children. *Nigerian Med J* 1976;6:63–8.
6. CEMUBAC. Rapport pour l'année 1983 concernant les activités de la mission médicale CEMUBAC en République du Zaire, notamment auprès du Département Médical de l'IRS et des hôpitaux ruraux de Kirotshe, Masisi et Rutshuru. *Lwiro* 1983;60.
7. Dubowitz L, Dubowitz V, Goldberg C. Clinical assessment of gestational age in the newborn infant. *J Pediatr* 1970;77:1–10.
8. Buekens P, Delvoye P, Wollast E, Robyn C. Epidemiology of pregnancies with unknown last menstrual period. *J Epidemiol Community Health* 1984;38:79–80.
9. Olowe SA. Standards of intrauterine growth for an African population at sea level. *J Pediatr* 1981;99:489–95.
10. Rooth G, Meirik O, Karlberg R. Estimation of the normal growth of Swedish infants at term. *Acta Paediatr Scand* 1985; Suppl. 319:76–9.
11. Pecorari D, Costa L, Barbone F. Practical application of the Bristol perinatal growth chart to Mediterranean populations. *Acta Paediatr Scand* 1985;Suppl. 319:80–3.
12. Stein H, Ellis U. The low birthweight African baby. *Arch Dis Child* 1974;49:156–9.
13. Villar J, Belizan JM. The relative contribution of prematurity and fetal growth retardation to low birthweight in developing and developed societies. *Am J Obstet Gynecol* 1982;143:793–8.
14. World Health Organization. World malaria situation 1984. *World Health Stat Q* 1988;41:64–73.
15. Meuris S, Mavoungou D, Polliotti P. Malaria: la fin d'un règne multimillénaire. *Pathol Biol* 1986;34:886–92.
16. Wickramasuryia GAW. Clinical features of malaria in pregnancy. In: Wickramasuryia GAW, ed. *Malaria and ankylostomiasis in the pregnant woman*. London: Oxford University Press, 1937;5–90.

17. Le Van Hung. Paludisme et grossesse à Saigon. *Rev Paludisme Med Trop* 1951;83:75–112.
18. Menon R. Pregnancy and malaria. *Med J Malaysia* 1972;27:115–9.
19. Clark HC. The diagnostic value of the placental blood film in aestivo-autumnal malaria. *J Exp Med* 1915;22:427–45.
20. Blacklock DB, Gordon RM. Malaria infection as it occurs in late pregnancy: its relationship to labour and early infancy. *Ann Trop Med Parasitol* 1925;19:327–65.
21. Brabin BJ. An analysis of malaria in pregnancy in Africa. *Bull WHO* 1983;61:1005–16.
22. Bray RS, Sinden RE. The sequestration of plasmodium falciparum infected erythrocytes in the placenta. *Trans R Soc Trop Med Hyg* 1979;73:716–9.
23. Trager W, Rudzinska MA, Bradbury P. The fine structure of Plasmodium falciparum and its host erythrocytes in natural malarial infections in man. *Bull WHO* 1966;35:883–92.
24. Perrin LH, Mackey LM, Miescher PA. Hematology of malaria in man. *Semin Hematol* 1982;19:70–81.
25. McGregor IA. Epidemiology, malaria and pregnancy. *Am J Trop Med Hyg* 1984;78:1–8.
26. Brabin BJ, Nagel J, Hagenaars AM, Ruitenberg E, Van Tilborgh AMJC. The influence of malaria and gestation on the immune response to one and two doses of adsorbed tetanus toxoid in pregnancy. *Bull WHO* 1984;62:919–30.
27. McGregor IA, Rowe DS, Wilson ME, Billewicz WZ. Plasma immunoglobulin concentrations in an African (Gambian) community in relation to season, malaria and other infections and pregnancy. *Clin Exp Immunol* 1970;7:51–74.
28. Bray RS, Anderson MJ. Falciparum malaria and pregnancy. *Trans R Soc Trop Med Hyg* 1979;73:427–31.
29. Gilles HM, Lawson JB, Sibelas M, Voller A, Allan N. Malaria, anaemia and pregnancy. *Ann Trop Med Parasitol* 1969;63:245–63.
30. Maroulis GB, Buckley RH, Younger JB. Serum immunoglobulin concentrations during normal pregnancy. *Am J Obstet Gynecol* 1971;109:972–6.
31. Galbraith RM, Faulk WP, Galbraith GMP, Holbrook TW, Bray RS. The human materno-foetal relationship in malaria: 1. Identification of pigment and parasites in the placenta. *Trans R Soc Trop Med Hyg* 1979;74:52–62.
32. Walter P, Garin Y, Blot P. Placental pathologic changes in malaria: a histologic and ultrastructural study. *Am J Pathol* 1982;109:332–44.
33. Covell G. Congenital malaria. *Trop Dis Bull* 1950;47:1147–67.
34. McGregor IA, Wilson ME, Billewicz WZ. Malaria infection of the placenta in the Gambia, West Africa: its incidence and relationship to stillbirth, birthweight and placental weight. *Trans R Soc Trop Med Hyg* 1983;2:232–44.
35. Watkinson M, Rushton DI. Plasmodial pigmentation of placenta and outcome of pregnancy in West African mothers. *Br Med J* 1983;287:251–4.
36. Bruce-Chwatt LJ. Malaria in African infants and children in Southern Nigeria. *Ann Trop Med Parasitol* 1952;46:173–200.
37. Archibald HM. Influence of malarial infection of the placenta on the incidence of prematurity. *Bull WHO* 1956;15:842–5.
38. Archibald HM. Influence of maternal malaria on newborn infants. *Br Med J* 1958;2:1512–4.
39. Cannon DSH. Malaria and prematurity in the Western Region of Nigeria. *Br Med J* 1958;2:877–8.
40. Spitz AJW. Malaria infection of the placenta and its influence on the incidence of prematurity in Eastern Nigeria. *Bull WHO* 1958;21:242–4.
41. McLaren DS, Ward PG. Malaria infection of the placenta and foetal nutrition. *East Afr Med J* 1962;39:182–9.
42. Jelliffe EFP. Low birthweight and malarial infection of the placenta. *Bull WHO* 1968;38:69–78.
43. Jilly P. Anaemia in parturient women, with special reference to malaria infection of the placenta. *Ann Trop Med Parasitol* 1969;63:109–11.
44. Kortmann HFCM. Malaria and pregnancy. M.D. Thesis, University of Amsterdam. Utrecht: Drukkerij Elinkwijk, 1972.
45. Reinhardt MC, Ambroise-Thomas P, Cavallo-Serra R, Meylan C, Gautier R. Malaria at delivery in Abidjan. *Helv Paediatr Acta* 1978;33:65–84.
46. Walter P, Garin JF, Blot Ph. Placenta et paludisme: étude morphologique, parasitologique et clinique. *J Gynecol Obst Biol Reprod* 1981;10:535–42.
47. Brody S, Carlström G. Immuno-assay of human chorionic gonadotropin in normal and pathologic pregnancy. *J Clin Endocrinol* 1962;22:564–74.

48. Chandra RK. Fetal malnutrition and postnatal immunocompetence. *Am J Dis Child* 1975;129: 450–4.
49. McLaren DS. Records of birth weight and prematurity in the Wasukuma of Lake Province Tanganyika. *Trans R Soc Trop Med Hyg* 1959;53:173–8.
50. McGregor JD, Avery JG. Malaria transmission and fetal growth. *Br Med J* 1974;3:433–6.
51. Watkinson M, Rushton DI, Lunn PG. Placental malaria and foetoplacental function: low plasma oestradiol associated with malarial pigmentation of the placenta. *Trans R Soc Trop Med Hyg* 1985;79:448–50.
52. Mavoungou D, Walter P, Gass R, Billiault X, Meuris S, Collet M, Roth-Meyer C, Polliotti B. Umbilical serum levels of steroid hormones in relation to spontaneous labour and vaginal delivery: influence of malaria. In: Proceedings of the 5th World Congress on Human Reproduction, 1985.
53. Polliotti B, Meuris S, Mavoungou D, Walter P. Influence of placental malarial lesions on maternal serum levels of human chorionic gonadotrophin, placental lactogen and estriol. *Placenta* 1986;7:490.
54. Taufa T. Malaria and pregnancy. *Papua New Guinea Med J* 1978;21:197–206.
55. Antonov NA. Children born during the siege of Leningrad, 1942. *J Pediatr* 1947;30:250–5.
56. Smith CA. Effect of wartime starvation in Holland upon pregnancy and its product. *Am J Obstet Gynecol* 1947;53:599–608.
57. Gebre-Medhin M, Gurovsky S, Bondestam L. Association of maternal age and parity with birth weight, sex ratio, still birth and multiple births. *J Trop Paediatr Environ Child Health* 1976;22: 99–102.
58. Gebre-Medhin M, Sterky G, Taube A. Observation on intrauterine growth in urban Ethiopia. *Acta Paediatr Scand* 1978;67:781–9.
59. Gebre-Medhin M, Gobezie A. Dietary intake in the third trimester of pregnancy and birth weight of offspring among non-priviledged women. *Am J Clin Nutr* 1975;28:1322–9.
60. Naeye RL, Dozer A, Tafari N, Ross SM. Epidemiological features in perinatal death due to obstructed labour in Addis Ababa. *Br J Obstet Gynaecol* 1977;84:747–50.
61. Morley D, Knox G. The birth weights of Yoruba babies. *J Obstet Gynaecol* 1960;67:975–80.
62. Tafari N, Naeye RL, Gobezie A. Effects of maternal undernutrition and heavy physical work during pregnancy on birthweight. *Br J Obstet Gynaecol* 1980;87:222–6.
63. Naeye RL, Tafari N. Biologic bases for international fetal growth curves. *Acta Paediatr Scand* 1985; Suppl. 319:164–9.
64. Taggart NR, Holliday RM, Billewicz WZ, Hytten FE, Thompson AM. Changes in skinfold thickness during pregnancy. *Br J Nutr* 1967;21:439–51.
65. Royston E. The prevalence of nutritional anaemia in women in developing countries: a critical review of available information. *World Health Stat Q* 1985;38:52–75.
66. Bégué P, Capochichi D. Les nouveaux-nés de petit poids de naissance au Togo. I. Classification en fonction de l'âge gestationnel, à partir de 888 cas. *Ann Pediatr* 1979;26:639–51.
67. Kessel E, Sastrawinata S, Mumford SD. Correlates of fetal growth and survival. *Acta Paediatr Scand* 1985;Suppl. 319:120–7.
68. Rodriguez MH, Jungery M. A protein on plasmodium falciparum-infected erythrocytes functions as a transferrin receptor. *Nature* 1986;324:388–91.
69. Flint J, Hill AVS, Bowden DK, et al. High frequencies of alpha-thalassaemia are the result of natural selection by malaria. *Nature* 1986;321:744–50.
70. Pasvol G. The interaction between sickle haemoglobin and the malarial parasite plasmodium falciparum. *Trans R Soc Trop Med Hyg* 1980;74:701–5.
71. Brabin BJ, Perrin L. Sickle-cell trait and plasmodium falciparum parasitaemia in pregnancy in Western Province, Kenya. *Trans R Soc Trop Med Hyg* 1985;79:733.
72. van Dongen PWJ, van't Hof. Sickle cell trait, malaria and anaemia in pregnant Zambian women. *Trans R Soc Trop Med Hyg* 1983;77:402–4.
73. Serjeant GR. Sickle haemoglobulin and pregnancy. *Br Med J* 1983;287:628–30.
74. Roopnarinesingh S, Ramsewak S. Decreased birthweight and femur length in fetuses of patients with the sickle-cell trait. *Obstet Gynecol* 1986;68:46–8.
75. Hoff C, Wertelecki W, Dutt J, Hernandez R, Reyes E, Sharp M. Sickle-cell trait, maternal age and pregnancy outcome in primiparous women. *Human Biol* 1984;55:763–70.
76. Bwibo NO. Birthweights of infants of teenage mothers in Nairobi. *Acta Paediatr Scand* 1985;Suppl. 319:89–94.

77. Rehan NE, Tafida DS. Low birthweight in Hausa infants. *Nigerian Med J* 1976;6:324–6.
78. Latham MC, Robson JRK. Birthweight and prematurity in Tanzania. *Trans R Soc Trop Med Hyg* 1960;60:791–6.
79. Fadahunsi O. Low birthweight and maturity in the Nigerian infant. *Nigerian Med J* 1976;6:324–6.
80. Nylander PPS. Perinatal mortality in Ibadan. *Afr J Med Sci* 1971;2:173–8.
81. Bégué P, Assimadi K, Capochichi D. Les nouveau-nés de petits poids de naissance au Togo. II. Essai d'appréciation de différents facteurs étiologiques. *Ann Pediatr* 1979;26:647–51.
82. Adelusi B, Lapido OA. Preterm and other babies with low birthweights in Ibadan. *Trop Geogr Med* 1976;28:316–22.

Intrauterine Growth Retardation, edited by
Jacques Senterre. Nestlé Nutrition Workshop
Series, Vol. 18. Nestec Ltd., Vevey/Raven Press,
Ltd., New York © 1989.

Intrauterine Growth Retardation in India and Bangladesh

Cipriano A. Canosa

Department of Pediatrics, Children's Hospital "La Fe," 46009 Valencia, Spain

INTRODUCTION

The birthweight (BW) of a newborn infant is probably the most important single factor that affects his/her survival and quality of life (1–8). Birthweight is determined by two factors: the duration of gestation and the amount of intrauterine growth; therefore birthweight can be modified by variation in combinations of these factors (9–11). The birth of a baby at less than 37 weeks of gestation (preterm), and poor intrauterine growth [intrauterine growth retardation (IUGR)], are responsible for low birthweight (LBW) (12–14). The various possible combinations of gestational length and rate of intrauterine growth (preterm, term, and post-term; appropriate, small, or large for the gestational age) produce nine well-defined and characterized clinical pictures (7,9,10). The duration of gestation and intrauterine growth are determined by the health and nutritional status of the mother. Maternal malnutrition, ill health, and physical and emotional stress are the most frequent causes of prematurity and IUGR (13). These phenomena occur during the most critical and vulnerable period of life, the perinatal period (5,14–17).

Until 1976, prematurity was defined as less than 37 weeks gestation with a birthweight of 2,500 g or less. After 1976 LBW was defined as a birthweight of less than 2,500 g (up to and including 2,499) regardless of gestational age (9,13).

The World Health Organization (WHO) strategy to attain the objective "Health for All by the Year 2000" (HFA 2000), unanimously acclaimed by all members states in Alma Alta in 1978 (18), identified 12 health indicators. The eighth health indicator states that the nutritional status of children is adequate if:

1. At least 90% of newborn infants have a birthweight of at least 2,500 g
2. At least 90% of children have a weight appropriate for his/her gestational age.

Eleven years are left for these goals to be achieved. The developing countries are characterized, among other factors, by low income, low literacy rate, poverty, poor environmental conditions, high fertility rates, population explosion, elevated indices of LBW and IUGR, and high perinatal, neonatal, and infant mortality and morbidity rates (7,19–24). Another characteristic of these countries is the limited amount of reliable health statistics and epidemiological information. The values and figures available are in some instances estimated guesses. However, to attain the "HFA 2000" goal, it becomes imperative not only to know the incidence and prevalence of LBW, but also to document and periodically monitor the effectiveness of the action programs to be implemented. In the developed countries, the situation is just the opposite: high income and literacy, low fertility rates, stagnation of the population growth, and low IUGR and infant mortality rates (25,26).

It has been estimated that in 1979, there were 21 million LBW infants born in the world, representing 17% of all births, the vast majority of which were born in the developing countries (13,21). Negative consequences and serious handicaps among LBW infants are often found and could be irreversible. These are responsible for the high morbidity and mortality rates in the infants (4,7,9,11,20,23,27–32,37). Numerous pathological conditions are the direct consequence of LBW: respiratory distress syndrome, broncho-pulmonary dysplasia, cardiovascular disorders, neonatal infections, retarded physical growth and development, and impairment of the central nervous system (1–3,8,33–41). The alterations in the brain are responsible for abnormalities which affect behavior, personality, and mental development.

In the developing countries, it is imperative to reduce drastically the LBW, IUGR, and perinatal and infantile mortality rates, and, in the developed world, to further reduce IUGR and to secure the quality of life of survivors.

MATERIAL AND METHODS

India has the second largest population of any country in the world, after the Republic of China (21). Indian health statistics and demographic information are in most cases estimated guesses. In 1973 India had an estimated population of 500 million people; in 1983, 730 million; and it is expected to reach 1 billion by the year 2000 (21). Almost 20 million births occur every year. It is believed that 7 to 10 million LBW infants are born every year in India (29).

India has a wide variety of races, climates, languages, and cultural, social, and economic classes. The caste system still exists in many parts of the country. All these factors make it impossible to generalize about information on health statistics, and specifically on LBW. Most of the data come from hospital records which are in some cases of dubious validity. The birth rate is 32:1000 (22), the infant mortality rate 123:1000, and the illiteracy rate 70%. Approximately 80% of the population lives in rural settings and it is estimated that 90% to 95% of all deliveries are attended by untrained and mostly illiterate traditional birth attendants (12,42). Annual income per capita is $180 in United States currency. The main causes of neonatal mortality are birth asphyxia, LBW, infections, and neonatal tetanus (13,19,32,33, 37,39,43–47).

Bangladesh is among the poorest countries in the world, with the lowest socio-cultural, economic, and health indicators (13,48,49). It is one of the most densely populated countries in the world, with an uncontrolled and explosive population growth. As there is no civil registry, it is impossible to obtain reliable information on health statistics. It was estimated that at the time of a perinatal survey in 1983 Bangladesh had a population of 94 million inhabitants, and in 1986 it was estimated at 100 million. Its capital, Dhaka, has approximately 5.5 million inhabitants. The country has a predominantly tropical climate, with mean temperatures oscillating between 15 and 45°C, and a relative humidity during monsoon months of 85% to 95%. It is estimated that 85% to 90% of the population live in rural areas and are mainly engaged in primitive rice monoculture throughout the year. The illiteracy rate is estimated at 65% to 70% of the population, with wide differences between males and females. Over 90% of the population is Moslem and the remaining are mainly of Hindu origin. Home deliveries in rural areas are believed to account for 85% to 90% of all births, mostly attended by untrained and illiterate traditional birth attendants.

The first source of information was the MEDLINE search from 1966 through 1987, and an EMED search from 1973 through 1985, aimed at identifying all Indian and Bangladesh perinatal studies related to birthweight. MEDLINE provided a list of 191 publications, and EMED 187. The publications from the two sources were not similar. The second source of information was provided by the Advance MCH Centre, Department of Community Medicine, Chandigarh, India, 1986, ''Low Birthweight, Incidence and Mortality, 1954–1986.'' A total of 121 publications was identified. The third and final source was the WHO *World Health Statistics Quarterly* which also provided valuable information. A systematic effort was made to incorporate all reliable information published in Indian as well as in other international journals. From the three sources, a selection of 176 Indian and Bangladeshi publications were scrutinized. Only 38 Indian references were selected, and these form the basis of the Indian data in this chapter.

Only three publications from Bangladesh were available, incorporating a small number of infants (13,48,49). A perinatal survey was organized in 1983 to obtain a larger sample of newborns from urban and rural settings. The outcome of this survey is the basis of the Bangladesh data.

Obviously there were different objectives, methodologies, and types of analyses in these publications, which gave rise to difficulties in achieving a coherent analysis and interpretation of the data. A determined effort was made to incorporate the widest possible geographical representation, standardization of methodology, and easy comparison of the results. Publications with fewer than 100 reported cases were not incorporated. Source, year, mean birthweight, standard deviation, sample size, gestational age, newborn characteristics, morbidity, and perinatal, early neonatal, neonatal, and infant mortality rates were reported when available. An attempt was also made to follow up etiological factors of LBW and IUGR in newborns in order to determine patterns of physical growth and development. In some publications, when this information was not specified as such, it was possible to calculate it from tables and graphs. Numerous Indian authors defined LBW as those with birthweight less than or equal to 2,250 g. However, they provided the BW distribution, which allowed us to draw up these tables. In some instances definitions of perinatal, early neonatal, neonatal, and infant mortality rates were also confusing. Birthweight surrogates were also investigated.

Numerous personal visits to widely distributed departments of obstetrics and pediatrics, public health institutions, and rural health facilities in India and Bangladesh were resolutely carried out in order to interpret the available information in the best possible way. This approach provided the insight that made us aware of the existence of numerous difficulties: lack of equipment and trained personnel and logistical obstacles which had to be solved in order to be able to collect and interpret LBW and IUGR data and to overcome socio-cultural taboos. The difficulties of obtaining BW within the first 24 hr of birth in isolated and primitive rural communities where no available health facilities or personnel are available must be considered before unwarranted and superficial criticisms are made. Important socio-cultural barriers to carrying out these studies exist among the vast majority of rural, illiterate, poor, and isolated families and communities.

Bangladesh lacks reliable health statistics. There are only three references on neonates in the medical literature, and they involve 193 infants (2,13,49). In 1983, during a 3-month period, a perinatal survey was conducted to obtain information on birthweight. All mothers delivering live newborns during this period were examined 7 days a week throughout the study by one person (C. A. Canosa). Ten public health midwives (PHM) were selected, trained, and supervised. These midwives, who worked in attendance with the principal investigator, were responsible for all rural home deliveries and also acted as interpreters. Male observers were not allowed to be present during deliveries. "Ad hoc" questionnaires were drawn up for the survey, collecting 50 quantifiable variables. Following standard procedures, all newborns were examined naked during the first 24 hr of life. In spite of the low socio-cultural background of the mothers, their last menstrual period was accurately obtained using patient questioning. Beam scales with ± 100 g sensitivity were used. Standardization of scales was observed daily. Fiberglass tapes were utilized and changed every 30 days. Anthropometric examination of the mothers was carried out in upright position within 24 hr of delivery. Mothers' weight was always obtained when they were fully clothed in their normal dress. Twenty-five representative local women's garments were weighed, but these weights were not subtracted from the reported maternal weights. An attempt was made to study the same ethnic group. Various socio-cultural backgrounds, as well as urban and rural populations, were incorporated. Great efforts were made to collect the following variables: delivery identification and classification; hospital, urban, rural, and home delivery; gestational age; fertility history; economic status; identification of factors affecting BW; mother's illnesses during gestation; and the anthropometry of mothers and newborns obtained with 24 hr of birth.

RESULTS

India

From a total of 176 reviewed publications, only 38 are quoted; 138 were excluded because they were not considered suitable for this presentation, mainly because the methodology, identification and definition of variables, standardization procedures, and quality control were of dubious quality and/or confusing. In some reports no specifications were made as to how the samples had been obtained, or for how long, or what type of sample had been studied (total, random, etc.).

In Table 1, the 38 studies are presented, incorporating 125,816 cases. The studies are chronologically organized from 1960 to 1984. The following variables are docu-

TABLE 1. *India incidence of low birthweight, 1960–1986*

Region	Ref.	Year	Source	No. of births	L-S	GA week	Mean BW	SD	$\leq 2,000$	$\leq 2,500$	$\leq 3,000$	$> 3,000$
Delhi	61	1960	H	1,000	L	37	2,520	—	11.4	40.4	—	—
Agra	51	1961	H	500	L-S	—	3,069	590	13.0	26.4	41.0	20.0
Gwalior	53	1961	H	2,927	L	—	2,893	—	3.7	18.6	57.4	20.3
Delhi	42	1962	H	2,695	L-S	—	2,730	—	8.0	29.3	62.7	—
Madras	19	1962	HT	5,298	L-S	—	2.736	—	—	29.5	45.0	—
Pondicherry	58	1962	H	106	L	—	2,750	—	5.2	28.1	66.7	—
Bombay	59	1963	HR	1,270	L	37	2,578	—	—	22.6	—	—
Punjab	62	1963	H	8,023	L	—	2,900	—	—	24.1	—	—
Delhi	12	1963	H	1,000	L-S	—	—	—	—	40.4	—	—
Calcutta	24	1964	H	1,785	S	—	2,870	550	4.5	28.0	62.0	4.5
Goa	56	1965	H	3,851	—	—	2,780	410	5.7	23.0	63.0	8.3
Agra	63	1968	H	1,398	L	—	2,780	200	6.6	26.5	59.6	7.3
Kanpur	64	1967	HT	1,009	L	—	2,488	485	13.8	44.5	41.7	—
Varanasi	50	1967	H	447	L	—	2,493	580	21.0	33.6	28.2	17.0
Assam	27	1967	HT	1,086	—	—	2,535	508	13.6	31.8	39.4	15.2
Bombay	20	1967	H	10,000	L	37	2,560	—	11.9	31.1	41.4	15.6
North India	65	1968	H	1,470	L	—	—	—	8.8	28.2	36.5	26.5
Delhi	55	1968	H	4,100	L-S	37	2,680	—	6.1	30.0	—	—
Hyderabad	66	1968	H	3,124	L-S	37	2,710	—	10.3	33.3	34.9	21.5
10 states	67	1969	H	10,756	L-S	37	2,748	536	7.8	30.5	49.5	12.2
Kanpur	64	1969	HT	900	L	37	2,725	340	13.3	31.1	42.3	13.2
Tirupati	68	1969	H	1,000	L	37	2,730	545	7.6	24.7	65.5	2.2
Delhi	69	1970	H	9,000	L-S	37	2,547	—	11.3	48.2	—	—
Bombay	46	1970	H	1,000	—	—	2,636	467	7.0	31.2	42.3	19.5
Rajastan	70	1970	HT	1,651	L	37	2,777	483	6.2	24.5	45.6	23.7
Delhi	71	1971	HT	8,146	L	37	2,648	530	7.6	35.5	—	—
Varanasi	68	1971	H	510	L	—	2,423	325	—	60.5	—	—
Ahmedabad	47	1972	HT	12,811	L	—	—	—	—	24.5	—	—
Calcutta	45	1975	H	1,165	L-S	—	2,541	560	9.9	45.0	35.0	10.1
Pondicherry	58	1976	H-HOM	558	L	—	2,625	498	5.0	22.2	72.8	—
Delhi	72	1977	H	6,026	L	37	2,829	—	2.7	22.9	68.7	5.7
Bokaro	43	1978	H	5,340	—	—	—	—	9.5	45.4	—	—
Delhi	60	1978	H	4,325	—	—	2,812	284	5.5	22.7	36.5	35.3
Agra	40	1980	H	925	L-S	37	2,497	284	—	31.4	8.2	—
Ahjmer	52	1981	HT	2,931	—	37	—	—	—	80.5	—	—
Delhi	73	1982	H	6,222	L	—	2,745	380	—	27.5	—	—
Wardha	33	1984	H	1,461	L	—	2,684	450	9.8	34.9	—	—

BW, birthweight; GA, gestational age; H, hospital delivery; H-HOM, hospital-home; HR, hospital-rural; HT, total hospital sample; L, live; L-S, live-single; S, single.

TABLE 2. *Intrauterine growth retardation (IUGR) among low birthweight (LBW) newborns*

Ref.	Region	Year	Source	L-S	No.	Mean BW	LBW (%)	IUGR (%)
55	Delhi	1970	H	L-S	4,100	2,652	35.5	78.3
17	Hyderabad	1970	H	L-S	860	2,741	36.9	80.0
54	Delhi	1973	H	L	9,000	2,542	48.2	81.1
28	Chandigarh	1975	H	L	5,465	2,647	25.7	67.2
56	Agra	1980	H	L	925	2,494	36.2	76.4

L-S, live-single; BW, birthweight; H, hospital delivery; L, live.

TABLE 3. *Delivery distribution by gestational age*
[data from Bhargava et al., 1985 (21)]

	Author				
	Sheth	Ghosh	Singh	Sheth	Babson
Year	1972	1979	1974	1972	1970
Place	Bombay	Delhi	Delhi	Bombay	USA
Source	Hospital	Urban	Hospital	Hospital	Hospital
	Low SE	community	High SE	High SE	
n	5,336	6,023	3,550	1,242	40,000
GA (week)					
28	0.22	0.12	—	0.48	0.19
29	0.16	0.02	—	0.24	0.10
30	0.34	0.08	0.59	0.32	0.20
31	0.64	0.10	—	0.32	0.17
32	1.09	0.32	—	0.64	0.26
33	1.89	0.86	1.04	1.21	0.57
34	2.34	1.78	1.24	1.37	0.79
35	4.05	2.62	1.18	2.42	2.10
36	11.60	4.10	3.32	8.37	3.75
37	37.01	7.90	5.18	16.59	9.40
38	26.26	15.11	14.37	41.87	16.52
39	9.48	22.55	18.08	25.76	39.23
40	4.87	21.07	38.56	—	15.12
41	—	11.26	10.20	—	7.86
42	—	5.08	4.37	—	2.20
43	—	2.82	1.46	—	0.57
44	—	4.22	—	—	—
≤ 36	22.33	10.00	7.37	7.1	5.35
37–41	77.67	77.88	86.80	92.9	84.02
≥ 42	–	12.12	5.83	—	10.63

SE, socioeconomic level; GA, gestational age.
Data from refs. 57–60, 74.

mented: region, year, source, number of cases, and characteristics of newborns (gestational age, mean birthweight, standard deviation and its distribution). All were hospital cases except for one reference which incorporated home deliveries. Sample size varied between 106 and 12,811 newborns. The lowest reported mean birthweight was 2,423 g in Varanasi in 1971 (50); the highest was 3,069 g in Agra in 1961 (51). The highest incidence of LBW was 80.5%, reported from Ajmer in 1981 (52), and the lowest was 22.3% in Gwalior in 1961 (53).

Table 2 shows the reported incidence of IUGR among LBW newborns from five reports (17,28,54–56). The sample size was 20,350 cases. LBW incidence varied between 25.7% and 48.2%, and among these the IUGR rate varied between 67.2% and 81.1%. Many of the unquoted publications showed that the vast majority of LBW newborns were suffering IUGR. However, precise figures were not given.

In Table 3, birthweight distribution by gestational age is represented by five different samples between 1970 and 1979, involving 56,151 infants. Two Bombay samples are reported by the same author [Sheth (57)] during the same year, one belonging to a high socioeconomic group and the other to a low social group. There are also two studies from Delhi [Ghosh (58), Singh (59)], one representing an urban community of low socioeconomic status, the other a hospital sample of high social class. A U.S.A. reference [Babson (60)] is also shown. Prematurity was highest (22.3%) among the lowest socioeconomic groups and lowest (7.1%) in the high social class group (which was similar to the control group from the U.S.A.).

Table 4 presents data on early neonatal mortality collected from 22 centers between 1962 and 1986. A total of 123,154 neonates are included. In seven of the reporting centers there was 100% early neonatal mortality in infants weighing 1,000 g or less and in 18 centers mortality was over 80% in this weight category. Early neonatal mortality in the weight group 2,500–3,000 g was between 0.3 and 4.5% of the total population.

Figures 1 and 2 show weight and height gains from birth to 6 years of age. It can be seen that both weight and height are lowest in the IUGR group, followed by the preterm group. The Indian control group is lighter and shorter than the group from the U.S.A. The curves are parallel to each other, showing no evidence of the catch-up phenomenon (29).

Table 5 shows a correlation matrix between birthweight; head, chest, and abdominal circumferences; and length. It can be seen that the highest correlation coefficient observed is between birthweight and chest circumference, $r = 0.87$, and between mid-arm circumference and chest circumference, $r = 0.90$. Correlation between head circumference and chest circumference was also high ($r = 0.74$). The highest correlation coefficients observed among all neonatal anthropometric variables were related to chest circumference (61).

Bangladesh

Between February 18th and April 22nd, 1983, a perinatal survey was carried out in four different Bangladeshi institutions, which were identified with the help and

TABLE 4. *Indian birthweight vs. early neonatal mortality (%), 1962–1986*

Place	Year	Source	No.	L-S	≤ 1,000	≤ 2,000	≤ 2,500	≤ 3,000	> 3,000
Delhi	1962	H	2,695	L-S	96.5	48.4	2.6	0.4	
Delhi	1963	H	1,000	L-S	100.0	38.2	2.0	0.7	
Lucknow	1966	H	1,000	L-S	—	—	—	3.9	2.3
North India	1968	H	1,470	L	100.0	22.2	5.4	4.5	—
Kanpur	1969	H	7,357	L	—	35.7	4.3	—	4.9
10 states	1969	H	10,756	L-S	—	28.4	4.8	—	
Ahmedabad	1969	HT	1,000	—	—	56.0	4.9	4.4	
Delhi	1969	R	1,910	L	44.8	14.3	3.4	0.9	
Hyderabad	1970	H	270	L	46.7	35.5	14.0	—	—
Hyderabad	1972	H	3,792	L	100.0	7.43	29.6	3.5	
Delhi	1973	H	9,000	L	86.2	12.3	9.1	3.0	
Gulbarga	1974	H	1,600	L	100.0	60.4	6.5	—	
Chandigargh	1975	H	5,465	L	88.5	48.3	3.9	0.8	
Pondicherry	1976	H	558	L	—	21.4	4.8	3.6	
Delhi	1977	H	25,878	L	96.5	48.0	2.2	0.7	0.9
South India	1978	H	10,691	L-S	—	24.0	1.2	0.6	
Delhi	1979	H	5,598	—	100.0	26.4	1.2	0.3	
Ajmer	1981	HT	2,931	L	—	47.2	22.1	1.0	
Delhi	1982	H	6,222	L-S	54.6	4.1	1.4	1.2	
Allahabad	1982	HT	2,500	—	82.0	24.3	6.3	1.6	
Warha	1984	HR	1,461	L	100.0	71.4	27.4	2.9	
Madras	1986	HT	20,000	L	100.0	47.5	7.1	0.9	

H, hospital delivery; HR, hospital-rural; HT, total hospital sample; L, live; L-S, live-single.

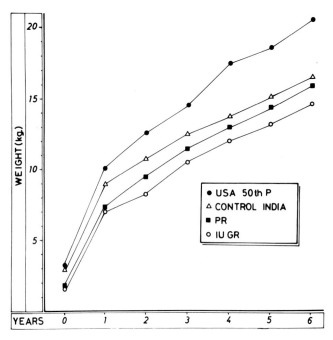

FIG. 1. Weight gain in control, preterm, and intrauterine growth retarded newborns. (From ref. 29.)

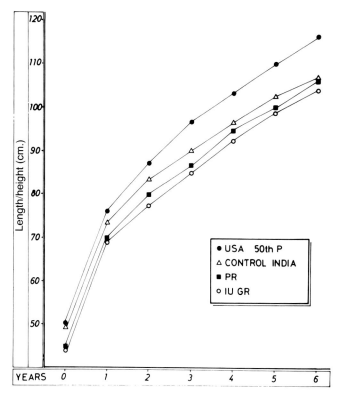

FIG. 2. Length/height gain in control, preterm, and intrauterine growth retarded newborns. (From ref. 29.)

TABLE 5. *Correlation matrix between anthropometric variables in newborns in hospital sample (n = 520)*

	Mid-arm circumference	Birthweight	Head circumference	Chest	Length
Birthweight (g)	0.8110				
Head circumference (cm)	0.6240	0.7264			
Chest circumference (cm)	0.8998	0.8696	0.7243		
Length (cm)	0.6808	0.8023	0.7417	0.7869	
Abdomen (cm)	0.7113	0.7705	0.5963	0.8052	0.6505

From ref. 29.

collaboration of the Authorities of the Ministry of Health, the Institute of Public Health Nutrition (IPHN), and Dhaka Medical College. The collaboration of the personnel at all levels from all institutions was outstanding and was responsible for the successful implementation of the survey.

The survey was performed in the following institutions:

1. Holy Family Hospital in Dhaka, a private 300-bed hospital, "the best in the country," caring for upper-middle-class families. The daily hospital bed cost was $70 in United States currency. A total of 114 consecutive mother-infant pairs (100%) of the deliveries during the survey period were studied by the same observer (CAC).
2. Azimpur Maternity Hospital in Dhaka, a public health facility catering to lower-middle-class citizens. Prenatal, delivery, and neonatal care is carried out only by female obstetric personnel in this hospital. A total of 365 consecutive mother-live born infant pairs were examined (100%). The principal researcher (CAC) was not allowed to be present during the deliveries.
3. The Manikganj Thana Health Complex. Manikganj is an isolated and primitive rural community, located 45 miles northeast of Dhaka, with a population of approximately 8,000 inhabitants, mostly engaged in agricultural activities. The health complex has six obstetric beds. During the period of observation, all consecutive mother-live born infant pairs were studied by the same observer (CAC). A total of 41 pairs were studied (100%).
4. Home deliveries were also included. These were drawn only from the surrounding Manikganj rural area. The population probably belongs to the lowest social group of Bangladesh. Six specially trained public health midwives are responsible for the identification and examination of mothers and live-born infants within 24 hr of birth. The collaboration and participation of local traditional birth attendants was fundamental for carrying out this survey, and without their help and advice it would not have been possible. Portable beam scales were used by the midwives to weigh the babies in the homes. Scale standardization was done *in situ* before each determination. A total of 104 mother-infant pairs were studied by the public health midwives.

Validation of the Sample

The number of deliveries at the different institutions during the 3-month study period was similar to the numbers delivered during the equivalent 3-month period in the previous year. The proportion of the total yearly deliveries in the various study centers was 35.7% for the high social class urban group, 28.7% for the mid-low social class urban group, and 41.5% for the higher class rural group (Health Center deliveries). It is not known how representative the home deliveries were of the total home delivery population. On average, 6.5 neonates were examined daily at Azimpur Hospital, 2.3 at Holy Family Hospital, 1.1 home deliveries, and 0.4 at Mankiganj Thana Health Complex. That is 10.3 mother-infant pairs daily.

TABLE 6. *Bangladesh perinatal survey, 1983: socioeconomic classification*

Social group	n	Income per capita (U.S. $)		Years of school			Age of marriage	
		Mean	SD	0	Mean	SD	Mean	SD
1. High urban	114	140.8	101.5	4.3	10.4	3.6	19.8	13.1
2. Low urban	365	45.4	50.1*	54.8	3.3	4.0*	15.4	3.1*
3. High rural	41	45.7	36.5*	41.5	5.1	5.0*	15.6	2.8*
4. Low rural	104	32.04	28.6*	60.6	2.1	3.1*	15.2	2.3*
Total	624							

*$p < 0.001$.

Of the 50 variables collected, only 15 are analyzed in this paper. Insoluble difficulties were encountered that made it impossible to collect the required information in all cases, particularly in the rural areas. Pre-delivery weight, blood pressure, and hemoglobin were only rarely obtained in the rural cases.

Sample Characteristics

Of the 624 newborns, 324 were males (52%) and 300 females (48%). Mean male birthweight was $2,633 \pm 464$ g; $2,545 \pm 510$ g for females. The differences are statistically significant, $p<0.05$.

Socioeconomic Classification

Table 6 shows the socioeconomic classification for the four groups. Income "per capita" in U.S. dollars, mother's years of schooling, and age at marriage were selected as socioeconomic indicators. Mean values, standard deviation (SD), and statistical significance are shown. Income "per capita" was 3.5 times higher in the high social class urban group compared with the other groups. Illiteracy was 4.3% in the high social class urban group and 60.6% in the lowest rural social class group. Years of school attendance were also markedly different between the two groups: 10.4 years and 2.1 years for the high and low social class groups, respectively. Mean age of marriage was 19.8 years for the high social class urban group and 15.2 years for the low social class rural group. The differences for these three variables between the high and low socioeconomic groups are all statistically significant, $p<0.001$.

Table 7 shows the cumulative frequency distribution of mothers' age at marriage. At 16 years of age, 29.6 of the high social class urban mothers were married versus 78.8% for the low social class rural mothers. It is not known exactly when the marriages were consummated; however, it was common to find that the "first seen"

TABLE 7. Bangladesh perinatal survey, 1983: mothers' age at marriage (years), cumulative frequency distribution

Social group	n	≤ 10	10.1– 12	12.1– 14	14.1– 16	16.1– 18	18.1– 20	20.1– 22	22.1– 24	24.1– 26	26.1– 28	≥ 28.1	Mean	SD
1. High urban	114	2.6	3.4	9.5	29.6	52.4	71.7	86.6	91.8	92.6	97.8	100	19.8	13.5
2. Low urban	363	6.1	17.9	33.6	68.6	89.0	95.1	98.4	99.8	100	—	—	15.4	3.1
3. High rural	41	7.3	12.2	29.3	53.3	92.3	100	—	—	—	—	—	15.6	2.8
4. Low rural	104	4.8	8.6	31.7	78.8	94.2	98	100	—	—	—	—	15.2	2.3
Total	622	5.3	13.3	28.6	62.2	83.4	91.6	96.6	98.4	99.0	100	—	16.2	6.6

menstrual period occurred several years after the mother already had had 2 to 3 pregnancies. The difference in age of marriage between the high social class urban mothers and the other three groups was statistically significant, $p<0.001$.

Table 8 shows maternal anthropometry results: weight before and after delivery, height and arm circumference. Mean dress weight for all groups was 1.3 kg, which has to be deducted from the mean reported weight. No information was available for pre-delivery weight in the rural women since they did not attend prenatal clinics. Pre-delivery weight in the high social class urban group was 58.6 ± 9.5 kg, and 49.7 ± 6.2 in the low social class urban group. The differences are statistically significant, $p<0.001$. The mothers' weight after delivery was 51.9 ± 9.4 kg in the high social class urban group, and 41.0 ± 5.8 kg in the lowest rural social group ($p<0.001$).

The mothers' stature was 151.9 ± 5.5 cm in the high social class urban group and 149.2 ± 5.5 cm in the lowest rural social group ($p<0.001$).

TABLE 8. Bangladesh perinatal survey, 1983: mothers' anthropometry

Social group	n	Weight before delivery[a] (kg)		Weight after delivery[a] (kg)		Height (cm)		Arm circumference (cm)	
		Mean	SD	Mean	SD	Mean	SD	Mean	SD
1. High urban	112	58.6	9.5	51.9	9.4	151.9	5.5	23.4	2.9
2. Low urban	357	49.7	6.2*	44.2	6.7*	150.4	9.1	21.4	1.8*
3. High rural	41	—	—	44.1	5.9*	147.2	21.8*	22.0	2.0
4. Low rural	102	—	—	41.0	5.8*	149.2	5.5*	21.0	1.9*
Total	612	53.4	7.4	45.4	7.9	150.3	9.5	22.6	2.0

[a]Weight includes clothing.
*$p < 0.001$.

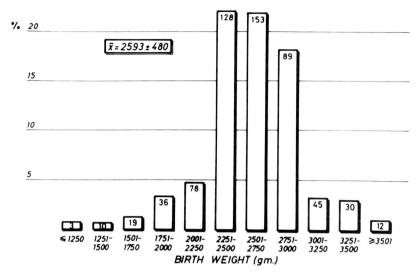

FIG. 3. Bangladesh birthweight distribution, 1983. n = 603.

The mothers' arm circumference was 23.4 ± 2.9 cm in the high social class urban group, and 21.0 ± 1.9 cm in the lowest rural social group ($p < 0.001$).

Figure 3 shows a birthweight frequency distribution plot (n = 603). Mean birthweight is $2,593 \pm 480$ g, and 474 infants were of low birthweight (45.4%).

Figure 4 shows maternal age plotted against infant birthweight (n = 624). Birthweight increased with age from 14 to 31 years. From 32 years onwards it decreased

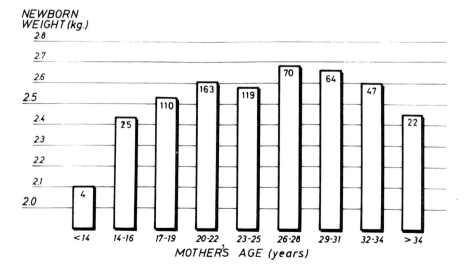

FIG. 4. Mother's age versus newborn birthweight in Bangladesh, 1983. n = 624.

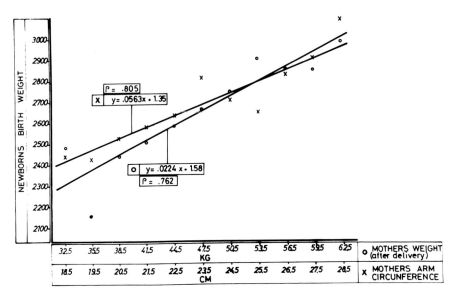

FIG. 5. Bangladesh perinatal nutrition survey, 1983. Birthweight versus mother's weight and mother's arm circumference.

again. All mothers aged less than 16 years or more than 34.1 years had low birth-weight infants. The highest mean birthweight occurred in women between 26 and 31 years of age.

Figure 5 shows maternal weight and arm circumference versus infant birthweight, expressed as linear functions. Between 32.5 and 62.5 kg, maternal weight was

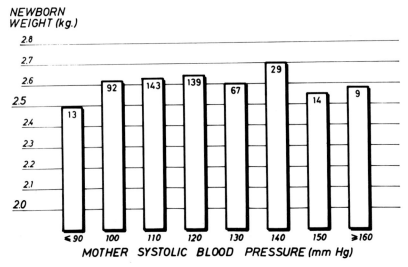

FIG. 6. Post-delivery mother's systolic blood pressure versus birthweight in Bangladesh, 1983. n = 506.

highly correlated with infant birthweight, appearing as a straight linear function with a correlation coefficient of 0.81. All women whose post-delivery weight was less than 41 kg had low birthweight infants. Maternal arm circumference and infant birthweight were also highly correlated. The smallest arm circumference corresponded to the highest incidence of low birthweight and the correlation coefficient was 0.76. All mothers with arm circumference measurements less than 20 cm had low birthweight infants.

Figure 6 compares maternal post-delivery systolic blood pressure with infant birthweight. Women with systolic blood pressures less than 90 mm Hg had low birthweight infants. There was a trend for birthweight to increase with increasing blood pressure up to a (systolic) value of 140 mm Hg. Above 150 mm Hg there was a tendency for birthweight to decrease.

DISCUSSION

Birthweight is probably one of the most sensitive and precise indicators of the health status of a population (18). Low birthweight is a negative health indicator affecting 21 million children in the world yearly (21). Of these, 7 to 10 million occur in India (29) and probably 2 to 3 million occur in Bangladesh.

In the developed countries, there is ample and precise information on birthweight because the vast majority of deliveries occur in well-equipped hospitals with highly qualified personnel. In the developing countries, there is little information on birthweight, mainly because most of the population live in rural areas, qualified health personnel and facilities are limited, and home deliveries are the norm, usually attended by untrained and illiterate traditional birth attendants.

In India there is ample information on birthweight, most of it coming from hospital records, but information on rural and home-based deliveries is practically nonexistent. Therefore, hospital data and their relevance to the national situation deserve cautious interpretation.

In Bangladesh, there is an almost complete lack of data on birthweight, the only available information being three original publications describing 112 infants (13,48,49).

India

From 1960 to 1984, in spite of general improvements in the socio-cultural status of the population and the country's capacity to produce enough food to feed its population, there has been no clear tendency to show significant improvements in the incidence of LBW. The lowest incidence was observed in Gwalior, 18.6% in 1961, and the highest was in Ajmer, 80.5% in 1981. This lack of improvement can probably be explained on the basis that the rural areas have not yet benefited from the higher income and food availability, that heavy work loads for women remain practically unchanged, and that prenatal care is not yet established.

Except for home-based data from Pondicherry in 1976 (62) and Bombay rural studies in 1963 (63), all remaining publications were from hospitals. From these two rural studies, it appears that the incidence of low birthweight was not different from hospital-based studies. There may therefore be no need to consider urban and rural low birthweight data separately.

The lowest mean birthweight was obtained in Varanasi ($2,423 \pm 325$ g) in 1971, and the highest was $3,069 \pm 590$ g in Agra in 1961. The low birthweight incidence in Varanasi was 54.6% in 1967 and 75% in 1971. Is it possible to see such large differences in low birthweight incidence in the same population during such a short period of time? Data for singleton liveborn infants were reported in only 10 of the 38 studies, so some of the results could be modified by the inclusion of multiple births.

In Indian studies, it always appears that the majority of infants are affected by intrauterine growth retardation, though in most studies precise figures are not reported. In five studies in which reliable information is available (17,28,54–56), the IUGR rate varied between 67.2% and 81.1% of the total population. These figures are in line with similar data from developing countries worldwide, and are much lower than figures reported from the developed countries.

Preterm deliveries occur more often in low socioeconomic groups in both developing and developed countries. The Indian data fit this pattern as is shown in four different studies and one control group (21). In a low social class population in Bombay, preterm deliveries occurred in 22.3% as opposed to only 7.1% in a high social class population. These samples were collected by the same investigator, at the same time, and using the same methodology. Preterm deliveries for the control group were 5.3%. Mother's age (too young or too old), frequent pregnancies, short birth intervals, anemia, bleeding, hypertensive diseases during pregnancy, infections, parasitic infestations, protein energy malnutrition, hard physical work, tobacco use, and emotional stress are among the most relevant etiological factors in the developing countries. In some areas of the world the role of heavy indoor smoke (carbon monoxide) could be an important factor in birthweight.

Early neonatal mortality is one of the outstanding negative factors of low birthweight. In newborn infants with weights less than 1,000 g, 100% mortality occurred in 32% of the centers and more than 80% in 55% of them. In the BW group 1,000 to 2,000 g, early neonatal mortality varied between 4.1 and 71.4%. These figures probably reflect limited facilities, lack of trained personnel, lack of equipment, and a generally poor infrastructure of obstetric and pediatric care. No figures are known for home-based rural deliveries; however, it is likely that the early neonatal mortality would be even higher than reported for hospital deliveries.

The catch-up phenomenon is a well-known feature of LBW and IUGR infants. If adequate nutrition is provided and the infectious diseases prevented, catch-up occurs in 1,000 g infants between 12 and 36 months. However, a follow-up study of Indian LBW infants from birth to 6 years of age showed that the catch-up phenomenon did not occur (29).

In the majority of developing countries, mainly in rural areas, it is difficult to obtain birthweight because of lack of trained personnel and equipment, as well as distances and terrain difficulties. Numerous efforts were, and still are, being made to find alternative solutions which could provide accurate and reliable surrogates for birthweight. Head, chest, and abdominal circumferences, and height are being explored as alternatives. Recent reports consistently show that the best birthweight surrogate is chest circumference (40,55,61,64). If this proves true, great progress should soon be achieved in obtaining an anthropometric surrogate for birthweight which could be easily implemented by public health workers in developing countries.

Bangladesh

Significant characteristics of the Bangladesh program were that: (a) the study was completed by the same observer who collected all the data; (b) all consecutive mother-infant pairs were studied in three different institutions, two urban and one rural; home deliveries were examined by six well-trained public health midwives; (c) over 98% of mothers were Moslem. (See Tables 9 through 11.)

Among the low social class rural mothers, it was shown that at 16 years of age 79% of women were married versus 30% in the high social class urban group. In the perinatal survey, all women who were less than 16 years of age at the time of the delivery had LBW infants, regardless of socioeconomic status. Highest birthweight was observed among mothers who were between 26 and 31 years of age. In Bangladesh, marriage is determined by a combination of religious, economic, and cultural factors decided among family members of the bride and groom. Young girls may be married at 6 to 7 years of age, though the marriage is not usually consummated until they reach the age of puberty. We have seen several mothers of 11 years of age who always delivered low birthweight infants. This complex sociocultural-economic family situation will be rather difficult to overcome in the near future. Therefore, the LBW rate will probably remain high in Bangladesh for some time to come.

An important and valuable indicator of favorable progress in pregnancy is weight gain, unless due to edema. Weight gain during pregnancy for the high social class urban group was 6.7 kg, and 5.5 kg for the low social class urban group. Considering that the women's stature was 151.9 and 150.4 cm, respectively, it is clear that in both groups there was insufficient weight gain during pregnancy, as would be ex-

TABLE 9. *Bangladesh perinatal survey, 1983: Post-delivery systolic and diastolic blood pressure (BP) (mmHg)*

Social group	n	Systolic BP (mmHg)		Diastolic BP (mmHg)	
		Mean	SD	Mean	SD
1. High urban	112	120	14	84	16
2. Low urban	355	118	15	79*	13
3. High rural	37	102	9	66*	14
4. Low rural	—	—	—	—	—
Total	504	117	15	79	14

*$p < 0.001$ vs. high urban.

TABLE 10. *Bangladesh perinatal survey, 1983: birthweight (g) frequency distribution*

Social group	n	≤ 1,250	1,251–1,500	1,501–1,750	1,751–2,000	2,001–2,250
1. High urban	108	1.8	1.8	1.8	0.9	6.5
2. Low urban	354	0.8	0.8	4.2	6.2	8.7
3. High rural	39	5.1	0	5.1	5.1	7.7
4. Low rural	102	0	1.0	1.0	10.0	16.7
Total	603	1.1	1.0	2.5	6.6	9.6

*$p < 0.001$ vs. high urban.

pected from the high incidence of LBW. Allowing for the mean clothing weight of 1.3 kg, the lowest social class rural group weighed only 39.7 kg after delivery. It is therefore not surprising that 70.8% of all newborns in this socioeconomic group were low birthweight infants. Arm circumference was a valuable index of the mother's nutritional status. Regardless of age, height, and social status, women with an arm circumference of less than 20 cm always produced LBW infants. From this study it can be stated that, at the time of delivery, a 20 cm maternal arm circumference is the cutoff point below which she will certainly produce a low birthweight infant.

Blood pressure plays a decisive role in placental perfusion and, therefore, on fetal nutrition. Mean systolic and diastolic pressures were low among the low social class rural women and there was a clear tendency for blood pressure to be correlated with birthweight, such that the lower the systolic pressure the lower the birthweight. High blood pressures (≥140 mm Hg) also resulted in a decreased birthweight. The optimum range of blood pressure with respect to birthweight was (systolic) 120 to 140 mm Hg.

Among the population sample of LBW infants, IUGR was present in 48.2% of the high social class urban group and in 81.5% of the low social class rural group. These findings are consistent with those in the current literature from both developed and developing countries.

An excellent and highly significant statistical correlation was observed at delivery between maternal weight and arm circumference and the birthweight of the infant. The almost perfect correlation found in this study between these two maternal variables and birthweight is remarkable. This phenomenon has also been shown in similar studies. This raises the possibility that a simple chart could be developed, including mother's arm circumference and birthweight, which perhaps could be of help in isolated and primitive rural areas of the developing world, which lack expensive and cumbersome equipment and facilities, and well-qualified health personnel.

Some of the estimated demographic characteristics of Bangladesh are as follows: 80% of the population live in poor and isolated rural areas; 60% to 70% of its inhabitants are illiterate; 90% of the deliveries occur at home, and the vast majority are attended by untrained and illiterate traditional birth attendants. Based on these fac-

Table 10. *(Continued)*

2,251–2,500	2,501–2,750	2,751–3,000	3,001–3,250	3,251–3,500	> 3,501	Mean	SD
11.0	17.6	29.6	10.2	13.9	4.6	2.85	0.510
23.2	22.9	19.2	6.8	4.8	2.0	2.63*	0.540
15.4	41.0	5.1	5.1	10.2	0	2.55*	0.520
42.1	21.6	5.9	2.0	0	0	2.40*	0.300
23.7	22.9	18.1	6.5	6.0	2.0	2.59	0.480

TABLE 11. *Bangladesh perinatal survey, 1983; low birthweight (LBW) and intrauterine growth retardation (IUGR)*

Social group	n	LBW (%)	IUGR (%)
1. High urban	108	23.8	48.2
2. Low urban	354	43.9*	64.9*
3. High rural	39	38.4*	63.8*
4. Low rural	102	70.8*	81.5*
Total	603		

*$p < 0.001$ vs. high urban.

tors, it is evident that the most representative of the four samples studied is the home-delivery rural group. This group had an incidence of low birthweight of 70%, and among these infants, 81% suffered IUGR. If a more comprehensive and representative sample confirms these figures, the situation appears to be among the worst in the world affecting the health and well-being of the great majority of the population. The role of women in society, the uncontrolled population growth, and the poor state of food production and availability during the last 10 years have compounded the situation. It is difficult to envision a rapid or even a medium-term improvement in this situation.

CONCLUSION

Our experience in Southeast Asia, and specifically in India and Bangladesh, demonstrates that as far as birthweight is concerned there are numerous difficulties to be overcome before the HFA-2000 goal can be achieved, and only 11 years are left to attain it. It is a dream rather than an objective. Religious, socioeconomic, and cultural factors have to be overcome in most of the developing countries before this goal can be achieved. Numerous positive changes are occurring in India, including higher literacy among women, better family planning and population control, availability of mass media (particularly radio and television), higher family income, and better food production and distribution. One hopes that these factors will ameliorate the fate of millions of pregnant women and children.

This staggering challenge is here and it must be the resolve of governments to face it forcefully and ultimately to solve it. With firm determination this can and will be done.

REFERENCES

1. Habicht JP, Lechtig A, Yarborough C, et al. Maternal nutrition, birth weight and infant morbidity. In: *Size at birth*, Ciba Symposium no. 27, London, 1974. Amsterdam Oxford, New York: Elsevier, 1974;353–78.
2. Habicht JP et al. Relationship of birth weight, maternal nutrition and infant mortality. *Nutr Rep Int* 1973;7:533–46.
3. Kaminski M, Gousaro S, Rumeau-Rouquette C, et al. Prediction of low birthweight and prematurity by a multiple regression analysis with maternal characteristics known since the beginning of the pregnancy. *Int J Epidemiol* 1973;2:195–204.
4. Lechtig A, et al. Low birth weight babies: worldwide incidence, economic cost and program needs. In: Rooth G, Engstrom L, eds. *Perinatal care in developing countries*. Uppsala: Perinatal Research Laboratory and World Health Organization, 1977.
5. Mata LJ, Urrutia JJ, Uronmal RA, Joplin C, et al. Survival and physical growth in infancy and early childhood; study of birth weight and gestational age in a Guatemalan Indian village. *Am J Dis Child*, 1975;129:561–6.
6. Petros-Barvazian A, Behar M. Low birth-weight: a major global problem in SAREC. Birth weight distribution—an indicator of social development. In: Sterky G, Mellander L, eds. SAREC/WHO Workshop Report no. 2. Stockholm: SAREC, 1978.
7. Serrano CV, Puffer RR. Utilization of hospital birth weights and mortality as indicators of health problems in infancy. *Bull Pan Am Health Organ* 1974;8:325–46.
8. World Health Organization. Social and biological effects on perinatal mortality. Volume 2. Geneva: WHO, 1978.
9. Bergman RE, Vaughan VC. *Nelson textbook of pediatrics*. Philadelphia: W.B. Saunders Co, 1983.
10. Statistics Canada. Health division. Vital statistics. Births, Ottawa: Statistics Canada, 1979.
11. Chamberlain G, Philipp E, Howlet B, Master SK, et al. British births, 1970. A survey under the joint auspices of the National Birthday Trust Fund and the Royal College of Obstetricians and Gynaecologists. London: William Heineman Medical Books Ltd., 1978.
12. Ghosh S, Vaga S. Comparison of gestational age and weight as standards of prematurity. *J Pediatr* 1967;71:173–5.
13. World Health Organization, Division of Family Health. The incidence of low birthweights: a critical review of available information. *World Health Stat Q* 1980;33:197–224.
14. Yusof ZA. Economic aspects of health and human development. Part II. Tokyo: South-East Asian Medical Information Center, 1979:chap. 5.
15. France. Ministère de la Santé et de la Sécurité Sociale. Institut National de la Santé et de la Recherche Médicale. *Naître en France. Enquête nationale sur la grossesse et l'accouchement* (1972–1976). Paris: INSERM, 1979.
16. Martell M, Falkner F, Bertolini LB, Diaz JL, et al. Early postnatal growth evaluation in full term, preterm, and small-for-dates infants. *Early Hum Devel* 1978;4:313–23.
17. Surainer YA, Prasad SK, Hemavaty V. A study of gestational age and birth weight. *Indian Pediatr* 1970;7:338–46.
18. World Health Organization. Global strategy for health for all by the year 2000. Geneva: WHO, 1981.
19. Achar ST, Yankauer A. Studies on the birth weight of South Indian infants. *Indian J Child Health* 1962;11:157–67.
20. Aiyar R, Agarwal JR. Observation on the newborn: a study of 10,000 consecutive live births. *Indian Pediatr* 1969;6:729–42.
21. Bhargava SK, Sachdev HPS, Iyer PU, Ramji S. Current status of infant growth measurements in the perinatal period in India. *Acta Paediatr Scand* 1985; Suppl 319:103–10.

22. Cravioto J, Birch HG, DeLicardie ER, Rosales L, et al. The ecology of infant weight gain in a pre-industrial society. *Acta Paediatr Scand,* 1967;56:71–7.
23. Morley DC, Woodland M, Martin WJ, et al. Heights and weights of West African village children from birth to the age of five *West Afr Med J* 1968;17:8.
24. Srivastava BC, Maheswari BB, Gupta RD. The effect of various biological factors on birth weight. *Indian J Pediatr* 1971;38:202–7.
25. United Nations. *Demographic yearbook,* 1975.Table 30, New York: United Nations, 1976.
26. United States Department of Health, Education and Welfare. Public Health Service. Vital and Health Statistics Publication Series 21 no 30. Characteristics of Births United States, 1973–1975. Hyattsville, Md.: US DHEW, 1978.
27. Agarwal S, Bharochi GR, Kaur A, Jain S. Perinatal mortality in an industrial hospital. *Indian Pediatr* 1978;15:1001–6.
28. Bhakoo ON, Narang A, Kulkarni KN, et al. Neonatal morbidity and mortality in hospital born babies. *Indian Pediatr* 1975;12:443–50.
29. Bhargava SK. Outcome of low birth weight infants. *Acta Paediatr Scand* 1984;73:406–7.
30. Bhatia VP, Katiyar GP, Agarwal KN. Effect of intrauterine nutritional deprivation on neuromotor behaviour of the newborn. *Acta Paediatr Scand* 1979;68:561–6.
31. Dawson I, Golder RY, Jonas EG. Birthweight by gestational age and its effect on perinatal mortality in white and in Punjabi births: experience at a district general hospital in West London 1967–1975. *Br J Obstet Gynaecol* 1982;89:896–9.
32. Idnani N, Sharma U, Saxena S, et al. Effect of maternal factors on the clinical features. morbidity and mortality of the newborn. *Indian J Pediatr* 1979;46:75–86.
33. Bhatia BD, Mathur NB, Chaturvedi P, et al. Neonatal mortality pattern in a rural based medical college. *Indian J Pediatr* 1984;51:309–12.
34. Chandra RK. Fetal malnutrition and postnatal immunocompetence. *Am J Dis Child* 1975;129:450–4.
35. Ebrahim GJ. Care of the newborn. *Br Med J* 1984;289:899–901.
36. Ghosh S, Bhargava SK, Sharma DB, Bhargava V, Saxena HMK. Perinatal mortality—a preliminary report on a hospital based study. *Indian Pediatr* 1971;8:421–6.
37. Lal K, Lal J. Factors associated with perinatal mortality. *Indian Pediatr* 1974;11:743–7.
38. Martins J, Aristodermo J, Carvalho JF, Bueno RD, Paes De Frestas NA, Carvalho MB, Morals LP. Desnutricion intrauterine variation du poids a la naissance en fonction de la classe socio-economique dans une maternite de la ville de campinas. SP Brazile. Centre International de L'Enfance Courrier, 1974;24:122–9.
39. Patel IS, Patel SH, Mehta MJ, Ghodadra JK, Perinatal mortality—its incidence and causes in civil hospital—Ahmedabad. *Pediatr Clin India* 1969;4:159–67.
40. Prasad R, Pandey H, Mathur PP, Singh YR, Dayal RS. Anthropometric study of 925 newborns. *Arch Child Health* 1980;22:25–32.
41. Srinevasa DK, Danabalan M, Anand D. Certain aspects of infant mortality—a prospective study in an urban community. *Indian Pediatr* 1976;13:409–13.
42. Ghosh S, Beri S. Standard of prematurity for North Indian babies. *Indian J Child Health* 1962;11:210–5.
43. Agarwal VK, Gupta SC, Roy Choudhary S, Narula RK. Some observations on perinatal mortality. *Indian Pediatr* 1982;19:233–8.
44. Kumar S, Mathur BP, Surainder YA, Seetha T. Incidence and causes of perinatal mortality at the Ich-Niloufer Hospital, Hyderabad. *Indian Pediatr* 1972;9:99–106.
45. Rao PSS, Inbaraj SG. A prospective study of infant mortality and congenital malformations in relation to intra-uterine growth rates in South India. *Indian J Med Res* 1978;67:245–54.
46. Rao S, Talwalkar YB, Bharucha PE. Neonatal morbidity and mortality. *Indian Pediatr* 1970;7:271–5.
47. Shah HN. A study of 3,138 premature babies. *Arch Child Health* 1972;9:145–55.
48. Hussain MA, Khan AK, Abeden Z, Ferdoos Z, et al. Studies on nutritional status of expectant mothers and newborn babies. *Bangladesh Medical Research Council Bulletin* 1976;2:120–6.
49. Khan M, et al. Growth and development studies: Rural Meheran. Comilla. *Bangladesh Med J* 1979;7:74.
50. Pachauri S, Marwah SM. A study of the effect of certain maternal factors on birthweight. *Indian J Med Sci* 1970;24:650–60.
51. Kalra K, Kishore N, Dayal RS. Anthropometric measurements in the newborn. *Indian J Pediatr* 1961;34:73–82.

52. Bhargava H, Karna S, Pant N. Perinatal mortality. *J Obstet Gynaecol India* 1981;31:587–92.
53. Park JF, Chandra H. A study of the bearing of children in Gwalior City (Madhya Pradesh). *Indian J Pediatr,* 1964;3:217–22.
54. Gross SJ, David RJ, Durham NC, Bauman LMS, Tomarelli RM. Nutritional composition of milk produced by mothers delivering preterm. *J Pediatr* 1980;96:641–4.
55. Guha DK, Rashmi A, Kochar M. Relationship between length of gestation, birthweight and certain other factors. *Indian J Pediatr* 1973;40:44–53.
56. Ramaiah TJ, Narasimhan VL. Birth weight as a measure of prematurity and its relationship with certain maternal factors. *Indian J Med Res* 1967;5:513–24.
57. Sheth P, Merchant SM. Fetal growth in two socio-economic groups. *Indian Pediatr* 1972;9:650–7.
58. Ghosh S, Bhargava SK, Moriyama IM. Longitudinal study of the survival and outcome of a birth cohort; report of phase I of the research project of 01-658-2; funded by the National Center for Health Statistics, 3700 East West Highway, Hyattsville, Maryland 20782, USA, 1979.
59. Singh MB, Giri SK, Ramachandran K. Intrauterine growth curves of liveborn single babies. *Indian Pediatr* 1974;11:475–9.
60. Babson SG, Behrman E, Lessel R. Liveborn birthweights for gestational age of white middle class infants. *Pediatrics* 1970;45:937–42.
61. Bhargava SK, Ramji S, Kumar A, Mohan M, Marwah J, Sachdev HPS. Mid-arm and chest circumferences at birth as predictors of low birthweight and neonatal mortality in the community. *Br Med J* 1985;291:1617–9.
62. Srinivasa DK, Danabalan M, Gnanasujayam M. Influence of maternal care, parity and birthweight on neonatal mortality—a prospective study in an urban community. *Indian J Med Res* 1976;64:358–60.
63. Udani PM. Physical growth of children in different SE groups in Bombay; *Ind J Child Health* 1963;12:595–611.
64. Datta Banik ND. A study of incidence of different birthweight babies and related factors. *Indian Pediatr* 1978;15:327–34.
65. Walia BNS, Khetarpal SK, Mehta S, Ghai OP, Kapoor P, Taneja PN. Observations on 1,000 live born infants. *Indian J Child Health* 1963;12:243–9.
66. Nath S. Sex ratio, birthweight, and prematurity. *The Licenciate* 1963;12:313–7.
67. Srivastava JR, Saluja KK, Bai S, Samuel KC. Studies on perinatal mortality in medical college hospitals, Kanpur. *Indian Pediatr* 1969;6:374–82.
68. Saigal S, Srivastava JR. Maternal factors in relation to birthweight. *Indian Pediatr* 1969;6:773–82.
69. Datta Banik ND, Krishan R, Mane SIS, Raj L. Assessment of prematurity of North Indian babies. *Indian J Pediatr* 1968;35:135–9.
70. Chandra H. Birthweight of infants of different economic groups in Hyderabad. *Nutr Soc India* 1971;10:99–103.
71. Madhavan S, Taskar AD. Birthweight of Indian babies born in hospitals. *Indian J Pediatr* 1969;36:193–204.
72. Bahl L, Gupta SP, Vikshit SK. Study of maternal factors in relation to birthweight and gestational age of the newborn. *Indian Pediatr* 1971;8:707–11.
73. Ghai OP, Sandhu RK. Study of physical growth of Indian children in Delhi. *Indian J Pediatr* 1968;35:91–107.
74. Gupta BM, Sharda DC. A study of birth weights in Central Rajasthan. *Indian J Pediatr* 1972;30:144–9.
75. Pachauri S, Marwah SM. An anthropometric study of the newborn in a New Delhi urban community. *Indian J Pediatr* 1971;38:291–8.
76. Singh M, Tripathy K, Arya LS. Birthweight gestational age correlates of neonatal mortality. *Indian J Pediatr* 1982;49:511–7.
77. Ghosh S, Hooja V, Mittal SK, Verma RK. Biosocial determinants of birthweight. *Indian Pediatr* 1977;14:107–14.

Intrauterine Growth Retardation, edited by
Jacques Senterre. Nestlé Nutrition Workshop
Series, Vol. 18. Nestec Ltd., Vevey/Raven Press,
Ltd., New York © 1989.

Risk Factors Associated with Intrauterine Growth Retardation in Developed Countries: Italy as an Example

Antonio Marini and Chiara Vegni

Neonatal Division, Institute of Obstetrics and Gynecology "L. Mangiagalli,"
University of Milan, Milan, Italy

PATHOPHYSIOLOGY

Intrauterine growth retardation (IUGR) can result from a variety of environmental or genetic influences of fetal growth (1). However, the pathophysiology is still not completely understood, although the lack of transport of sufficient quantities of nutrients and oxygen to the fetus is commonly recognized as the endpoint causing IUGR (2). Genetic, metabolic, and nutritional factors cannot be viewed totally independently, but in some ways are interrelated (Fig. 1) (3).

From the studies of Naeye and Tafari (4), based on data collected in the U.S.A. (Collaborative Perinatal Project), several aspects appear to point towards a deficiency of utero-placental blood flow, due either to a lack of expansion of plasma volume during pregnancy or to an impairment of microcirculation at the placental level. This fact complicates pre-existing negative factors, like undernutrition or living at high altitude, and is further aggravated by exposure to a toxic environment.

Two examples substantiate the concept that the increase in plasma volume during pregnancy is very important in allowing good intrauterine growth. The first example

PATHOPHYSIOLOGY OF GROWTH RETARDATION

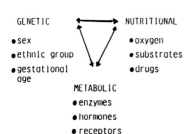

FIG. 1. The major factors that determine fetal growth and development. (From ref. 3.)

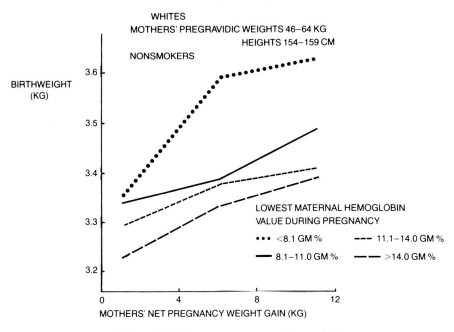

FIG. 2.   Risk factors in pregnancy. (From ref. 4.)

is that the degree of anemia in the third trimester of pregnancy, which can be viewed as a consequence of hemodilution, is inversely related to birthweight (BW) (Fig. 2). The second example is that the level of peak diastolic pressure during pregnancy (up to 95 Torr), which is in some ways correlated with the circulating blood volume, is directly related to BW, even in those cases with low net maternal weight gain (Fig. 3). The presence of maternal proteinuria and/or edema did not markedly influence intrauterine growth unless peak diastolic pressure was <85 Torr. These data are substantiated by the previous work of Räihä (5) which showed a close relationship between the lack of increase of blood volume in pregnancy and incidence of prematurity. This fact suggests that IUGR in pregnancies complicated by edema, proteinuria, and hypertension can be due to reduced blood volume. Thus, therapeutic strategies aimed at expansion of plasma volume and/or amelioration of the microcirculation may be effective in at-risk mothers (6,7).

However, as recently suggested by Warshaw (8), IUGR can also be viewed from the point of view of the fetus as an adaptation in which its own size may be appropriate to the availability of nutrients, including oxygen supply. An increase in oxygen consumption has been described after chronic glucose infusion in fetal sheep (9) and in a fetus with marginal oxygen delivery this may cause increased risk. Furthermore, mothers receiving high-protein supplementation in a nutritional intervention program had an excess of prematurity and IUGR (10).

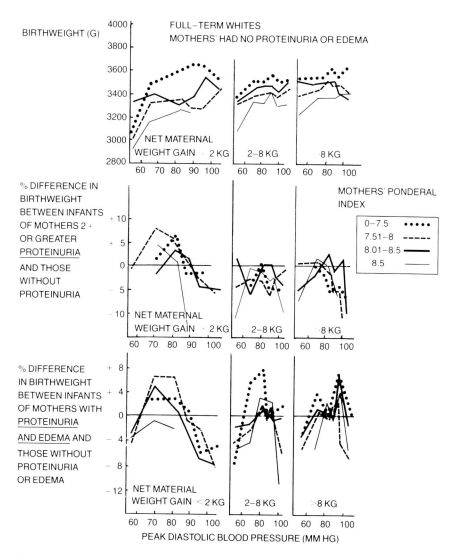

FIG. 3. Influence on birthweight of peak diastolic pressure during pregnancy. Values are referred to three classes of mothers: healthy (**top**), with proteinuria (**middle**), with proteinuria and edema (**bottom**). Values are also expressed considering mothers' ponderal index and net maternal weight gain in pregnancy. (From ref. 4.)

THE ITALIAN EXPERIENCE OR STUDY

In the Italian Perinatal Project (1973–78), the incidence of IUGR, calculated on the basis of our own intrauterine growth curves from the 32nd to the 43rd week of gestation (11–13), appeared to be 10% to 11% of all neonates, with no substantial differences between rural and industrialized areas. The causes of IUGR did not differ from those commonly recognized in other studies in well-developed countries

TABLE 1. *Risk factors for intrauterine growth*

Demographic
  Age (< 17 years, > 34 years)
  Unmarried
  Low socioeconomic[a]

Risk condition preceding pregnancy
  Low maternal weight[a]
  Small stature[a]
  Genital anomalies
  Diseases not pregnancy-related
  Nephritis
  Chronic hypertension
  Heart/cardiovascular disease
  Liver disease

Obstetric history
  Previous IUGR baby[a]
  Previous preterm delivery
  Previous fetal or neonatal deaths

Medical risks—current pregnancy
  High parity
  Multiple pregnancy
  Sexually transmitted infections
  Fetal anomaly
  Abruptio placentae
  Low diastolic blood pressure
  High systolic blood pressure[a]
  Toxemia[a]

Environmental risks—current pregnancy
  Smoking[a]
  Nutritional deprivation[a]
  Heavy alcohol use
  Drug abuse

Health care risk factor
  Inadequate prenatal care

Evolving concepts of risk stress
  Inadequate plasma volume expansion
  Selected environmental pollution exposure
  Selected genitourinary infections

IUGR, intrauterine growth retardation.
[a]Attributable risk values.
Adapted from ref. 19.

(Table 1) (14,15). Serious maternal diseases, especially preeclampsia, predomi-
nated as leading factors in severe IUGR. It must be pointed out that, in about 50%
of infants with a BW <2,500 g, pre-existing factors (e.g., the height of both parents
and the mother's pre-pregnancy weight) were responsible for a BW below the 10th
percentile, though in all these cases the BW was above the 3rd percentile.

Looking at the environmental factors, it clearly appeared that heavy smoking during pregnancy was responsible for reduced BW and birth length (Tables 2 and 3),
even when adjustment was made for other causes of a reduced BW, such as age and
parity of the mothers and low socioeconomic status (16). These data are in the line
of those reported by Naeve and Tafari (4) in the U.S.A. Perinatal Project (Fig. 4)
and these authors also demonstrated that the reduced growth persists up to at least 7
years of age (Table 4).

In the U.S.A. Perinatal Project, the effect of work during pregnancy on BW was
analyzed. BW was lower when women continued to work outside their homes after
the 28th week of gestation than when they quit work before this time. The only
exceptions were those mothers who had sit-down work and no children at home to
care for (Fig. 5). Both smoking and work aggravate the risks introduced by otherwise abnormal pregnancies.

From a clinical standpoint, the major problem consists in the care of neonates
with fetal growth retardation born before the 32nd week of gestation. Because of the

TABLE 2. *Influence of smoking on birthweight, head circumference, and crown-heel length*

	Nonsmokers	Stopped smoking	1–10 cigarettes / day	11 + cigarettes / day
Cases (%)	7,124 (63)	2,046 (18)	1,954 (17)	224 (2)
Birthweight (< 10th percentile) (%)	1,108 (16.0)	297 (15.0)	394 (20.8)	53 (24.2)
Odds ratios (95% int)	—	0.92 (0.80–1.06)	1.38 (1.21–1.56)	1.69 (1.23–2.32)
Odds ratios (95% int) adjusted for age, parity, socioeconomic class	—	0.90 (0.78–1.03)	1.39 (1.21–1.69)	1.73 (1.24–2.40)
Head circumference (< 10th percentile) (%)	587 (8.9)	165 (8.7)	214 (11.8)	19 (9.0)
Odds ratios (95% int)	—	0.97 (0.81–1.16)	1.37 (1.16–1.61)	1.01 (.63–1.63)
Crown-heel length (< 10th percentile) (%)	1,306 (19.8)	362 (18.9)	433 (23.8)	54 (25.6)
Odds ratios (95% int)	—	0.95 (0.83–1.08)	1.27 (1.22–1.44)	1.40 (1.02–1.91)

Sample selection: all high risk neonates, an equal number of normal neonates.
Cases are divided according to absence or presence (entity) of mothers' smoke. Numbers (and percentage)
of neonates with values < 10th percentile are indicated. Significant differences from nonsmokers are
underlined.
From ref. 16.

TABLE 3. *Influence of smoking on low birthweight (LBW) preterm deliveries, and perinatal deaths*

	Nonsmokers	Stopped smoking	1–10 cigarettes / day	11 + cigarettes / day
Cases (%)	7,124 (63)	2,046 (18)	1,954 (18)	224 (2)
LBW (%)	966 (13.6)	254 (12.4)	321 (16.4)	47 (21.0)
Odds ratios (95% int)	—	0.90 (0.78–1.05)	1.25 (1.09–1.44)	1.69 (1.22–2.35)
Odds ratios (95% int) adjusted for age, parity, socioeconomic class	—	0.95 (0.82–1.11)	1.35 (1.17–1.55)	1.74 (1.25–2.44)
Preterm deliveries (%)	1,077 (15.1)	287 (14.0)	258 (13.2)	38 (17.0)
Odds ratios (95% int)	—	0.92 (0.77–1.18)	.85 (0.74–0.99)	1.15 (0.80–1.64)
Perinatal deaths (%)	263 (3.7)	68 (3.3)	70 (3.6)	4 (1.8)
Odds ratios (95% int)	—	90 (0.68–1.18)	.97 (0.74–1.27)	0.47 (0.17–1.28)

Sample selection: all high risk neonates, an equal number of normal neonates.
Cases are divided according to absence or presence (entity) of mothers' smoke. Significant differences from non-smokers are underlined.
From ref. 16.

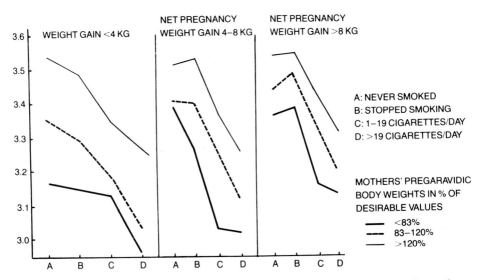

FIG. 4. Influence of tobacco smoking on birthweight. Values are expressed according to the entity of smoke (**A,B,C,D**), to mothers' pregravidic nutritional status and to net maternal weight gain in pregnancy. (From ref. 4.)

TABLE 4. *Intrapair comparisons of full-term siblings whose mothers smoked in one but not the other of their pregnancies*

	Birth	7 years of age	No. pairs of siblings
Body weights			
Stopped smoking	3,341 ± 440 g	24.3 ± 4.6 kg	140
Continued smoking	2,898[c] ± 384 g	22.9[c] ± 3.1 kg	
Body lengths			
Stopped smoking	50.9 ± 2.2 cm	121.2 ± 5.0 cm	
Continued smoking	50.3[a] ± 2.4 cm	119.5[c] ± 4.6 cm	
Head circumferences			
Stopped smoking	34.4 ± 1.2 cm	51.6 ± 1.3 cm	
Continued smoking	33.8[c] ± 1.3 cm	51.4 ± 1.4 cm	
Placental weights			
Stopped smoking	458 ± 88 g		
Continued smoking	431[b] ± 84 g		

All values ± 1 SD. [a]$p < 0.02$ compared with value in stopped-smoking category; [b]$p < 0.01$; [c]$p < 0.001$.
From ref. 4.

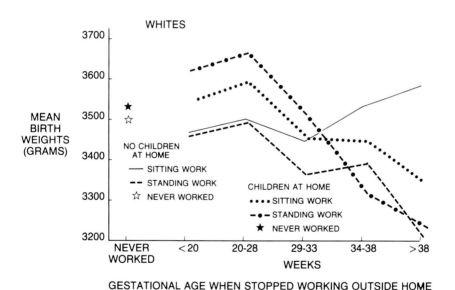

FIG. 5. Influence of work during pregnancy on birthweight. Data are analyzed according to type of work (sitting or standing) and presence or absence of other children at home to care for. (Data from ref. 4.)

TABLE 5. *Mean birthweight of liveborn infants from the whole population (WP) compared with interventive deliveries (ID)*

| | Gestation (weeks) | | | | |
	27	28	29	30	31
WP[a]	1,047	1,119	1,360	1,516	1,702
ID[a]	647	846	904	1,123	1,257
WP[b]	1,022	1,162	1,242	1,382	1,551
ID[b]	1,018	1,077	1,150	1,280	1,458

[a]Data from ref. 18.
[b]Data from ref. 17.

relative lack of accurate intrauterine growth curves below this gestational age, it is not easy to define IUGR in such infants. Only recently have two reports (17,18) provided data on "normal" growth for babies born highly preterm, and what is more, the data offered in these studies do not entirely coincide (Table 5). However, it appears clear that after subtracting those babies suspected of being sick *in utero* and born with an "interventive" delivery, precise intrauterine growth curves can be drawn, which then become a useful tool to classify IUGR in the very preterm group. Furthermore, considering that IUGR seldom appears before the 24th week of gestation and that early ultrasound evaluation of gestational age is highly reliable, we shall in the near future be able to define IUGR accurately in babies born from the 25th to 32nd week of gestation (Figs. 6–8).

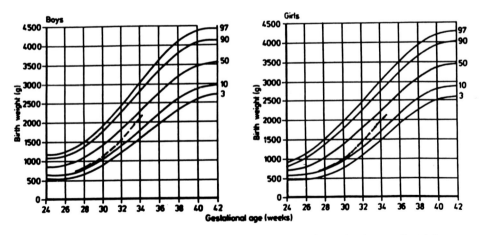

FIG. 6. Mean values *(broken line)* for birthweight in babies born after interventive delivery from 27 to 34 weeks of gestation (cesarean section or induction of labor for maternal or fetal-intrauterine growth retardation causes). Birthweight centiles for all the babies studied are also shown. (From ref. 18.)

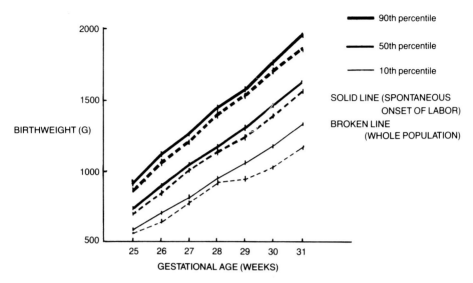

FIG. 7. 10th, 50th, 90th percentiles (not smoothed) for birthweight between 25 and 31 weeks gestation (whole population and spontaneous onset of labor). (From ref. 17.)

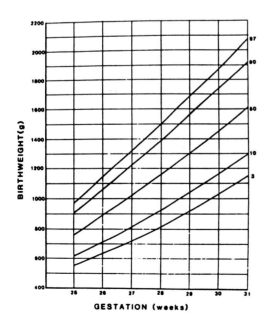

FIG. 8. Smoothed birthweight centile chart for infants 25 to 31 weeks gestation delivered spontaneously (i.e., excluding "interventive" deliveries). (From ref. 17.)

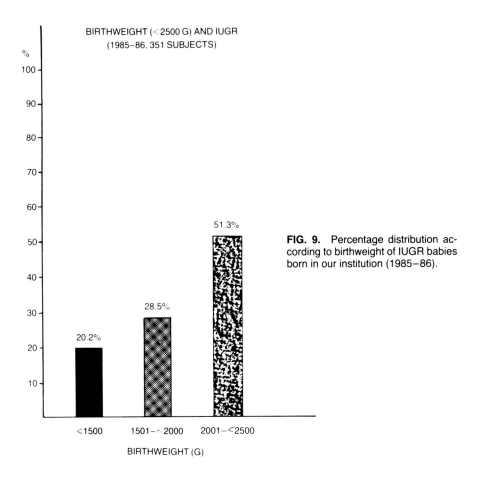

BIRTHWEIGHT (<2500 G) AND IUGR
(1985–86, 351 SUBJECTS)

FIG. 9. Percentage distribution according to birthweight of IUGR babies born in our institution (1985–86).

BIRTHWEIGHT (G)

With this background, we have recently reviewed etiological factors in a group of IUGR babies of BW <2,500 g, born in our institute in the last two years. Of 1,218 low birthweight (LBW) neonates, there were 351 cases of IUGR (31%).

Percentage distribution according to birthweight and gestational age is illustrated in Figs. 9 and 10. Analysis of etiological factors, subdivided into maternal, fetal, placental, and unknown reasons, indicates the following (see Table 6, Fig. 11): (a) In the great majority of cases, it is possible to find a cause for IUGR; (b) maternal factors predominate in babies born with a BW <1,500 g; (c) preeclampsia is the leading cause of IUGR in babies born with BW <2,000 g; (d) maternal environmental factors (smoking, drug abuse) predominate in babies with a BW >2,000 g; (e) placental factors are almost equally distributed in these 3 categories of BW; (f) infections are scarcely represented, which contrasts with the previous findings of Naeye and Peters (19) but is in accord with more recent findings (20); (g) twinning, especially monozygous, is a leading cause among fetal factors; and (h) serious mal-

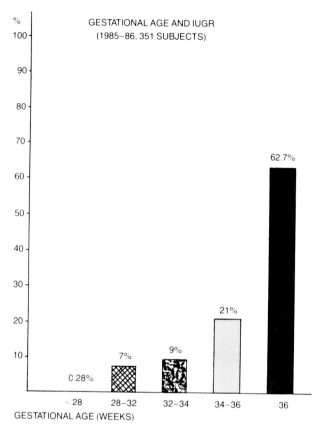

FIG. 10. Percentage distribution according to gestational age of IUGR babies born in our institution (1985–86).

TABLE 6. *Etiological factors for intrauterine growth retardation (IUGR)*

Maternal	Placental	Fetal
Cardiovascular	Small	Malformation
Infections	Abnormalities	Infections
Increase in weight ($\leq$ 6 kg)		Chromosome abnormalities
Smoking ($>$ 10 cigarettes / day)		Twinning
Alcohol		
Drug addiction		

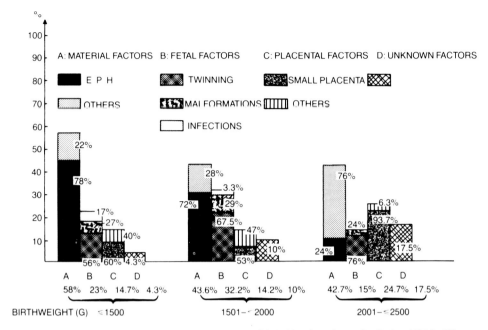

FIG. 11.   Percentage distribution of causes of IUGR babies born in our institution (1985–86).

formations, because of early intrauterine diagnosis followed by abortion, are rarely observed. Analysis of the ratio of placental weight to BW did not discriminate among the various etiological factors, agreement with earlier data of Molteni, Stys, and Battaglia (21).

If we take our findings as an indication of the causes of severe IUGR in a well-developed country with adequate antenatal care, and accept that maternal vascular factors together with placental abnormalities are the major causes of IUGR, then we may suggest that interventions aimed at cardiovascular control can be highly recommended. There is evidence that the evaluation and correction of abnormalities of plasma volume during pregnancy (6) and the early screening of pregnant women with a tendency to microvascular lesions (22) can be effective in reducing IUGR.

Obviously, another area of medical intervention is the prevention of infectious diseases, especially of the genito-urinary tract, because these can play a considerable role as causes of preterm delivery (19).

It has recently been pointed out (23) (Fig. 12) that abnormalities of glucose metabolism in pregnancy, leading to a tendency to hypoglycemia and to a lower release of insulin after glucose challenge, may be associated with some cases of IUGR. We do not yet know if this relationship is concomitant or causative. If the latter is true, we may expect that treatment causing increased plasma glucose levels in pregnancy would ameliorate growth failure associated with such abnormalities of glucose metabolism. However, experimental studies (9,24) and some clinical trials have not

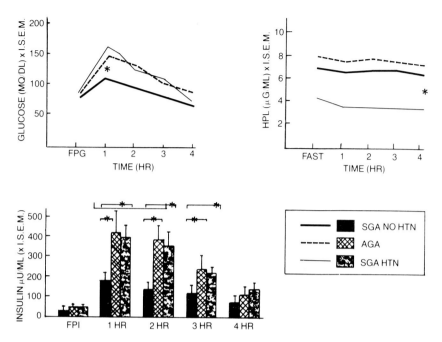

FIG. 12. Distribution of plasma glucose, human placental lactogen, and insulin levels after oral glucose load (OGL). HTN, Hypertensive; SGA, small for gestational age; AGA, appropriate for gestational age ($^*p<0.05$). (From ref. 23.)

been very effective, indicating that the increased supply of nutrients to the fetus must be coupled with an adequate oxygen delivery.

Socio-economic factors, including smoking and drug abuse, can be counteracted efficiently only by a more general approach to health care supported by wise politicians.

At the present time, we feel that in order to improve the long-term prognosis of IUGR babies (25), extremely careful monitoring during pregnancy, labor, and delivery is mandatory, since the affected fetus tolerates stressful conditions poorly. Good perinatal support, including efficient neonatal care given by qualified neonatologists, can minimize the long-term ill effects which have too often been described in the past.

REFERENCES

1. Gewolb IH, Warshaw JB. Influences on fetal growth. In: Warshaw JB, ed. *The biological basis of reproductive and developmental medicine*. New York: Elsevier, 1983;36.
2. Creasy RD, Resnick R. Intrauterine fetal growth retardation. In: Milunsky A, Friedman EA, Gluck L. *Advances in perinatal medicine* (vol 1). New York: Plenum, 1981;117.
3. Longo LD. Intrauterine growth retardation: a ''mosaic'' hypothesis of pathophysiology. *Semin Perinatol* 1984;8:662–72.

4. Naeye RL, Tafari N. Risk factors in pregnancy and diseases of the fetus and newborn. In: *Fetal growth*. Baltimore: William Wilkins, 1983;19.
5. Räihä CE. Prevention of prematurity. *Adv Pediatr* 1968;15:137.
6. Goodlin RC, Cotton DB, Haesslein HC. Severe EPH gestosis. *Am J Obstet Gynecol* 1978;132:595.
7. Wallenburg HCS, Dekker GA, Makovitz JW, Rotmans P. Low-dose aspirin prevents pregnancy-induced hypertension and pre-eclampsia in angiotensin-sensitive primigravidae. *Lancet* 1986;i:1.
8. Warshaw JB. Intrauterine growth retardation: adaptation or pathology. *Pediatrics* 1985;76:998.
9. Philipps AF, Dubin JW, Matty PJ, et al. Arterial hypoxemia and hyperinsulinemia in the chronically hyperglycemic fetal lamb. *Pediatr Res* 1982;16:653.
10. Rush O, Stein Z, Susser M. Diet in pregnancy: a randomized controlled trial of prenatal nutritional supplements. *Birth Defects* 1980;16:1.
11. Bossi A, Caccamo ML, De Scrilli A, Milani S. Standard del peso del neonato italiano (dalla 32a alla 43a settimana di gestazione). *Riv Ital Pediat* 1980;6:153.
12. Bossi A, Milani S. Crown-heel length and head circumference distribution at birth: a comparative study of results attained in five Italian centres. *Acta Medica Auxologica* 1980;12:181.
13. Bossi A, Milani S. Italian standards for crown-heel length and head circumference at birth. *Ann Hum Biol* 1987;14:321–35.
14. Committee to study the prevention of low birthweight. Preventing low birthweight. Washington: National Academy Press, 1985.
15. Ounsted M, Moar VA, Scott A. Risk factors associated with small-for-dates and large-for-dates infants. *Br J Obstet Gynaecol*, 1986;92:226.
16. De Scrilli A, Boracchi P, Paroi G, et al. Cigarette smoking in pregnancy: relationship to perinatal outcomes in six Italian centres. *Genus* 1986;42:37.
17. Lucas A, Cole TJ, Gandy GM. Birthweight centiles in preterm infants reappraised. *Early Hum Dev* 1986;13:313.
18. Yukin PL, Aboualfa M, Eyre JA, et al. Influence of elective preterm delivery on birthweight and head circumference standards. *Arch Dis Child* 1987;62:24–9.
19. Naeye RL, Peters RC. Amniotic fluid infections with intact membranes leading to perinatal death. A prospective study. *Pediatrics* 1978;61:171.
20. Chellam VG, Rushton DI. Chorioamnionitis and funiculitis in the placentas of 200 births weighing less than 2.5 kg. *Br J Obstet Gynaecol* 1985;92:808.
21. Molteni RA, Stys SJ, Battaglia FC. Relationship of fetal and placental weight in human beings: Fetal/placental weight ratios at various gestational ages and birth weight dimensions. *J Reprod Med* 1978;21:327.
22. Sant NF, Daley GL, Chand S, et al. A study of angiotensin II-pressor response throughout primigravid pregnancy. *J Clin Invest* 1973;52:2682.
23. Langer O, Damus K, Maiman M, et al. A link between relative hypoglycemia-hypoinsulinemia during oral glucose tolerance tests and intrauterine growth retardation. *Am J Obstet Gynecol* 1986;155:711.
24. Flake AW, Villa-Troyer RL, Scott AD, Zick N, Harrison MR. Transamniotic fetal feeding. III. The effect of nutrient infusion on fetal growth retardation. *J Pediat Surg* 1986;21:481.
25. Allen MC. Developmental outcome and follow-up of the small for gestational age infant. *Semin Perinatol* 1984;8:123.

Intrauterine Growth Retardation, edited by
Jacques Senterre. Nestlé Nutrition Workshop
Series, Vol. 18. Nestec Ltd., Vevey/Raven Press,
Ltd., New York © 1989.

Panel Discussion for B. Wharton, F. J. de Nóbrega, C. Robyn, C. A. Canosa, and A. Marini Chapters

Dr. Rachagan: It has been reported in the *British Journal of Obstetrics and Gynaecology* that oral correction of anemia in pregnancy is associated with a poor fetal outcome. Could Dr. Wharton comment on this please?

Dr. Wharton: I haven't read this particular article, but in general I think that we should be wary of automatically assuming that a low hemoglobin (Hb) is abnormal. In Britain there is more evidence that vitamin D should be given to pregnant women than iron, yet every pregnant woman automatically gets iron and folic acid supplements.

Dr. Rachagan: What do you think the ideal hemoglobin is?

Dr. Wharton: I really don't know. I shouldn't think there is an ideal value, as long as it does not start off too low, but I think an obstetrician would be better qualified to answer this.

Dr. Bossart: I don't think there is an ideal level. It will vary with the population, nutritional status, height above sea level, etc. In Lausanne the mean Hb is about 12 g per 100 ml, and this falls to about 11 g during pregnancy, in other words, a fall of about 8%. We regard this as our standard but I don't think we can have the same standard worldwide.

Dr. Marini: I agree that we cannot fix rules for pregnancy hemoglobin levels. However, it is well to remember that you could do harm. If you are not a wise obstetrician and you consider that a level of Hb of, say, 12 g per 100 ml is low because the normal should be 14 or 15 g, you will be tempted to try to increase the levels and you may well be successful. But then you run the risk of impairing the microcirculation in the placenta because of raised blood viscosity.

Dr. Priolosi: Dr. Wharton, in Sorrento, did you give a protein-supplemented diet to nutritionally deprived mothers who were at risk of having a baby with intrauterine growth retardation (IUGR)?

Dr. Wharton: We gave a balanced supplement, not a high-protein one. It consisted of 400 kcal per day, of which 10% were from protein.

Dr. Guesry: Our chairman asked us to be provocative, so I'm going to provoke Dr. Wharton! You showed very nicely that when you put Bengali women in a good environment with 5 o'clock tea, the birthweight of their babies increases by about 13 to 14 g per year. This to me seems to be a plea against the use of local or regional birthweight standards. With a good environment all babies should weigh more than 2,500 g.

Dr. Wharton: I do not find your comment provocative because I agree with it completely. Perhaps I could quote what I have previously written (1): "There seems little doubt that an internationally accepted fetal growth chart is required, based on internationally accepted reference data. Although as human biologists we study data from different individuals at different times, this does not mean we should translate the data into a plethora of standards. This argument is mirrored by similar discussions that have gone on concerning reference data and charts for growth after birth. The following arguments have been well-expounded elsewhere, by many authors including myself (2–8) but they bear repetition. The adoption of an international chart or set of reference data does not imply a standard of excellence—merely a standard of reference. The reference data when compared with another population should not necessarily be interpreted as optimal, normal, ideal, or a target to be achieved. The use of such charts and data allows international comparisons and presentation of new data in a comprehensive and easily comparable form. Furthermore, there are dangers that local standards will be interpreted as 'normal.' It seems probable, for example, that the population on which the Indian child growth standard is based contained a number of children with subclinical malnutrition (9). These and similar arguments have led to the adoption of an international standard for postnatal growth based on the

219

United States National Center for Health Statistics data (10)—not that all children should be the same size as American children, rather, that we should be able to compare children from wherever they are, easily. We now require an internationally accepted set of reference data against which we can compare our own babies. If they differ from it, we can then decide whether they are genetically smaller, or are small normals, i.e., no action is necessary. Or alternatively, we may decide that some of them are pathologically small, i.e., some intervention is desirable if effective, e.g., health education concerning smoking, less arduous work during pregnancy, dietary supplementation of selected mothers."

Dr. Toubas: If we continue to try to push up the birthweight of babies, will we cause an increase in the rate of hypertension in adult life?

Dr. Wharton: That is entirely speculative. I assume that there is some ultimate genetic potential for fetal growth in any particular woman, allowing for maternal size. We obviously don't want short women producing large babies, but after allowing for mother's height, which we can't alter during pregnancy, we do see improved mortality figures with increasing birthweight. There are some who would argue that all this attention to nutrition in pregnancy and improving fetal growth is misplaced and that instead it would be more effective to put our efforts into improvements in perinatal care. It has been suggested that these big nutrition supplementation programs around the world have been socially disruptive, that it has been impossible to carry them on, and so on. This is not a view I happen to agree with, but I have heard it argued very effectively.

Dr. Marini: From the practical point of view, there is no difference in caring for babies of 2,800 g and 3,000 g, so I see no point in putting a lot of effort into increasing birthweight by 100 g or so. I think the biggest effort should be put into prolonging gestation, because then we can avoid a lot of perinatal problems which cause morbidity and mortality.

Dr. Guesry: Obviously everyone here will agree that a baby of 2,800 g is essentially the same as one of 3,000 g, but we are not speaking of individual babies. We are speaking of an overall increase of 200 g in a population. This is quite a different matter. It would mean that 10% fewer babies would be less than 2,500 g at birth, which is a very important effect.

Dr. Pearse: Almost all studies have shown that perinatal mortality and morbidity are higher in IUGR with one major exception, which is Boersma's Tanzania study. In this study mortality was lowest in the partially growth-retarded infant and higher in the very small ones and in the large ones.

Dr. Guesry: I have a question for Dr. Robyn. I was puzzled by what you said about the coincidence between malarial infection in pregnant women and the peak of gonadotropic hormone production. I wonder if this is really true. Do you have any explanation, or do you think it is just a coincidence? Perhaps the reason is that you have started to inquire about malaria in your pregnant population at around 3 months. After all, it is quite improbable that you would be informed of pregnancy before this time, but maybe the rate of malarial infection is even more important in very early pregnancy.

Dr. Robyn: I agree that this could be a coincidence. But such findings should stimulate studies on possible relationships. For example, it would be interesting to know whether human chorionic gonadotropin (hCG) has any influence on growth of the Plasmodium. The explanation that depressed immunity is responsible for the increased incidence of malaria during pregnancy is not a very solid one. Immune functions decline progressively throughout pregnancy and even after delivery, and yet malarial infection rate is highest rather early in pregnancy.

Dr. Guesry: The immune response to malaria is cell-mediated, but is not the decline in immune competence during pregnancy related to humoral immunity?

Dr. Robyn: A definitive answer cannot be given. There are data showing that titers of antibodies to malarial antigens do not decrease during pregnancy. There is however a change in the distribution of T and B cells of about 100 days of gestational age. Whether this would mean a decrease in cellular immunity is not easy to say. Anyway, the immunity of the mother is not broken down since congenital malaria is extremely rare in endemic conditions. This is in contrast with the frequent congenital malaria seen in regions where epidemic conditions prevail. Finally, the newborn is protected for about 6 months against malaria. This is considered to be related to the transfer of anti-malarial antibodies.

Dr. Guesry: I thought the main reason for resistance in the neonate was the persistence of fetal hemoglobin.

Dr. Robyn: The paludeostatic effect of fetal hemoglobin is considered as complementary to that of passive immunity transmitted by the mother (11). The injection of IgG extracted from serums of adults to African infants with clinical signs of *Plasmodium falciparum* infection resulted in the reduction of the parasitemia (12).

Dr. Toubas: Are the lesions you observe in malarial placentas specific for malaria?

Dr. Robyn: No, these placental lesions are not very specific, with the exception, of course, of the malarial pigment. Thickening of the trophoblastic basal lamina is likely to have consequences on the exchanges between mother and fetus. This may be of importance in the etiology of IUGR related to malaria.

Dr. Desai: Obviously all mothers with malaria will also be anemic. What effect does this have on birthweight?

Dr. Robyn: Yes indeed. And I consider this possibly in the manuscript. The peak of hemolytic anemia according to Brabin follows by some 6 to 8 weeks the peak of parasitemia (13). Secondary megaloblastic anemia appears later in pregnancy.

Dr. Bossart: It looks as though there is a very high mortality in infants with IUGR if pregnancy proceeds to 39 or 40 weeks. I should like to ask Dr. Desai whether she thinks that if all her growth-retarded babies had been delivered by 36 weeks, perhaps three or four stillbirths would have been avoided?

Dr. Desai: If intervention could have been carried out at the right time, I agree that some of these babies might have been saved. The problem is that the mothers may not agree to being admitted for a preterm delivery, rendering us powerless to act.

Dr. Bossart: I should like to suggest that if IUGR is highly likely or certain, then the pregnancy should not be allowed to proceed beyond 36 weeks. In this way we should be able to prevent the deaths of many infants and also avoid a lot of handicap.

Dr. Desai: I agree with this, but such a policy is bound to increase the number of preterm babies who get into difficulty because of immaturity.

Dr. Cédard: There is always the problem of being sure of the exact term of gestation. I think this would be a serious limitation of any policy to deliver babies early deliberately.

Dr. Desai: In my experience, if you understand local events and the local calendar you will find that most women have a very accurate knowledge of their last menstrual period.

Dr. Chessex: I should like to ask Dr. Desai whether the small babies born of mothers weighing less than 45 kg really had IUGR, or whether they were just constitutionally small babies.

Dr. Desai: The mothers' weight was not the only parameter. They were also very short—less than 145 cm—and had very low Hb values. We defined these babies by our own standards and since they were below the 10th percentile, we considered them all to have IUGR.

Dr. Chessex: It seems to me there is a problem in defining what you mean by IUGR. These babies might be limited only by the size of the mother. I saw a recent paper in the *Indian Journal of Pediatrics* (14) in which three reference growth curves were described, one for mothers below 45 kg, one for 45 to 55 kg, and a third one for mothers over 55 kg. A baby born in the over 55 kg maternal weight category could be small-for-gestational-age (SGA), but would be appropriate-for-gestational-age (AGA) if born in the under 45 kg category.

Dr. Desai: I know about these charts. However, in the women I was describing low weight was not the only feature; they were also very anemic, as I have said. Taking all the factors into account I am convinced that they were SGA, even allowing for their mothers' small size.

Dr. Pearse: My feeling is that what has just been said strengthens the case for an international standard, which would enable us to compare your babies with those of other countries. I suspect that a rather high proportion of your babies would be SGA on our charts. It is not surprising to me that mothers who are very short give birth to a lot of very small babies. They probably come from the poorest classes of society and are underfed. I am sure you are right that the bottom 10%

of babies born to these women genuinely have IUGR, but by other criteria it might be a considerably larger proportion.

Dr. Toubas: A question for Dr. Canosa. What was the diastolic blood pressure of the women in your study, and how old were they? Were they very young adolescent girls? Blood pressure (BP) in adolescents is not the same as in adults.

Dr. Canosa: The mean age of the mothers in the study was 25.6 years. We did not study distribution of BP as a function of age, but even taking into account the mean age of the rural mothers their systolic and diastolic blood pressures were still very low in comparison with the urban group.

Dr. Marini: Was the level of non-pregnant blood pressure in the rural area lower than it was in the urban area? If so, it could be related to life style or diet.

Dr. Canosa: Absolutely. There are so many factors which we simply have no information about. I was only talking about blood pressure globally and it is of course very difficult to interpret this as a function of birthweight without having information on hemoglobins, plasma proteins, smoking, and so on.

Dr. Toubas: I'd like to ask Dr. Marini whether he has used thiocyanate as an index of smoking.

Dr. Marini: Thiocyanates can be used as an index of active or passive smoking, though if I remember correctly the levels are higher in pipe or cigar smokers than in cigarette smokers. Also, it is not so stable as cotinine, which is the stable metabolite of nicotine. I have had no experience of its use, but, in theory, I should prefer cotinine.

REFERENCES

1. Wharton BA. Sorrento studies of birthweight. *Acta Paediatr Scand* 1985; Suppl 319:171–9.
2. Clarson CL, Barker MJ, Marshall T, Wharton BA. Secular change in birthweight of Asian babies born in Birmingham. *Arch Dis Child* 1982;57:867–71.
3. Wharton BA. Food, growth and the Asian fetus. In: McVicar J, McFadyen I, eds. *Obstetric problems of the Asian community in Britain.* London: Royal College of Obstetricians and Gynaecologists, 1982.
4. Wolsanski NL. Biological reference systems in the assessment of nutritional status. In: Roche AF, Falkner F, eds. *Nutrition and malnutrition.* New York: Plenum Press, 1974;231–69.
5. Waterlow JC. Classification and definition of protein energy malnutrition. In: Beaton GH, Bengoa JM, eds. *Nutrition in preventative medicine.* Geneva: WHO, 1976;530–55.
6. Neumann GG. Reference data. In: Jelliffe JB, Jelliffe EP, eds. *Human nutrition. Vol 2. Nutrition and growth.* New York: Plenum, 299–328.
7. Waterlow JC. Letter: Child growth standards. *Lancet* 1980;1:717.
8. Graciter PL, Centry EM. Measuring children: one reference standard for all. *Lancet* 1981;2:297–9.
9. Neumann CG, Sharker H, Uberoi IS. Nutritional and anthropometric profile of young rural Punjabi children. *Indian J Med Res* 1969;57:1122–5.
10. National Center for Health Statistics NCHS, Growth Charts Monthly Vital Stat. Rep. 1976;25. Suppl No.3 Rockville: US Government Printing Office.
11. Bruce-Chwatt LJ. Les rapports entre la mère et l'enfant dans le paludisme endémique africain. *Arch Fr Pediatr* 1985;42:911–6.
12. Cohen S. Immunity to malaria. *Proc R Soc Lond (Biol)* 1979;203:323–45.
13. Brabin BJ, van den Berg H, Nijmeyer F. Folacin, cobalamin, and hematological status during pregnancy in rural Kenya: the influence of parity, gestation, and Plasmodium falciparum malaria. *Am J Clin Nutr* 1986; 43(5):803–15.
14. Bhargava V, Chatterjee M, Prakash A, Bhatia B, Mishara A. Fetal growth varuatuibs—I. Influence of maternal size and nutrition on identification of fetal growth retardation. *Indian Pediatr* 1983;20:549–59.

Intrauterine Growth Retardation, edited by
Jacques Senterre. Nestlé Nutrition Workshop
Series, Vol. 18. Nestec Ltd., Vevey/Raven Press,
Ltd., New York © 1989.

Food Supplements During Pregnancy

Jorge Suescun* and José O. Mora**

*Department of Paediatrics, Medical School of Colombia; and **Senior Medical
Nutritionist, LTS International Nutrition Unit, Bogotá, Colombia*

There is general agreement among experts in human growth on the importance of
the intrauterine period and early childhood up to the age of 6 years as basic critical
stages in the development of man. Indeed, it is at these stages of life that the child's
body and, more specifically, his central nervous system are the most flexible. It is a
well-known biological fact that the body's vulnerability to hostile environmental effects is directly related to the speed of the growth and development process.

The results of animal research on the effects of nutritional deprivation during
pregnancy on the fetus have been confirmed by the findings of human "natural experiments" (1–3). Acute malnutrition of the mother during the second half of pregnancy results in a smaller body and lower weight at birth (4,5). Low weight-for-
gestational-age has traditionally been considered a consequence of the mother's
malnutrition and is of special importance because it is closely related to perinatal
and neonatal mortality and, therefore, with the chances of survival of the newborn
baby. In addition, in those who survive, there is a risk of growth and subsequent developmental disorders, which is why this factor is a crucial variable for the newborn
baby's prospects (6,7). In general terms, the intrauterine period cannot escape the
harm caused by poverty or by the effects of adverse environmental factors. But, although animal studies have produced conclusive proof of a close relation between
nutritional deprivation during pregnancy and retardation of fetal growth, studies carried out on humans have shown contradictory results. For moral reasons, the
normally used pattern of deprivation in animal research cannot be applied to humans
but, on the other hand, the major differences between these two species make it impossible to generalize about the findings.

The data which are available on the human species are based on three kinds of
study: (a) The so-called "natural experiments" in which calamities such as war un-
intentionally mimic conditions of the pattern of deprivation used in animal experiments (1–3); (b) epidemiologic studies, involving large samples of the population,
on the relationship between the diet followed during pregnancy and fetal growth and
development (8–12); (c) clinical studies on a small scale (13–15). Although there
have been some inconsistencies in these studies, the following general conclusions
have been drawn:

a. Severe nutritional deprivation during the second half of pregnancy results in delayed fetal growth and greater perinatal mortality.
b. When less energy and/or protein than recommended is consumed, there is a definite relationship between such reduced consumption and fetal growth.
c. Weight at birth, which is the most generally accepted fetal growth criterion, is clearly related to perinatal mortality and to the child's later growth and development (16–21).
d. A large energy and/or protein intake during the second half of the last trimester of pregnancy can increase the weight at birth of babies whose mothers' diets were deficient during the first half of pregnancy.

These conclusions justified the drawing up of programs to provide food supplements during pregnancy for populations at risk from malnutrition. Experimental studies have, however, in some cases failed to show that such measures are effective. The effects of prenatal food supplements on weight at birth indicate in some cases that we cannot conclude that such measures are invariably efficient in increasing fetal growth (22,23); this has led to some skepticism, which appears to be justified.

The risk of dismissing too lightly nutritional measures because of the apparent inconsistency of their results makes it necessary to consider some aspects connected with their efficiency, so that we can determine the conditions under which such measures really are effective. It should be pointed out that the apparent failure of some prenatal food supplementation programs to affect weight at birth in a major way does not imply an absence of a direct relation between maternal nutrition and fetal growth. Apart from the problems inherent in the design of such studies or relating to assessment of the programs, it is essential to consider in practice at least two very important aspects which help explain the differences between the results obtained.

INITIAL NUTRITIONAL STATUS

It is logical to assume that any nutritional measures will have effects which can be proved only if they are designed to correct deficiencies which really are found in the target population involved. Food supplementation should therefore be aimed at pregnant women whose nutritional deficiencies can be proved. Unfortunately, there are no indicators of the nutritional status of pregnant women which are sufficiently valid and reliable to be used in field conditions. The search for indicators which are sensitive and easy to apply when assessing the nutritional status of a pregnant woman and which can be used in community programs is a pressing need which should be met as a priority in nutritional research.

The variations in the effects obtained with prenatal food supplementation are partly due to the fact that the target populations have varying levels of nutritional deficiencies of an ill-defined extent. Thus, for example, discouraging effects have been recorded in industrial countries with groups with marginal or unproved nutritional deficiencies. Thus, some studies have provided supplements of specific nutrients, either without previous documentation of the presence of the respective deficiencies, or in pregnant women with generalized nutritional deficiencies, as happens in most developing countries. The type of initial deficiency would, for example, explain why some studies relate an increase of weight at birth to energy supplementation whereas others relate it to increased protein consumption.

THE REAL SUPPLEMENTATION LEVEL ACHIEVED

It is to be expected that there would be a direct relationship between the effects and the extent to which the initial deficiency is corrected. The correction level depends both on the quality and on the quantity of the supplements given, and also on their actual consumption and on the behavior of the recipients in relation to their usual diet.

a. *The quality and quantity of supplements* is important in relation to the type and extent of the deficiencies which are meant to be corrected; various studies have supplied varying quantities of supplements of varying nutritional content which are bound to have covered varying proportions of the nutritional deficiencies involved.

b. *The consumption of the supplements* may vary with their quantity and quality, the extent to which they fit into the population's eating patterns, the distribution systems and checking methods and the nutritional education imparted. It also appears to depend on the mothers' perception of their nutritional needs compared with those of the other members of their families. It is obvious that, when supplements are distributed for consumption at home, they may not be used by the intended person, but instead may be sold or exchanged, or diluted within the family. Consumption problems are reduced when the supplements are given directly at food centers but this system is not practical in programs covering large areas; problems are aggravated where the distribution systems involve coupons or vouchers.

c. *The behavior of recipients regarding their usual diets* is generally characterized by the substitution of usual foods by those given as supplements, which therefore become substitutes instead of supplements. This substitution is a genuine problem which is often underestimated and which affects the results of the programs a great deal. This means that the food supplement programs, rather than constituting a purely nutritional measure, are really transfer-of-income programs—due to the changes they bring about in the distribution of the family budget—with marginal nutritional effects.

IMPACT OF FOOD SUPPLEMENTATION DURING PREGNANCY ON MOTHER AND CHILD

The previously explained concepts have been confirmed by the results of a study of measures carried out in the marginal urban areas of Bogotá, as part of a longitudinal investigation of nutrition, stimulus, and mental development, carried out jointly by the Colombian Institute for Family Well-Being and Harvard University. The data being reported are those of the prenatal and perinatal phase of this study, for which families from the poor districts in the southern part of the city were selected according to the following criteria: (a) mothers in the first or second third of pregnancy; and (b) malnutrition found in at least 50% of children under 5 years (malnutrition was defined as less than 85% of the proper weight for age).

The population of the whole area was counted four times, at six monthly intervals; 456 families were selected and allocated at random to six experimental groups, as shown on Figs. 1 and 2. Until confinement, groups A, B, and A1 may, between them, be considered the control group who did not receive supplements, whereas groups C, D, and D1 represent the sample given supplements. All families involved in the study received a full health care program, including the free distribution of drugs prescribed by the doctors involved in the program. All families were subjected to the same assessments, regarding social class, health, physical growth, and intellectual development, for the entire duration of the study.

Food supplements were started in families from groups C, D, and D1 at the beginning of the third quarter of pregnancy. The supplements were distributed in suf-

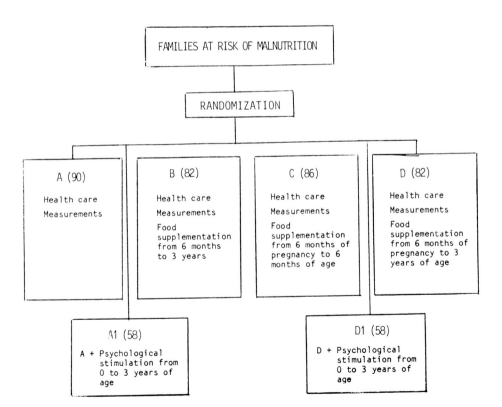

FIG. 1. Experimental design.

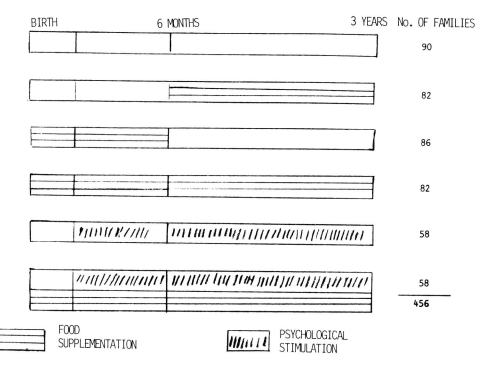

FIG. 2. Study groups according to the interventions and duration.

ficient quantities to meet a substantial part of the daily energy and nutrient intake recommended for pregnant women and other family members (Table 1). The foods were distributed weekly from premises resembling a neighborhood shop, away from the Health Center where the medical program was carried out, so as to reduce contact between the supplemented and unsupplemented groups to a minimum. The pregnant women being given supplements were instructed on the importance of continuing their usual diet as well as the supplement. As a means of checking on this, they were asked to return the empty packs when being handed the food for the following week. In addition, the correct use of the foods was checked by means of unexpected home visits by project staff. The food intake of the pregnant women was measured by means of a general survey recording consumption as recalled over 24 hr, at the beginning of the study and 2 months later.

Gestational age was calculated from the first day of the last period. In 12 cases, gestational age had to be estimated by successive measurements of uterine height, since the timing of the last period was vague. All the women were weighed at the beginning of the study, i.e., at roughly 25 weeks' gestation, and every month during pregnancy. In 117 women, the mother's weight was obtained during labor and before rupture of the membrane. The first and last measurement obtained during the study were used to estimate average weekly weight gain.

TABLE 1. *Composition of food supplements proposed for the mothers during the last trimester of pregnancy*

Food supplement	g	kcal	Protein (g)	Vitamin A (I.U.)	Iron (mg)
Skim milk powder	60	214	21.6	18	0.4
Enriched bread	150	466	16.8	6	2.6
Vegetable oil	20	176	—	—	—
Vitamin C—mineral complement	—	—	—	6,000	15.0
Total	230	856	38.4	6,024	18.0
Percentage of the recommendations	—	40	60	100	100

Quantities are per person per day.

Two-thirds of the women in the sample were delivered at the Hospital of San Juan de Dios where previously hired project staff had been instructed on how to collect information on the confinement and to take anthropometric measurements of the newborn baby. Weight at birth was determined by using a gauged balance (Toledo) with a capacity of 13,500 g and a sensitivity to 20 g. The rest of the sample had their babies in other maternity hospitals or at home, where it proved impossible to obtain the weight at birth.

Out of a total of 456 families, 7 were lost during the rest of pregnancy. There were 10 cases of stillborn babies and 6 sets of twins. We thus obtained a sample of 433 singleton births from our study. Two hundred ninety-seven babies were weighed at the hospital immediately after birth and again 25 and 31 hr after birth, and at age 15 days. One hundred ten of the remaining 136 were weighed by project staff: 13 at age 25 hr, 8 at 31 hr, and 89 when 15 days old. So as to estimate the weight at birth of these 110 babies, a regression equation was calculated with the data from the 242 babies who had complete data, i.e., at birth, at ages 25 hr, 31 hr, and 15 days. The correlation of weight at birth with the other weighings was 0.98, 0.98, and 0.87, respectively. Thus, data on the weight at birth were obtained for 407 babies, either directly or indirectly. The results of the study were not distorted when the subsample of babies of estimated weight was included.

RESULTS

Random allotment produced groups with comparable relevant socio-economic and biologic variables such as size of family, income, food expenditure, the mother's age, height, weight, and gestational age on admission, initial calorie and protein intake, number of previous pregnancies, and educational level (Table 2).

TABLE 2. *Initial comparison of relevant socioeconomic and biological variables in the groups*

Variable	Control group (n = 230)	Supplemented group (n = 226)
Size of family	5.8 ± 2.5	5.2 ± 2.0
Number of rooms in house	1.7 ± 0.9	1.6 ± 0.9
Area of house (m² per person)	3.2 ± 1.8	3.5 ± 1.9
Monthly family income (in US $)	50.9 ± 25.4	46.9 ± 20.5
Monthly income per capita (in US $)	9.7 ± 6.1	9.9 ± 4.8
Family expenses for food (in US $)	27.7 ± 13.4	26.2 ± 12.6
Characteristics of mother		
age (years)	26.6 ± 6.1	25.8 ± 5.4
height (cm)	149.9 ± 5.3	149.9 ± 5.5
daily consumption of energy (kcal)	1,621 ± 655	1,623 ± 635
daily consumption of protein (g)	37.0 ± 22.9	35.6 ± 19.2
number of previous pregnancies	4.2 ± 3.2	3.6 ± 2.6
number of years of education (average)	2.96	3.01

Impact on the Mothers' Diets

Tables 3 and 4 show average daily calorie and protein consumption by the pregnant women before and during the program, both in absolute quantities and in percentages of adequate quantities. Starting with a low initial consumption rate (around 1,600 kcal and 36 g protein), the reference group did not change their consumption during the program, whereas the group receiving supplements only increased their total intake by 150 kcal and 20.6 g protein, contrasting with the 856 kcal and 38.4 g protein provided. In terms of recommended quantities, the net increase was only 6% in terms of energy and 30% in terms of protein (24).

Figure 3 shows the results, with the origin of the energy and protein consumed. Real supplementation was below expectation due both to lower consumption of the supplements and to the presence of "substitution" to the normal diet; the latter was lower for proteins than for calories, showing that low-protein foods were substituted

TABLE 3. *Average daily consumption of energy and protein at the 6th and 8th month of pregnancy*

Groups	Energy (kcal)		Protein (g)	
	6 months[a]	8 months	6 months[a]	8 months
Control group	1,621 ± 655	1,573 ± 656	37.0 ± 22.9	35.5 ± 21.2
Supplemented group	1,623 ± 635	1,773 ± 568	35.6 ± 19.2	56.2 ± 22.0

[a]Before starting supplementation.

TABLE 4. *Daily intake of energy and protein in the supplemented group (percent of standard recommended intake)*

	Energy (kcal)	Protein
Before	74.8 ± 28.6	56.1 ± 30.3
After	80.9 ± 25.9	86.3 ± 34.0
Increase	6.1 ± 29.5	30.2 ⊥ 37.7

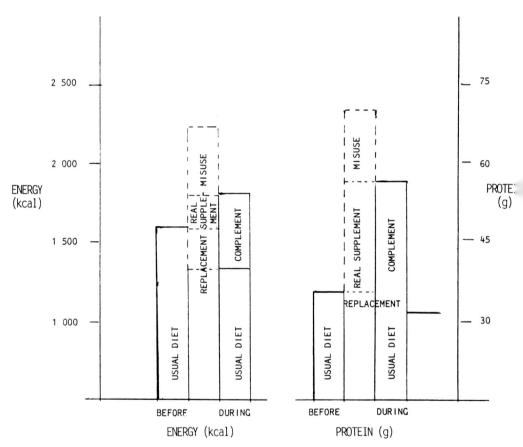

FIG. 3. Consumption of energy and protein in supplemented mothers before and during the program. Expected consumption during the supplementation period.

TABLE 5. *Weight gain during the last quarter of pregnancy by supplementation group*

Supplementation group	n	Weight gain (g)	p^a
A. Control	183	3,461 ± 1,731	—
B. Supplemented	190	4,205 ± 1,759	0.0005
< 13 weeks	75	3,940 ± 1,940	0.025
≥ 13 weeks	115	4,378 ± 1,616	0.0005
C. Total sample	373	3,840 ± 1,782	—

[a]One-tail *t*-test.

by the food supplements which were rich in proteins. In this program, the low consumption rate of supplements by the pregnant women was due more to misuse than to dilution, since they were given foods for the whole family. The substitution level was highly correlated with initial consumption in both energy ($r = 0.71$, $p < 0.001$) and protein ($r = 0.67$, $p < 0.001$).

Impact on Mothers' Weight Gain

The food supplements had a significant effect on the weight gain of mothers during the last trimester and weight gain was greater in those who took part in the program for 13 weeks or more (Table 5). On the other hand, weight gain correlated significantly with birthweight both in the control group ($r = 0.18$, $p < 0.001$) and in the group receiving supplements ($r = 0.28$, $p < 0.001$), and in the total sample ($r = 0.24$, $p < 0.001$). Similarly, in the group receiving supplements, the duration of supplementation significantly correlated with the mother's weight gain ($r = 0.18$, $p < 0.01$).

Impact on the Baby's Weight at Birth

Food supplements given for 13 or more weeks significantly affected the babies' weight at birth; the difference between the weight of the supplemented group and that of the control group was 90 g (Table 6); supplements given for less than 13 weeks did not produce significant results. The difference between the total group receiving supplements and the control group was only 63 g (25). The time during which supplements were given correlated significantly with weight at birth ($r = 0.19$, $p < 0.01$). The relation between quantity and response in terms of supplementary calories was about 50 g for every 10,000 kcal; this response is better than that found in a similar study carried out in Guatemala (26), which was 30 g for every 10,000 kcal, and it is within the range estimated for various ranges of energy/protein consumption (26). It should be noted that the real supplementation achieved was rel-

TABLE 6. *Birthweight in term infants by supplementation group*

| Supplementation group | n | Birthweight (g) | | p^a |
		Mean	SD	
A. Control	165	2,940	318	—
B. Supplemented	177	3,003	354	< 0.05
< 13 weeks	76	2,967	344	NS
≥ 13 weeks	101	3,030	364	< 0.025
C. Total sample	342	2,973	338	—

[a]One-tail *t*-test.

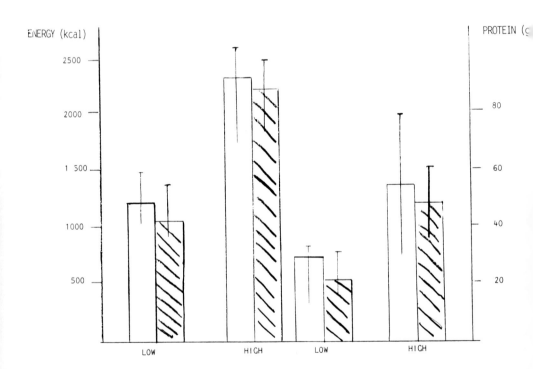

FIG. 4. Initial consumption of energy and protein by pregnant women according to consumption categories.

atively greater in terms of protein than in terms of energy in a group where protein deficiency is greater (45%) than energy deficiency (25%).

In order to study the effects of giving supplements to pregnant women with varying initial consumption levels, the sample was divided into subgroups with high and low initial consumption, using a cutoff point somewhere near the average, i.e., 1,500 kcal and 30 g protein (27). Figure 4 shows that the mean initial intakes in the low and high consumption categories did not differ between the supplemented and unsupplemented groups; the low consumption categories had an average initial intake of about 1,100 kcal and 20 g protein; the high consumption category had an intake of 2,100 kcal and 50 g protein.

The first interesting finding was the absence of differences in average consumption of supplements between the low and high initial consumption categories. Second, in the group receiving supplements, those with a low initial consumption increased their consumption considerably, taking up to 1,600 kcal and 50 g protein, whereas the large consumers increased their protein consumption (up to 60 g), but not their calorie consumption, due to a high proportion of substitution in their diet (Fig. 5).

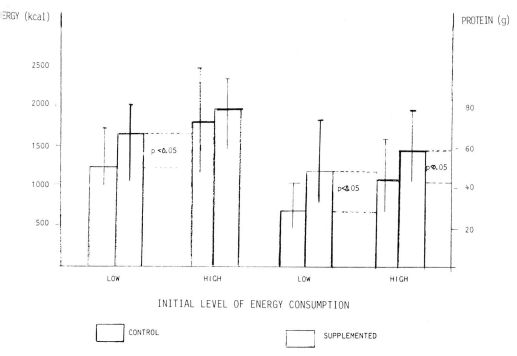

FIG. 5. Final consumption of energy and protein by pregnant women according to the consumption categories.

TABLE 7. *Birthweight by supplementation group according to initial consumption levels of energy and protein*

Initial consumption level	Control group			Supplemented group			Difference (g)	p^a
	n	Mean (g)	SD	n	Mean (g)	SD		
Energy (kcal)								
> 1,500	102	2,910	418	107	3,018	391	108	< 0.025
< 1,500	98	2,945	363	99	2,924	344	− 21	NS
Protein (g)								
> 30	106	2,916	410	144	3,031	362	115	< 0.025
< 30	94	2,939	371	92	2,901	371	− 38	NS

[a]One-tail *t*-test

Last, there were significant differences in weight at birth between the control group and the high category of the supplemented group, but not the group with low initial consumption (Table 7). This effect on weight at birth was specifically associated with a greater intake of protein without an increased calorie consumption, contrary to the findings of the study in Guatemala; this discrepancy can partly be attributed to the fact that the Bogotá sample had a greater initial protein deficiency (average daily consumption in Guatemala 45 g versus 36 g in the Bogotá sample), while calorie deficiencies were similar (around 1,600 kcal per day).

The absence of effects on fetal growth in the lower consumption subgroup—in spite of the fact that the supplementation achieved was greater in terms of both protein and calories—suggests the existence of a minimum or threshold level of consumption which must be exceeded if there are to be effects on fetal growth. This level could be expressed either in terms of daily consumption or in terms of duration of supplementation of the amount achieved. It should be noted that, although the mothers' weight gain was greater in the high consumption category, the differences between the control group and the group receiving supplements were significant in

TABLE 8. *Perinatal and neonatal mortality by supplementation group*

	Control group		Supplemented group		Total	
	No.	Rate	No.	Rate	No.	Rate
Stillbirth[a]	8	36.0	2	9.0	10	22.6
Perinatal mortality[a]	14	63.1	7	31.7	21	47.4
Neonatal mortality[b]	9	42.1	5	22.8	14	32.3

[a]Rates of stillbirths and perinatal mortality per 100 pregnancies.
[b]Rates of neonatal mortality per 1,000 live births.

both categories. This suggests that nutritional supplementation in chronically under-fed pregnant women first restores the depleted reserves of the mother and *then* results in increased fetal growth.

Impact on Perinatal Mortality

The greatest differences between newborn babies whose mothers had received supplements and those who had not showed in the rates of stillbirth and perinatal and neonatal mortality (28). Indeed, all three rates were at least twice as high in the group who had not received supplements (Table 8). Both perinatal and neonatal mortality rates were generally more than ten times as high in premature babies than in those born after full gestation, while both figures were about three times lower in premature babies whose mothers had received supplements (Table 9) (29).

Impact on Duration of Breast-Feeding

As shown in Table 10, the supplementation program did not act as a brake on the mothers' milk production; on the contrary, there was a tendency to prolong breast-feeding in the group who received supplements, compared with the control group. The average duration of breast-feeding was 6 months in the control group, and 7.2 months in the group who received supplements. The fact that the food supplements also significantly increased the mother's weight gain in the last 3 months of pregnancy suggests that the difference in the duration of breast-feeding could be connected with the mothers' improved nutritional status in the group receiving supplements (30).

TABLE 9. *Perinatal and neonatal mortality in premature and term infants by supplementation group*

	Control group		Supplemented group		Total	
	No.	Rate	No.	Rate	No.	Rate
Perinatal mortality[a]						
Preterm infants	9	360.0	3	136.4	12	255.3
Term infants	5	28.6	4	21.4	9	24.9
Total	14	63.1	7	31.7	21	47.4
Neonatal mortality[b]						
Preterm infants	6	285.7	2	95.2	8	190.5
Term infants	3	15.5	3	15.2	6	15.3
Total	9	42.1	5	22.8	14	32.3

[a]Perinatal mortality rate per 100 pregnancies.
[b]Neonatal mortality rate per 1,000 live births.

TABLE 10. *Duration of breast-feeding in a sample of 1,977 mothers by supplementation group*

	Control group			Supplemented group		
	n	%	Cum %	n	%	Cum %
Duration (months)						
< 3	50	29.8	29.8	45	27.1	27.1
3–5	34	20.2	50.0	30	18.1	45.2
6–11	39	23.2	73.2	40	24.1	69.3
≥ 12	45	26.8	100.0	51	30.7	100.0
Total	168	100.0	—	166	100.0	—
Average duration	6 Months			7.2 Months		

Cum %, cumulative percentage.

SUMMARY

There appear to be few doubts about the direct connection between prenatal nutrition, expressed in terms of energy and protein consumption, and fetal growth; or about the effectiveness of suitable food supplements during pregnancy for pregnant women with nutritional deficiencies. The important practical question is to define the most efficient means by which to achieve adequate energy and protein intakes in pregnant women belonging to the large masses of marginal populations in the developing countries. The answer to this question should consider not only the possibilities of acting directly and temporarily as a palliative measure, but—and this is more important—a search for final solutions to the problem of poverty whose ultimate eradication would relegate studies such as the present one to mere academic speculation.

REFERENCES

1. Stein Z, et al. Famine and human development: The Dutch Hunger Winter of 1944/45.
2. Smith CA. Effect of maternal undernutrition upon the newborn infant in Holland (1944–1945). *J Pediatr* 1947;30:229.
3. Antonov AN. Children born during the siege of Leningrad in 1942. *J Pediatr* 1947;30:250.
4. Winick M. Malnutrition and brain development. *J Pediatr* 1969;74:667.
5. Dobbing, J. The later growth of the brain and its vulnerability. *Pediatrics* 1974;53:2.
6. Bergner L, Susser MW. Low birthweight and prenatal nutrition: an interpretative review. *Pediatrics,* 1972;46:946.
7. Lechtig A, et al. Causas de bajo peso al nacer en Latinoamerica. *Arch Latinoam Nutr* 1971;27:320.
8. Burke BS, Beal VA, Kirkwood SB, Stuart HC. The influence of nutrition during pregnancy upon the condition of the infant at birth. *J Nutr* 1943;26:569.
9. Ebbs J. The influence of prenatal diet on the mother and child. *J Nutr* 1941;22:515.
10. McGanity WR, Cannon RO, Bridgeforth EB, Martin MP, Densen PM, Darby WJ. The Vanderbilt Cooperative Study on maternal and infant nutrition. Relationships of obstetric performance to nutrition. *Am J Obstet Gynecol* 1954;67:501.

11. Sontag LW, Wines J. Relation of mothers' diets to status of their infants at birth and in infancy. *Am J Obstet Gynecol* 1947;54:994.
12. Thomson AM. Diet in pregnancy, III. Diet in relation to the course and outcome of pregnancy. *Br J Nutr* 1959;13:509.
13. Kasius RV, Randall A, Tompkins WT, Wiehl DG. Maternal and newborn studies at Philadelphia Lying-in Hospital. Newborn Studies. I. Size and growth of babies of mothers receiving nutrient supplements. In: *The promotion of maternal and newborn health*. New York: Milbank Memorial Fund, 1955:153.
14. Venkatachalam PS. Maternal nutritional status and its effect on the newly born. *Bull WHO* 1962; 26:193.
15. Iyenger L. Effects of dietary supplements late in pregnancy on the expectant mother and her newborn. *Indian J Med Res* 1967;55:85.
16. Churchill JA, Neff JW, Caldwell DF. Birth weight and intelligence. *Obstet Gynecol* 1966;28:425.
17. Wiener G, Rider RV, Oppel WC, Harper PA. Correlates of low birth weight: psychological status, at eight to ten years of age. *Pediatr Res* 1968;2:110.
18. Yerushalmy J. Relation of birth weight, gestational age, and the rate of intrauterine growth to perinatal mortality. *Pediatr Clin N Am* 1970;17:114.
19. Puffer RR, Serrano CV. Patterns of mortality in childhood. Washington D.C.: Pan American Health Organization (PAHO) Scientific. Publication No. 262, 1973.
20. Davies PA, Stewart AL. Low birth-weight infants: neurological sequelae and later intelligence. *Br Med Bull* 1975;3:85.
21. Committee on Maternal Nutrition, Food and Nutrition Board, National Research Council. Nutritional supplementation and the outcome of pregnancy. Washington, D.C.: National Academy of Sciences, 1973.
22. Blackwell RQ, Chow BF, Chinn KSK, Blackwell BN, Hsu SC. Prospective maternal nutrition study in Taiwan: rationale, study design, feasibility, and preliminary findings. *Nutr Rep Int* 1973;7:517.
23. Lechtig A, Habicht JP, Delgado H, Klein RE, Yarbrough C, Martorell R. Effect of food supplementation during pregnancy on birth weight. *Pediatrics* 1975;56:508.
24. Mora JO, de Paredes B, Wagner M, de Navarro L, Suescún J, Christiansen N, Herrera MG. Nutritional supplementation and the outcome of pregnancy. I. Birthweight. *Am J Clin Nutr* (in press).
25. Mora JO, de Navarro L, Clement J, Wagner M, de Paredes B, Herrera MG. The effect of nutritional supplementation on calorie and protein intake of pregnant women. *Nutr Rep Int* 1978;17:217.
26. Lechtig A, Yarbrough C, Delgado H, Habicht JP, Martorell R, Klein RE. Influence of maternal nutrition on birth weight. *Am J Clin Nutr* 1975;28:1223.
27. Christiansen N, Mora JO, de Navarro L, de Paredes B, Herrera MG. Effects of nutritional supplementation during pregnancy upon birth weight: the influence of pre-supplementation diet. (In preparation.)
28. Mora JO, Clement J, Christiansen N, Suescún J, Wagner M, Herrera MG. Nutritional supplementation and the outcome of pregnancy. III. Perinatal and neonatal mortality. Enviado para publicación, 1976.
29. Mora JO. Complementacion alimentaria durante el embarazo impacto sobre la madre y el nino. ICBF (Columbian Institute for Family), cuadernillo número 6.
30. Mora JO, de Navarro L, Suescún J, Wagner M, Herrera MG. Situación actual y tendencia de la lactancia materna en la zona urbana de Bogotá. ICBF, cuadernillo número 8.

DISCUSSION

Dr. Senterre: In the literature, there are very divergent findings and views on the effects of maternal food supplementation during pregnancy on birthweight. Dr. Wharton, at Sorrento Maternity Hospital, Birmingham, showed a differential effect of supplementation during pregnancy according to the nutritional state of the mothers and reviewed recent pregnancy supplemention studies (1). I would like to get his opinion about the problem of dietary supplementation in pregnancy.

Dr. Wharton: The table shows my own analysis (Table 1) of 8 trials of nutritional supple-

TABLE 1. *Summary of recent pregnancy supplementation studies*

Study design and controls	Subgroups, if any	Supplement regimen			Results		
		Per day				Effect compared to controls	
		Energy kcal	Protein (g)	Duration	Number	Birth wt	Wt for gestation
Guatemala: Prospective, not random, all mothers offered supplement. Controls: poor attenders consuming small amounts	Atole supplement	163	11	2nd, 3rd trimester	219	+ 131 g	
	Fresco supplement	59	Nil		186	+ 87 g $p < 0.01$	
Colombia: Prospective, randomized. Controls: contemporary, same program, no supplement	Boys	155	20	3rd	200	+ 107 g $p < 0.10$	
	Girls	155	20	3rd	207	− 7 g NS	
Aberdeen: Prospective. Controls: contemporary, matched mother also likely to produce light baby, no supplement		300	16	3rd	180	+ 37 NS	Increased with amount of supplement supplied $p < 0.03$
Harlem: New York Prospective randomized. Controls: contemporary, same clinic given multivitamins	Supplement	470	40	Before 30 wks	248	− 32 g NS	More preterm
	Complement	322	6		256	+ 41 g NS	

Study	Group						
Taiwan: Prospective. Controls: contemporary, given low energy supplement. Historical comparison with mother's previous baby	Compared with contemporary controls						
	Boys	800	80	From birth of previous baby	110	+ 55 NS	
	Girls	800	80		103	+ 32 NS	
	Compared with previous births to mother						
	Boys	800	80		111	+ 161 $p < 0.05$	
	Girls	800	80		105	− 49 g NS	
Sorrento: Birmingham Prospective, randomized. Controls: contemporary same clinic given multivitamins	Unselected	273	8	2nd, 3rd	142	− 40 g NS	+ 0.1 SD NS
	Nutritionally at risk	425	11	3rd	45	+ 330 g $p < 0.05$	+ 0.8 SD $p < 0.01$
	Nutritionally adequate	425	11	3rd	83	− 180 g NS	− 0.03 SD NS
Gambia: Prospective, not random, all mothers given supplement. Controls: historical comparison with mothers observed in previous 4 years	Wet season	900	35	2nd, 3rd	146	+ 225 g $p < 0.01$	+ 224 g $p < 0.01$
	Dry season	900	35	2nd, 3rd	126	+ 2 g NS	− 32 g NS

Adapted from ref. 1.

mentation during pregnancy (2–9). They are divided into three groups, i.e., those where there has been a positive effect on intrauterine growth (trials 1–3), no effect (trials 4,5) or a differential effect (trials 6–8). Very recent studies of maternal nutrition have been published from Kenya (10) and India (11). The comment made earlier on the importance of considering energy balance may explain these apparently conflicting results. There is a need to select mothers for supplementation, i.e., it should be targeted. At Sorrento, supplementation enhanced fetal growth in mothers at nutritional risk but had no effect or possibly an adverse effect in the adequately nourished ones. The Gambian findings published later have similarities. In mothers supplemented during the wet season, when food was limited and work in the fields arduous (i.e., when energy balance was less satisfactory), fetal growth was enhanced compared with the historical controls. However, in mothers supplemented during the more affluent dry season, fetal growth was not enhanced—indeed, it was slightly below control levels. Like all therapeutic maneuvers, dietary supplementation should be targeted only at those who require the therapy. Increment in triceps skinfold was an effective method of selection. Probably in Guatemala, Colombia, and in Gambia during the wet season, where supplementation had a positive effect, the mothers were nutritionally at risk. The Aberdeen mothers selected for supplementation had adverse nutritional features associated with poor intrauterine growth (e.g., weight, height, and weight gain below the 25th percentile). Concerning the Taiwan results, if the safer contemporary controls are used for comparison, then supplementation had no effect, but then "before supplementation there was little evidence of gross abnormality with respect to . . . fetal growth." The New York study supplementation was aimed at mothers with a low weight, low weight gain or low dietary intake but no evidence was produced that these factors were good predictors of poor intrauterine growth in that population. We did not find poor intrauterine growth to be associated with poor nutritional status in our European population, so we did not supplement them.

Dr. Seeds: I'd like to ask Dr. Villar if there was a difference in defined IUGR between his supplemented and unsupplemented groups. Also, was there any difference in fetal distress in labor?

Dr. Villar: I do not have data on labor. With regard to IUGR, the increase in birthweight which we observed was mainly due to intrauterine growth and not to longer gestation, after allowing for maternal height and parity. The effect on gestational age was very minor—only 2 to 3 days.

Dr. Canosa: Did you make adjustments for physical work in the mothers?

Dr. Villar: The results I showed were adjusted for several confinding variables including S.E.S. We did not have specific indicators of work during pregnancy.

Dr. Canosa: From my experience in Southeast Asia, heavy work is an important variable which must be accounted for before making recommendations about norms for pregnancy weight gain and so forth. Another variable that might be worth considering is carbon monoxide (CO). Women who spend most of the day inside the house cooking may be exposed to significant levels of CO.

Dr. Belizan: We studied a rural population in Guatemala and showed an effect of CO contamination and birthweight. This was in women who lived in one-room homes where they cooked, lived, and slept (12).

Dr. Villar: The percentage of women who cook and live in the same room in Guatemala City is very small. The main contaminant in this urban population is reported to be lead. However, we did a longitudinal study of lead levels among pregnant women but found low levels. I suspect the main reason is that they have a very high calcium intake, so there is competition between calcium and lead which reduces lead absorption from the gut.

Dr. Wharton: One of the major criticisms of the Guatemala study has been that the women were self-selected for treatment. What is your comment about this, Dr. Villar?

Dr. Villar: This is always a possibility. Several pieces of evidence can be present against the self-selection effect. In the first place, the association was between total supplementation and birthweight and not with the number of visits to the clinic. Second, it was the poorest section of the population who had the highest supplementation levels. If there had been a significant number of more educated and highly motivated women in the highly supplemented population, this would certainly have had a confounding effect, because you would have expected their infants to weigh more. But that was not the case. These are the two main arguments that the results were a genuine reflection of the effects of the supplement.

Dr. Marini: How reproducible are the biometric impedance measurements? We have had some experience in growing preterm infants which seems to show that even small changes in the position of the electrodes can alter the values. Is the method reliable?

Dr. Villar: Since there are no standards, it is difficult to talk about reliability. There is good agreement between the impedance method and other methods of known accuracy. For example, the correlation between impedance and densitometry in our pregnant and post-partum women is about 0.80, and there have been several studies in non-pregnant women showing good argeement with results of body composition using deuterium. However, I think you were referring more to standardization than to reliability. I agree that the method is sensitive to electrode position, but this requires standardization of procedures just like any other method, skinfold measurement, for example. We use only one person in each clinic to do the measurements and the techniques are standardized.

REFERENCES

1. Wharton BA. Sorrento studies of birthweight. Case for international reference data. *Acta Paediatr Scand* 1985;suppl 319:170–9.
2. Lechtig A, Habicht JP, Delagodo H, Klein RE, Yarbrough C, Martorell R. Effect of food supplementation during pregnancy on birthweight. *Pediatr* 1975;56:508–19.
3. Mora JO, de Paredes B, Wagner M, de Navarro L, Suescún J, Christiansen N, Hera MB. Nutritional supplementation and the outcome of pregnancy. 1. Birthweight. *Am J Clin Nutr* 1979;31:455–62.
4. Campbell-Brown M. Protein energy supplements in primigravid women at risk of low birthweight. In: Campbell DM, Gillmer MDG, eds. *Nutrition in pregnancy.* London: Royal College of Obstetricians and Gynaecologists, 1983;85–98.
5. Rush D, Stein Z, Susser M. A randomized controlled trial of prenatal nutritional supplementation in New York City. *Pediatr* 1980;65:687–97.
6. McDonald EC, Pollitt E, Mueller W, Hsueh AM, Sherwin R. The Bacon Chow study: maternal nutritional supplementation and birthweight of offspring. *Am J Clin Nutr* 1981;34:2133–44.
7. Viegas OAC, Scott PH, Cole TJ, Mansfield HN, Wharton P, Wharton BA. Dietary protein energy supplementation of pregnant Asian mothers at Sorrento, Birmingham. I: Unselective during second and third trimesters. *Br Med J [Clin Res]* 1982;285:589–92.
8. Viegas OAC, Scott PH, Cole TJ, Eaton P, Needham PG, Wharton BA. Dietary protein energy supplementation of pregnant Asian mothers at Sorrento, Birmingham. II: Selective during third trimester only. *Br Med J [Clin Res]* 1982;285:5925.
9. Prentice AM, Whitehead RG, Watkinson M, Lamb WH, Cole TJ. Prenatal dietary supplementation of African women and birthweight. *Lancet* 1983;1:489–92.
10. Kusin JA, Jansen AA. Maternal nutrition and birthweight: selective review and some results of observations in Machakos, Kenya. *Ann Trop Paediatr* 1986;6:3–9.
11. Tyagi NK, Bhatia BD, Sur AM. Low birthweight babies in relation to nutritional status in primipara. *Indian Pediatr* 1985;22:507–14.
12. Belizan et al. *J Trop Med Hyg* 1981;84:243.

Intrauterine Growth Retardation, edited by
Jacques Senterre. Nestlé Nutrition Workshop
Series, Vol. 18. Nestec Ltd., Vevey/Raven Press,
Ltd., New York © 1989.

Maternal Parenteral Alimentation and Intra-Amniotic Nutrition

J. M. Ernest

Department of Obstetrics and Gynecology, Bowman Gray School of Medicine, Wake Forest University, Winston-Salem, North Carolina 27103

Adequate nutrition during pregnancy is a common goal of physicians and pregnant patients. While general guidelines and common sense about diet usually suffice, some pregnant women require extended counseling and therapy to prevent undernutrition or malnutrition. The physician rarely resorts to enteral or parenteral alimentation, the subject of this chapter, to deliver adequate nutrients to the pregnant patient and her fetus. In this chapter, a brief review of the effects of maternal malnutrition and supplementation will precede general guidelines regarding components of the diet. Next, conclusions obtained from a review of case reports involving total parenteral nutrition (TPN) during pregnancy will be followed by an outline of indices which are useful in the evaluation of the undernourished patient. Individual components of TPN and their safety will be discussed before concluding with information about TPN and intra-amniotic nutrition used to treat the fetus at risk.

MATERNAL MALNUTRITION AND SUPPLEMENTATION

In 1965 Berg (1) restricted pregnant laboratory rats to decreasing percentages of normal food intake. At 75% of normal intake, the mothers gained weight and mean fetal weight was normal. At 50% of normal intake, an 8% loss of baseline weight was noted, coupled with a decrease in fetal weight of 12%. Embryonic death occurred in 23% of cases. With maternal diet restricted to 25% of normal, 26% to 32% of maternal body weight was lost, but mean fetal weight was 50% of control and an embryonic death rate of 64% to 92% was found. In pigs fed a low-protein diet during pregnancy, 17% of their initial weight was lost and fetuses weighed 33% less than controls (2). In humans, protein restriction has been shown to reduce plasma volume significantly (3). Reduction in plasma volume during pregnancy correlates with reduced fetal size and other pregnancy complications (4). Human experience with severe maternal nutritional deprivation indicates that some maternal adaptation occurs, but the threshold value is poorly defined. During the 7 month Dutch famine in 1944–1945, maternal caloric intake was estimated to have reached a low of 1,200

TABLE 1. Parenteral nutrition during pregnancy, 1972–1986

Authors (year)	Cases	Underlying complication	TPN Gestational age (weeks)	TPN Duration (days)	Gestational age at delivery (weeks)	IUGR suspected at onset of TPN	IUGR present
Cox et al. (1981) (21)	1	Severe Crohn's disease	32	42	38	Y	Y
Di Constanzo et al. (1982) (22)	1	Corrosive burn of upper GI	28	49	35	N	N
Dudrick et al. (1979) (23)	2	Brain dead	2d–3d trimester	8–12 weeks	NA	?	NA
Gineston et al. (1984) (24)	1	Severe acute pancreatitis	22	83	34	N	N
Hatjis and Meis (1985) (25)	1	Duodenal jejunostomy, posterior gastrojejunostomy	31	24	36	N	N
Hew and Deitel (1980) (26)	1	Severe hyperemesis	12	14	38	N	N
Klein et al. (1983) (27)	2	Crohn's disease	2nd trimester		Term	N	N
	1	Severe pancreatitis	35	14	37	Y	Y
	1	Cerebal palsy, esophagitis, hiatal hernia	33	14	35	Y	Y
Lakoff and Feldman (1972) (20)	1	Hyperemesis, diabetic ketoacidosis	33	21	36	Y	Y
	1	Anorexia nervosa	32	12	40	Y	Y
Lavin et al. (1982) (28)	1	Narcotic addiction, hemorrhagic gastritis, diabetes	27	44 (14 antepartum)	29	Y	Y
Lee et al. (1986) (29)	1	Class D diabetes, anorexia	21	24	26	N	Stillborn
LeGrix et al. (1978) (30)	1	Hemorrhagic rectocolitis	22	63	36	N	N
Lipkin et al. (1985) (31)	1	Small bowel venous occlusion	8	189	35	N	N
Loiudice and Chandrakaar (1980) (32)	1	Intractable nausea and vomiting, diarrhea, jejunoileal bypass	25	21	40	Y	N
Main et al. (1981) (33)	1	Crohn's disease	27	63	36	N	Y

Martin (1982) (34)	1	S/P hepatic lobectomy and splenectomy, diabetes	22	12	30	N	N
Rivera-Alsina et al. (1984) (35)	1	Nausea/vomiting	9	175	34	N	N
	1	Recurrent pancreatitis	31	28	35	N	N
	1	Intractable nausea and vomiting, weight loss, jejunoileostomy, twins	29	28	35	N	Y
	1	Regional enteritis	19	112	35	Y	N
	1	Chronic diarrhea, jejunoileal bypass, large weight loss	33	10	35	N	N
Schoenbeck and Segerbrand (1973) (36)	1	Severe hyperemesis	8	56	38	N	N
Herbert et al. (1986) (37)	1	Esophageal stricture	31	20	34	Y	Y
Seifer et al. (1985) (38)	1	Acute cholecystitis	37	10	39	N	Z
	1	Promyelocytic leukemia	26	10	34	?	Y
Stowell et al. (1984) (39)	1	Acute pancreatitis	31	42	39	N	Y
Tresadern et al. (1984) (40)	1	Severe Crohn's disease	Before conception	365	37	N	N
Webb (1980) (41)	1	Embryonal cell carcinoma on chemotherapy	28	32	32	N	N
Weinberg et al. (1982) (42)	1	Hyperlipidemic pancreatitis	35	14	37	Y	Y
Young (1982) (43)	1	Recurrent acute pancreatitis	30,36	7,1	36	N	N
	2	Recurrent pancreatitis	14,24	17,8	34,37	N,N	N/?
Rayburn et al. (1986) (44)	1	S/P decompression of brain tumor, need for ventilatory support	15	2	16	N	N
	1	Severe hyperemesis	10	4	41	N	N
	1	Severe hyperemesis, diabetic ketoacidosis	14	7	37	?	?
	1	Major burn	27	9	38	N	N

IUGR, intrauterine growth retardation; TPN, total parenteral nutrition.

kcal per day. A significant decrease in birthweight of 250 g was noted in infants born to women affected by the famine during the last two trimesters of pregnancy (5). This study and others indicate the influence of malnutrition on fetal growth, and question the old concept of "fetal parasitism" during periods of starvation.

In supplementation studies, pre-pregnancy nutritional status appears to be a critical determinant of the effects that improved nutrition may have on neonatal outcome (6). Supplementation studies have also demonstrated the importance of balanced supplementation. In New York City, Rush et al. (7) noted a possible link between a high protein supplement given prenatally and an increase in preterm and growth-retarded infants in a study population. Similar results with lower birthweights were reported in Scotland in women consuming a high-protein, low-calorie diet during pregnancy (8) compared to controls.

GENERAL NUTRITION GUIDELINES DURING PREGNANCY

The first two trimesters of pregnancy represent an anabolic state marked by increasing maternal protein and fat stores. During the third trimester catabolism prevails as fetal demands increase and are met by mobilizing maternal muscle protein stores. Increased lipolysis also occurs in gestation and free fatty acids are mobilized (9). While optimal nutrition during gestation is debatable because of these and other changes, recommendations do exist to guide the physician in nutritional support of the pregnant patient. Traditional teaching estimates the caloric cost of pregnancy to be approximately 80,000 kcal and can be met by increasing daily energy intake by 300 kcal per day (10). The Harris-Benedict equation (11) (see Table 4) can be used to estimate energy needs, with additional calories added for pregnancy, or the guideline of 36 kcal/kg-day (12) may be used to estimate optimal caloric intake. However, recent studies dispute the need for an additional 300 kcal per day and suggest fewer supplemental calories may be adequate during normal pregnancy (13). Dietary carbohydrate and fat provide the bulk of energy for most metabolic processes during pregnancy, including those of the fetus, and additional dietary protein is required to support increased maternal and fetal protein synthesis to offset the increased protein catabolism and gluconeogenesis.

Estimates of the increased protein requirements during pregnancy have either relied upon calculation of the total protein stores in mother and fetus, or on nitrogen balance studies. While estimates vary in early pregnancy between the two methods, both methods estimate nitrogen retention late in pregnancy to be approximately 1 g per day (14,15). In order to achieve this nitrogen balance, pregnant women need to consume 1.3 g/kg-day of protein, with additional allowances for adolescents (1.5 to 1.7 g/kg-day).

Maternal lipid metabolism is greatly altered during pregnancy, and plasma lipids increase appreciably during the latter half of pregnancy. Maternal fat ingestion should represent 20% to 25% of caloric requirements of normal pregnancy to supply fat for storage in early pregnancy, to supply essential fatty acids to the mother and fetus, and to decrease the dependence on a carbohydrate load to supply the increased energy requirements of pregnancy (16). Guidelines for minerals, trace elements, and vitamins during pregnancy have also been published (9).

With these concepts in mind, let us discuss the patient who is unable to maintain adequate nutrition and who is at risk for developing a nutritional deficiency. For this patient, the physician may consider intravenous or parenteral alimentation.

TOTAL PARENTERAL NUTRITION

Modern day intravenous nutrition began in 1913 when Henriques and Anderson (17) administered a protein hydrolysate intravenously to a goat. Development of total intravenous nutritional support was hindered by the inability to deliver adequate non-protein energy until the 1960s. Wretlind (18), developed in 1961 a non-toxic fat emulsion that could be given by peripheral vein, and Wilmore and Dudrick (19), in 1968, successfully administered hypertonic dextrose solution to an infant born with severe gastrointestinal (GI) atresia. In 1972, Lakoff and Feldman (20) reported the first patient to receive total parenteral nutrition during pregnancy. The last two decades have seen refinements in methodology, increased understanding of metabolic needs, and of special interest to this discussion, increased use of total parenteral nutrition during pregnancy.

Since 1972, 43 pregnant patients receiving central TPN as their sole energy source during a portion of or throughout pregnancy have been reported. Patients whose inadequate oral intake was supplemented by TPN or who received only peripheral TPN are not included in this discussion. Table 1 details each case and Table 2 summarizes the cases by specific medical condition and gives the number of patients in each group.

Gestational age and onset of therapy ranged from the preconceptional period to 37 weeks gestation. Duration of therapy ranged from 2 to 365 days.

TABLE 2. *Medical complications in pregnancy requiring TPN, 1972–1986*

Problem	No. of patients
Pancreatitis	8
Inflammatory bowel disease	7
Diabetes-related conditions	6
Hyperemesis gravidarum	5
Jejunoileal bypass	4
Long-term mechanical ventilatory support	3
Anorexia nervosa	2
Esophageal disease	3
Malignancy	2
Other (major burn, cholecystitis, small bowel obstruction)	3

TABLE 3. *TPN during pregnancy begun prior to 20 weeks gestation*

	GA begun (week)	Duration (days)	IUGR
Severe hyperemesis	12	14	No
Regional enteritis	19	112	No
Severe hyperemesis	8	56	No
Recurrent pancreatitis	14	17	No
Embryonal cell carcinoma, on chemotherapy before conception	Before conception	365	No
Severe hyperemesis	10	4	No
Severe hyperemesis	14	7	?
Small bowel occlusion	8	189	No

GA, gestational age; IUGR, intrauterine growth retardation; TPN, total parenteral nutrition.

Table 3 reviews TPN during pregnancy begun before 20 weeks gestation. While a number of case reports list intrauterine growth retardation (IUGR) occurring with TPN therapy during pregnancy, only two case reports (33,39) note the previously undiagnosed appearance of IUGR after beginning TPN, even when TPN was adminstered for the entire pregnancy. No report of IUGR exists when TPN was begun prior to 20 weeks gestation. One must assume that while IUGR frequently occurs in association with TPN during pregnancy, the underlying disease state and reason for the need for TPN is more likely the cause of the IUGR than the TPN.

INDICES OF NUTRITIONAL ASSESSMENT

In caring for a pregnant patient with nutritional problems, or at any time that a pregnant woman is at risk for undernutrition, nutritional assessment should be completed before TPN is implemented. Table 4 lists variables that may be useful to assess the extent of nutritional impairment and to determine the success of the therapy. When a patient becomes a candidate for TPN, the individual components of TPN—dextrose, amino acids and fat, as well as vitamins and trace minerals—must be determined.

COMPONENTS OF TPN

Carbohydrate

The carbohydrate in TPN is dextrose, which provides 3.7 kcal/g. The optimal rate of administration of parenteral glucose during TPN is 4 to 5 mg/kg-min or 400 to 500 g glucose in a 70 kg person per day. Above infusion rates of 7 mg/kg-min, Wolfe (45) and colleagues found no further increase in glucose oxidation. Rates of glucose administration in excess of energy requirements may cause significant rises in carbon dioxide (CO_2) production with increases in respiratory quotient, energy

TABLE 4. *Assessment of nutritional status*

Variable	Comments
1. Diet history/risk factors	
2. Physical examination	Emphasis on signs of malnutrition
Anthropometrics	
3. Height in cm	
4. Weight in kg	Weight loss > 10% significant
5. Triceps skinfold thickness	Index of fat stores
6. Mid-upper-arm circumference	Index of skeletal muscle mass
Energy requirements and balance studies	
7. Basal energy expenditure (BEE) (Harris-Benedict equation)	BEE for female = 655 + (9.6 × W) + (1.7 × H) − (4.7 × A) (W = actual weight in kg, H = height in cm, A = age in years)
8. Parenteral anabolic therapy	1.75 kcal × BEE
9. Protein requirements for pregnancy	1.2 − 1.5 × IBW (IBW = ideal body weight; ↑ with severe stress)
10. Estimate of net protein degradation/ synthesis	Nitrogen balance = (Protein intake/6.5) − (UUN + 4) (UUN = urinary urea nitrogen)
Somatic protein	
11. Lean body mass	Creatinine/height ratio = (Actual urinary creatine/Ideal urinary creatine) × 100 (Ideal urinary creatinine based on weight and height in standard tables)
12. Degradation product of muscle protein	3-methyl-histidine (research tool at present)
Visceral protein	
13. Serum albumin	Decreased in pregnancy
14. Serum transferrin	Dependent on iron stores
15. Retinol-binding protein	
16. Prealbumin	
Immunologic studies	
17. Total lymphocyte count	Altered by infection, sepsis
18. Cell-mediated immunity	

expenditure, or both. Minimum glucose supplied should be 400 kcal per day to supply fuel for brain, bone marrow, and injured tissue and to preserve protein stores. Dextrose concentrations above 10% must be supplied centrally rather than peripherally in order to avoid thrombophlebitis. The usual dextrose concentration for central TPN is 25%.

Protein

Because the placenta concentrates amino acids in the fetal circulation, the fetus is relatively protected from protein deficiency during periods of maternal deprivation (46). This occurs at the expense of maternal protein stores, however, and could lead to muscle breakdown, poor healing, and immunodeficiency. During short-term starvation, there is a continuous utilization of maternal body protein for gluconeogenesis because certain tissues such as brain have obligate glucose requirements, and carbohydrate reserves are depleted even more rapidly in the pregnant than the non-pregnant state. After carbohydrate depletion in the non-pregnant state (which may occur after 12 to 24 hr of starvation), the rate of protein breakdown is 60 to 75 g per day resulting in 10 to 12 g per day of urinary nitrogen loss. These large losses can be reduced to as little as 2 to 3 g nitrogen per day by providing a minimum of 100 g of carbohydrate daily. This protein-sparing effect is important to remember when deciding on the composition of fluids to be administered to patients who cannot eat for short periods of time or who are potential TPN candidates undergoing nutritional evaluation. A positive nitrogen balance (anabolism) cannot be obtained unless an exogenous protein source is supplied, however. Protein for TPN is supplied as mixed amino acid solutions with concentrations of 5% to 10%.

Fat

The non-protein energy in TPN may be supplied as glucose or lipid. Non-protein calories supplied from both glucose and lipid may promote better nitrogen retention than all-glucose systems alone. Optimal combinations supply 100 to 150 non-protein calories per g of nitrogen per day during pregnancy. Stressed patients may require up to 150 to 200 non-protein calories per g of nitrogen per day to maximize protein sparing. Lipid is supplied as a 10% or 20% phospholipid emulsion and is a ready source of the important fetal requirements for essential fatty acids. The most commonly used fat emulsion in the United States is Intralipid which is composed of 10% soybean oil, 1.2% egg yolk phospholipids, and 2.25% glycerin. The osmolarity is 280 mOsm/liter and the caloric content is 1 kcal per ml. The component fatty acids are linoleic (50%), oleic (26%), palmitic (10%), and linolenic (9%).

Vitamins

The three multivitamin preparations currently available in the United States provide adequate prenatal vitamin quantities in a 10 ml volume to be administered daily during TPN therapy. An example is given in Table 5. These preparations meet daily requirements during TPN by converting from oral to intravenous doses and assuming oral absorption to be 25% to 50%. Vitamin supplementation to prevent maternal hypovitaminemia is especially important in pregnancy because of evidence that not only is the placenta selective in the transport of vitamins to the fetus, but as a growing organ, the placenta has its own vitamin requirements and stores.

Trace Elements

Daily allowances for zinc, iron, copper, manganese, chromium, and cobalt have been established (9). Assuming 50% absorption rates of oral doses, several trace el-

TABLE 5. *Multivitamins (10 ml of solution daily)*

Ascorbic acid	100 mg
Vitamin A	1,000 μg
Vitamin D	5 μg
Thiamine HCl (81)	3 mg
Riboflavin (82)	3.6 mg
Pyridoxine HCl (B_6)	4 mg
Niacinamide	40 mg
Pantothenic acid	15 mg
Vitamin E	10 mg
Biotin	60 μg
Folic acid	400 μg
Cyanocobalamin (B_{12})	5 μg

ement preparations containing appropriate pregnancy doses are available for intravenous administration during TPN. Pregnant women require increased quantities of zinc (approximately 9–10 mg/day) which may be added to these preparations. Iodine is unnecessary for short-term hyperalimentation during pregnancy, but should be provided as 2 to 3 μg per kg body weight per day during long-term therapy. Iron may be supplied as periodic intramuscular administration during long-term TPN.

Electrolytes

Recommended dietary allowances for calcium, phosphorus, and magnesium are established (9), and wide ranges of doses of sodium, chloride, and potassium are usually well-tolerated if renal function is adequate. Periodic serum electrolyte level monitoring should prevent deficiencies or overdosages. During pregnancy, additional calcium is needed and may be supplied as a total daily dose of 20 mmol calcium per day. Phosphorus should be supplied in an amount of 2 mmol per g of nitrogen supplied per day, since tissue synthesis requires adequate phosphate. Hypokalemia may develop when the patient becomes anabolic; doses of 40 mmol/liter of TPN are usually sufficient.

Drugs

Heparin should be provided as 1,000 units per liter of solution to reduce fibrin formation around the catheter and to avoid phlebitis. Vitamin K (5 mg) should be supplied intramuscularly once a week for synthesis of vitamin K-dependent clotting factors. Regular insulin may be added to each liter of solution if glucose intolerance persists.

ENERGY AND PROTEIN REQUIREMENTS DURING TPN

After determining the actual caloric and protein requirements of the patient, the optimal balance of dextrose, protein, and fat must be determined. Most case reports of pregnant women receiving TPN describe 2,700 to 3,000 kcal/day administered. A daily combination of 2 liters of a standard central formulation using 25% dextrose with 500 ml of a 10% fat emulsion and 70 to 90 g of protein (1.2–1.5 g/kg body weight per day) approximates normal pregnant requirements. Additional fluids and electrolytes may be given as needed through a separate intravenous site. Non-protein energy intake per g of nitrogen per day should range between 100 and 150 kcal, and fat emulsion should not exceed 3 g/kg-day, or more than 60% of total calories, to avoid fat overload. High glucose loads may lead to overproduction of carbon dioxide and increased respiratory work (48). Excellent reviews describing the administration of TPN in pregnancy have been reported by Martin (12), Landon (16), Lee (29), and Rayburn (44).

USE OF HYPERALIMENTATION IN PATIENTS WITHOUT NUTRITIONAL RISKS FOR IUGR

Benny (49) and co-workers have described infusion of hypertonic dextrose and amino acids for 48 hr prior to delivery in six patients with low estriol excretion. Lecithin:sphingomyelin ratios were increased as were insulin levels in all patients following the infusion. There was a fall in amniotic fluid glucose and an increase in ammonia, amino acid nitrogen, and osmolarity. These findings suggest that amino acids may have crossed the placenta in increased quantities.

Beischer (50), in 1978, used TPN to treat pregnant women in whom IUGR was suspected because of low estriol excretion. He observed a lower incidence of growth retardation and perinatal mortality in treated patients when compared with control patients who had similar levels of reduced excretion of estriol. These studies suggest that subtle degrees of catabolism or malnutrition may affect late fetal development and are potentially amenable to nutritional or metabolic intervention.

SAFETY OF TPN DURING PREGNANCY

The safety of TPN during pregnancy has been questioned, both because of recognized hazards in the non-pregnant patient and because of concerns unique to pregnancy.

During the first trimester, TPN demands special attention because of the potential teratogenic effects of metabolic derangements such as hyperglycemia. Later in pregnancy, hyperglycemia due to hypertonic dextrose infusion could result in hyperstimulation of the fetal pancreas with complications similar to those noted in diabetic pregnancies.

Heller (51) has questioned the use of parenteral fat emulsions during pregnancy. High doses of fat infusion—over 50% of total calories—in rats caused fatty infiltration of the placenta. He also found an increase in uterine activity when infusing linoleic acid to pregnant rats near term. Neither of these findings has been observed in humans, and Seifer et al. (38) noted that the data associating preterm labor with fat emulsions were based on the use of Lipomul, a toxic fat emulsion no longer available.

The metabolic complications seen in neonates receiving TPN have also raised questions about the effects of long-term TPN in pregnancy. Because placental transfer mechanisms maintain a higher blood level of amino acids in the fetus than in the mother, maternal amino acid levels in excess are reflected in fetal levels. Maternal buffering systems should offset any metabolic acidosis due to the large amino acid load of TPN solutions. Protein hydrolysates contain large amounts of ammonia which has been linked to neonatal subclinical liver disease. In many cases of neonates receiving TPN who subsequently developed subclinical liver disease, however, underlying gastrointestinal disorders may have been responsible for the hepatic abnormality. While no definite reported neonatal risks are known with maternal TPN administration, theoretical concerns about the infusions remain.

INTRA-AMNIOTIC NUTRITION

While our knowledge of TPN and its effects on the developing fetus is limited, even less is known about fetal development and intra-amniotic nutrition. Numerous factors are responsible for normal fetal growth, and poorly understood aberrations of these factors play various roles in the development of intrauterine growth retardation. After excluding chromosomal and genetic factors and intrauterine infections, nutrient and oxygen delivery are felt to be essential determinants of fetal growth rates. In acute studies with fetal sheep, when umbilical blood flow is maintained, Wilkening and Meschia (52) have demonstrated that uterine oxygen delivery furnished by the normally high utero-placental blood flow in late pregnancy exceeds fetal needs and provides a large margin of safety for the fetus. These observations suggest that reductions in uterine blood flow resulting in fetal hypoxia are unlikely causes of intrauterine growth retardation. If these conclusions are confirmed in studies of more prolonged reductions of uterine blood flow and uterine oxygen delivery, the suggested role of *in utero* malnutrition as a causative factor of IUGR may be further supported. Studies linking *in utero* malnutrition to IUGR include reports of decreased maternal to fetal transfer of amino acid and glucose analogs in growth-retarded fetal animals (53,54) and autopsy similarities between growth-retarded human infants and infants dying of alimentary malnutrition (55).

Because of this apparent link between IUGR and *in utero* malnutrition, various investigators have explored the possibility of supplementing animal and human fetuses at risk for IUGR with intra-amniotic injections of nutrients. The rationale for intra-amniotic nutritional supplementation is that the fetus would swallow the nutrients in the amniotic fluid, fetal swallowing being well-documented. Several studies have estimated that the clearance of radioactively labeled protein from the amniotic sac has a half-time of 24 to 29 hr in late human pregnancy (56–58). Pitkin (58) estimated that amniotic fluid swallowing could provide the term fetus with 13% of its nitrogen requirements and suggested that fetal ingestion of protein may have nutritional and other important physiologic functions. Heller (59) and Saling et al. (60) injected amino acids into the amniotic cavity in the human and found a more rapid disappearance rate than Pitkin, suggesting absorption at the umbilical surface as well as in the alimentary tract. Amelioration of experimentally induced growth retardation in the fetal sheep occurred when Charlton (61) supplemented the fetus of the protein-calorie malnourished ewe with continuous intragastric infusions of 6.8% essential and non-essential amino acids and 4% glucose.

In addition to this basic research in amniotic fluid amino acids and proteins, researchers have used intra-amniotic amino acid solutions therapeutically in gestations with IUGR or severe feto-placental insufficiency. Renaud et al. (62) administered up to 14 injections of amino acid solution between 30 and 38 weeks gestation in patients at varying risk for IUGR and in control patients. No adverse effects were noted, and maternal 24-hr estriol excretion rates rose to normal in 4 of 5 patients in which estriol excretion was measured. Heller (59) in 1974 administered intra-amniotic injections of amino acids up to 12 times in patients with placental insufficiency diagnosed by cardiotocography, urinary estriol excretion, biparietal diameter measurements of the fetus, and/or human placental lactogen measurements. Normalization of low urinary estriol excretion rates in four cases and a disappearance of late decelerations of the fetal heart rate during an oxytocin challenge test in one case were noted after the intra-amniotic infusions. Massobrio (63), using fetal biparietal diameter measurements with maternal urinary estriol and pregnanediol excretion rates as indicators of severe feto-placental insufficiency, injected amino acid solutions intra-amniotically from one to eight times in five patients. He ascribed the survival of two of the fetuses to the repeated amino acid injections.

All investigators discussed in this chapter using intra-amniotic amino acid injections as therapy for high risk fetuses reported anecdotal benefits from their use. Universal caution was urged, however, and recommendations for more animal experimentation prior to further human fetal supplementation was repeatedly underscored by these investigators.

CONCLUSIONS

(1) Maternal total parenteral nutrition is an infrequently utilized but apparently safe method of supplementing the mother and fetus at high risk for malnutrition.
(2) While intrauterine growth retardation occurs frequently in association with TPN during pregnancy, the underlying disease state necessitating the TPN is more likely the cause of the IUGR than the TPN.
(3) Assessment of nutritional indices before and during TPN therapy may aid in treatment.
(4) While theoretical side effects of TPN specific to pregnancy are discussed, no actual side effects specific to pregnancy have been reported.
(5) Fetal malnutrition may be a major cause of IUGR, and intra-amniotic administration of nutrients has been suggested as a possible fetal treatment.
(6) Further studies in animals are needed to define the role of intra-amniotic nutrition as therapy for fetuses at risk for IUGR or placental insufficiency.

REFERENCES

1. Berg BN. Dietary restriction and reproduction in the rat. *J Nutr* 1965;87:344–48.
2. Pond WG, Strachnan DN, Sinha YN, et al. Effect of protein deprivation of the swine during all or part of gestation on birthweight, postnatal growth rate, and nucleic acid content of brain muscle of progeny. *J Nutr* 1969;99:61–7.
3. Blechner JN, Stenger VG, Prystowsky H. Uterine blood flow in women at term. *Am J Obstet Gynecol* 1974;120:633–40.
4. Croal J, Sheriff S, Matthews J. Nonpregnant maternal plasma volume and fetal growth retardation. *Br J Obstet Gynaecol* 1978;85:90–5.
5. Stein Z, Susser M, Saenger G, et al. Famine and human development: the Dutch Hunger Winter of 1944/45. Oxford, New York: Oxford University Press, 1975;87–118.
6. Mora JO, de Paredes B, Wagner M. Nutritional supplementation and the outcome of pregnancy—I. Birthweight. *Am J Clin Nutr* 1979;32:455–62.
7. Rush D, Stein Z, Susser M. A randomized controlled trial of prenatal nutritional supplementation in New York City. *Pediatrics* 1980;65:683–97.
8. Kerr JF, Campbell-Brown BM, Johnstone FD. Dieting in pregnancy. A study of the effect of a high protein low carbohydrate diet on birthweight in an obstetric population. In: Sutherland HW, Stowers JM, eds. *Carbohydrate metabolism in pregnancy and the newborn.* New York: Springer-Verlag, 1978;518–34.
9. *Recommended Daily Allowances,* 9th Rev. Ed. Washington, D.C.: National Academy of Sciences, 1980;25–7.
10. Harris JA, Benedict FG. *A biometric study of basal metabolism in man.* Washington, DC: Carnegie Institute of Washington, Publication No. 270, 1919;201–22.
11. Oldham H, Sheft BB. Effect of caloric intake on nitrogen utilization during pregnancy. *J Am Diet Assoc* 1951;27:847–54.
12. Martin R, Blackburn G. Hyperalimentation during pregnancy. In: Berkowitz R, ed. *Critical care of the obstetric patient.* Edinburgh, New York: Churchill Livingstone, 1983;133–63.
13. Durnin JVGA, Grant S, McKillop FM, Fitzgerald G. Is nutritional status endangered by virtually no extra intake during pregnancy? *Lancet,* 1985;66:823–6.
14. Hytten FE, Leitch I. *The physiology of human pregnancy,* 2nd ed. Oxford: Blackwell Scientific Publications, 1971;357–9.
15. King JC. Assessment of nutritional status in pregnancy—I. *Am J Clin Nutr* 1981;34:685–90.
16. Landon MB, Gabbe SG, Mullen JL. Total parenteral nutrition during pregnancy. *Clin Perinatol* 1986;13:57–72.
17. Henriques V, Anderson AC. Uber parenterale Ernährung durch intravenöse Injektion. *Z Physiol Chem* 1913;88:357–69.
18. Wretlind A. Development of fat emulsions. *JPEN* 1981;5:230–5.
19. Wilmore DW, Dudrick SJ. Growth and development of an infant receiving all nutrients exclusively by vein. *JAMA* 1968;203:860–4.
20. Lakoff KM, Feldman JD. Anorexia nervosa associated with pregnancy. *Obstet Gynecol* 1972; 39:699–701.
21. Cox KL, Byrne WJ, Ament ME. Home total parenteral nutrition during pregnancy: A case report. *JPEN* 1981;5:246–9.
22. Di Costanzo JD, Martin J, Cano N, et al. Total parenteral nutrition with fat emulsions during pregnancy—nutritional requirements: a case report. *JPEN* 1982;6:534–8.
23. Dudrick SJ, Copeland EM, Daly JM, et al. A clinical review of nutritional support of the patient. *JPEN* 1979;3:444–51.
24. Gineston JL, Capron JP, Delcenserie R, et al. Prolonged total parenteral nutrition in a pregnant woman with acute pancreatitis. *J Clin Gastroenterol* 1984;6:249–52.
25. Hatjis CG, Meis PJ. Total parenteral nutrition in pregnancy. *Obstet Gynecol* 1985;66:585–8.
26. Hew LR, Deitel M. Total parenteral nutrition in gynecology and obstetrics. *Obstet Gynecol* 1980;55:464–8.
27. Klein FS, Lin C, Lowensohn RI. Total parenteral nutrition during pregnancy. American Dietary Association 66th Annual Meeting, September 12–15, 1983;147.
28. Lavin JP, Gimmon Z, Miodovnik M, et al. Total parenteral nutrition in a pregnant insulin-requiring diabetic. *Obstet Gynecol* 1982;59:660–4.
29. Lee RV, Rodgers BO, Young C, et al. Total parenteral nutrition during pregnancy. *Obstet Gynecol* 1986;68:563–71.

30. LeGrix A, Colin R, Galmiche JP, et al. Acute outbreak of haemorrhagic rectocolitis in a pregnant woman treated with prolonged total parenteral nutrition (letter). *Nouv Presse Med* 1978;7:3044–5.
31. Lipkin EW, Benedetti T, Chait A. Normal fetal development in a patient maintained on total parenteral nutrition from the first trimester of pregnancy [Abstract]. *Clin Res* 1985;33:104A.
32. Loiudice TA, Chandrakaar C. Pregnancy and jejunoileal bypass. Treatment of complications with total parenteral nutrition. *South Med J* 1980;73:256–8.
33. Main AN, Shenkin A, Black WP, et al. Intravenous feeding to sustain pregnancy in patient with Crohn's disease. *Br Med J* 1981;283(603):1221–2.
34. Martin R. Hyperalimentation during pregnancy. *Clin Consult Nutr* 1982;2(Suppl):9.
35. Rivera-Alsina ME, Saldana LR, Stringer CA. Fetal growth sustained by parenteral nutrition in pregnancy. *Obstet Gynecol* 1984;64:138–41.
36. Schoenbeck J, Segerbrand E. Candida albicans septicaemia during first half of pregnancy, successfully treated with 5-fluorocytosine. *Br Med J* 1973;4:337–8.
37. Herbert WN, Seeds JW, Bowes WA, et al. Fetal growth response to total parenteral nutrition in pregnancy. A case report. *J Reprod Med* 1986;31:263–6.
38. Seifer DB, Silberman H, Catanzarite VA, et al. Total parenteral nutrition in obstetrics. *JAMA* 1985;253:2073–5.
39. Stowell JC, Bottsford JE, Rubel HR. Pancreatitis with pseudocyst and cholelithiasis in third trimester of pregnancy: management with total parenteral nutrition. *South Med J* 1984;77:502–4.
40. Tresadern JC, Falconer GF, Turnberg LA, et al. Maintenance of pregnancy in a home parenteral nutrition patient. *JPEN* 1984;8:199–202.
41. Webb GA. The use of hyperalimentation and chemotherapy in pregnancy. A case report. *Am J Obstet Gynecol* 1980;137:263–6.
42. Weinberg RB, Sitrin MD, Adkins GM, et al. Treatment of hyperlipidemic pancreatitis in pregnancy with total parenteral nutrition. *Gastroenterology* 1982;83:1300–5.
43. Young KR. Acute pancreatitis in pregnancy. Two case reports. *Obstet Gynecol* 1982;60:653–7.
44. Rayburn W, Wolk R, Mercer R, et al. Parenteral nutrition in obstetrics and gynecology. *Obstet Gynecol Surv* 1986;41:200–14.
45. Wolfe RR, O'Donnell TF, Stone MD, et al. Investigation of factors determining the optimal glucose infusion rate in total parenteral nutrition. *Metabolism* 1980;28:892–900.
46. Ghadimi H, Pecora P. Free amino acids of cord plasma as compared with maternal plasma during pregnancy. *Pediatrics* 1964;30:500–6.
47. Baker H, Frank O, DeAngelis B, et al. Role of placenta in maternal-fetal vitamin transfer in humans. *Am J Obstet Gynecol* 1981;141:792–6.
48. Silberman H, Eisenberg D, eds. *Parenteral and enteral nutrition for the hospitalized patient*. Norwalk, CT: Appleton-Century-Crofts, 1982;196–8.
49. Benny PS, Legge M, Aichim DR. The biochemical effects of maternal hyperalimentation during pregnancy. *NZ Med J* 1978;88:283–5.
50. Beischer N. Treatment of fetal growth retardation. *Aust NZ J Obstet Gynaecol* 1978;18:28–33.
51. Heller L. Clinical and experimental studies in complete parenteral nutrition. *Scand J Gastroenterol* 1968;4:Suppl. 4:7–16.
52. Wilkening RB, Meschia G. Fetal oxygen uptake, oxygenation, and acid-base balance as a function of uterine blood flow. *Am J Physiol* 1983;244:H749–51.
53. Nitzan M, Orloff S, Schulman J. Placental transfer of analogs of glucose and amino acids in experimental intrauterine growth retardation. *Pediatr Res* 1979;13:100–3.
54. Saintonge J, Côté R. Intrauterine growth retardation and diabetic pregnancy: two types of fetal malnutrition. *Am J Obstet Gynecol* 1983;146:194–8.
55. Naeye R. Malnutrition—probable cause of fetal growth retardation. *Arch Pathol* 1965;79:284–91.
56. Pritchard JA. Deglutition by normal and anencephalic fetuses. *Obstet Gynecol* 1965;25:289–97.
57. Gitlin D, Kumate J, Morales C, et al. The turnover of amniotic fluid protein in the human conceptus. *Am J Obstet Gynecol* 1972;113:632–45.
58. Pitkin RM, Reynolds WA. Fetal ingestion and metabolism of amniotic fluid protein. *Am J Obstet Gynecol* 1975;123:356–63.
59. Heller L. Intrauterine amino acid feeding of the fetus. In: Bode H, Warshaw J, eds. *Parenteral nutrition in infancy and childhood*. New York: Plenum, 1974;206–13.
60. Saling E, Dudenhausen JW, Kynest G. Basic investigation about intra-amniotic compensatory nutrition of the malnourished fetus. In: Persianinov L, Chervakova T, Presl J, eds. *Recent progress in obstetrics and gynecology*, Proceedings of the VII World Congress of Obstetrics and Gynecology. Prague: Excerpta Medica, 1974;227–33.

61. Charlton V. Fetal nutritional supplementation. *Semin Perinatol* 1984;8:25–30.
62. Renaud R, Kirschtetter L, Koehl C, et al. Amino acid intra-amniotic injections. In: Persianinov L, Chervakova T, Presl J, eds. *Recent progress in obstetrics and gynecology,* Proceedings of the VII World Congress of Obstetrics and Gynecology. Prague: Excerpta Medica, 1974;234–56.
63. Massobrio M, Margaria E, Campogravide M, et al. Treatment of severe feto-placental insufficiency by means of intraamniotic injection of amino acids. In: Salvadori B, ed. *Therapy of feto-placental insufficiency.* Berlin: Springer-Verlag, 1975;296–303.

DISCUSSION

Dr. Guesry: Dr. Ernest, I have a comment about the level of energy intake which you referred to as the energy cost of pregnancy. The figure of 80,000 kcal is a classic one but has been proved wrong. After Lawrence's work at Keneba in Gambia, the Nestlé Foundation (1) organized a multicenter study to check the true level of additional energy intake which is necessary for normal pregnancy, and it was found that adaptive phenomena reduce maternal energy expenditure so that the maximum requirement turns out to be less than 40,000 kcal (2).

Dr. Ernest: That is a good point. As you say, 80,000 kcal is the classic figure, and a lot also depends on the mother's pregravid weight. For example, a woman who is obese at the beginning of pregnancy may gain no weight during pregnancy but still have a larger body than a woman of 40 kg who gains a lot of weight. But it may well be that the values need to be revised.

Dr. Hay: I am amazed at how few of the papers from workers involved in maternal/fetal nutritional support have reported such obvious things as the maternal glucose concentrations during the periods of intravenous nutrition. You mentioned maternal hyperglycemia and fetal macrosomia, and you also talked of the potential for acidosis and other complications. In this regard the dose of glucose that you recommended (4-5 mg/kg per min) is almost twice the turnover rate of glucose that has been measured with stable isotopic studies in pregnant women in a number of centers (3,4). With regard to amino acids, there are many people who don't have an amino acid analyzer, but when you have the rare opportunity to find a patient who truly does benefit from this kind of support, then I think most people with such analyzers would be delighted to get their hands on some of the plasma and collaborate. You mentioned hyperaminoacidemia. This can be potentially a very serious problem, particularly with regard to phenylalanine. Levels of phenylalanine of 4 to 5 times normal have been observed in fetuses whose mothers were receiving parenteral supplements, and this is at least in part because we really don't know what dose to give the mother in this situation. I recommend that as people get interested in this subject and come up with more cases they should call up their colleagues and use the opportunities to do collaborative research, while also trying to develop animal studies.

Dr. Ernest: I am sure you are right about this. I hope it was obvious from my presentation that nobody has a lot of experience with these techniques and it is true that obstetricians have been rather unsophisticated in reporting their cases. There is only extremely cursory information in many of the published reports.

Dr. Chessex: It is amazing that with all the unknowns these babies have often been brought to term and seem to have done quite well.

Dr. Wharton: At least they weren't born with microcephaly, which would have been the effect if the fetus had been exposed to maternal phenylalanine levels as high as in maternal phenylketonuria.

Dr. Seeds: The outcome hasn't always been good. We observed a case of a woman with colonic interposition who ate quite well before she was pregnant, but for some reason completely lost her appetite when she became pregnant and would eat nothing. Her baby grew normally on ultrasound measurement up to about 24 weeks, but then growth ceased. We started total parenteral nutrition (TPN) in the mother and within 7 days fetal abdominal circumference had begun to accelerate dramatically. Unfortunately, within 2 weeks fetal distress developed, with late decelerations during spontaneous contractions. It occurred to us that we had stimulated the baby to outgrow his stunted placenta.

Dr. Ernest: There have been many complications reported, but I think these have usually been in babies who were already in difficulties and these came to a head after maternal TPN had been started. There have been a number of instances when babies have died during maternal TPN, but these have mainly been in women with diabetes, which seems to be the biggest risk factor for the baby in this situation. Such babies seem to do more poorly than babies in whom there were other reasons for requiring maternal TPN.

Dr. Bossart: Cases of pregnancy with maternal TPN seem to be rare, which I find surprising when you think of all the car accidents to pregnant women that there must be, and other reasons needing intensive care. I suppose the cases are simply not reported. What about intra-abdominal nutrition to the fetus? The abdominal cavity is a very useful cavity—almost everything you put into it disappears!

Dr. Ernest: The few cases of intra-abdominal nutrition I have found reported were more anecdotal than scientific in their approach. My feeling is that if you have the technical ability to provide intra-abdominal nutrition for the fetus, you probably have the facilities to take care of it outside the uterus unless it is so premature that it is not going to survive. I think the occasions when you diagnose IUGR of such severity that you need to consider intrauterine nutritional supplements before, say, 24 to 26 weeks must be pretty infrequent. If you diagnose this at 26 to 28 weeks or later, I think you'd be better off allowing your neonatologist to take care of the baby.

Dr. Bossart: I am glad you made that comment. It is important that some practical things come out of this discussion. As I understand it, you don't believe in intrauterine feeding of the fetus and advise that the best thing to do is to deliver it and look after it properly *ex utero*, if you can?

Dr. Ernest: I think you might be able to improve the fetus's condition by intrauterine nutrition, but I'm not sure that you cannot do it better by having the baby out. I also cannot remember many cases where we diagnosed such severe IUGR prior to viability. If you do diagnose it at this stage, then it is possible that intrauterine nutrition might be helpful to buy time, but I should also be thinking about other reasons for very early severe IUGR, such as chromosome abnormalities or fetal infection.

Dr. Hay: I think you would also want to know whether the fetal malnutrition is on the basis of poor maternal nutrition or a poor placenta. There is no reason to bypass a working placenta when the problem is with the mother, and in that case, maternal intravenous nutrition may have a place. Our caution in accepting the data you have presented doesn't mean that it is wrong to use these techniques under selected circumstances.

Dr. Toubas: If a baby is delivered at 26 weeks, we still have problems with nutrition. TPN in such infants is not easy, and about 30% of babies in neonatal intensive care units are in fact malnourished.

Dr. Ernest: I don't think either alternative is very good, but to do amniocentesis daily for a prolonged period to give the fetus intra-abdominal nutrients is putting both the mother and the fetus at risk from the point of view of the procedure per se.

Dr. Marini: In the early 1960s, when we were much involved with the Rh problem and were regularly placing intraperitoneal catheters in fetuses, we sometimes gave amino acid solutions and glucose as well as blood intraperitoneally. The results were catastrophic, so we had to stop doing it. I think that if you plan to give additional nutrients to the fetus because of placental problems, you must always combine such nutrients with an adequate supply of oxygen. If you increase nutrient supply to the fetus without increasing placental blood flow the fetus will not be able to utilize the nutrients.

Dr. Ernest: On the other hand, as Dr. Hay has already said, there is evidence that most fetuses have an overabundance of oxygen. If there is a problem with placental function, the active transport of amino acids, glucose, and other large molecules is much more likely to limit the fetus than the diffusion of oxygen; so in most cases oxygen delivery is likely to remain long after you lose the ability to transport nutrients.

Dr. Bossart: I agree with what you said about oxygen. Another problem, though, is that the fetus also has to excrete. The placenta is a two-way organ. Even if sufficient nutrients and oxygen can be provided, they will not be useful if the fetus is unable to dispose of metabolic waste adequately. What about placing a catheter in the fetal abdominal cavity for intrauterine nutrition?

Dr. Seeds: I have had considerable experience of the placement of intra-abdominal catheters. I am sure that if one end is attached outside the uterus there is not a chance in a thousand that the other end will stay in the fetal abdomen for any length of time. As soon as the fetus turns round it will pull out. Also, most of the plastics which are the right consistency for ease of placement become very soft at body temperature, which makes it even more likely that they will fall out.

REFERENCES

1. Lawrence M, Lawrence F, Lamb WH, Whiteheads RG. Maintenance energy cost of pregnancy in rural Gambian women and influence of dietary status. *Lancet* 1984;2:363–5.
2. Durnin JUGA, McKillop FM, Grant S, Fitzgerald G. Energy requirements of pregnancy in Scotland. *Lancet* 1987;2:897–900.
3. Kalhan SC, D'Angelo LJ, Savin SM, et al. Glucose production in pregnant women at term. *J Clin Invest* 1979;63:338–94.
4. Cowett RM, Susa JB, Sommer M, et al. Kinetic studies with ^{13}C-U-glucose in pregnant women and their offspring. *Pediatr Res* 1979;13:357.

Intrauterine Growth Retardation, edited by
Jacques Senterre. Nestlé Nutrition Workshop
Series, Vol. 18. Nestec Ltd., Vevey/Raven Press,
Ltd., New York © 1989.

Postnatal Experiences of Intrauterine Growth-Retarded Infants

*José Villar, **José Belizan, and †Vincent Smeriglio

*Prevention Research Program, National Institute of Child Health and Human
Development, NIH, Bethesda, Maryland 20892; and Department of Gynecology and
Obstetrics, The Johns Hopkins Hospital, Baltimore, Maryland 21218; **Centro Rosarino
de Estudios Perinatales, 2000 Rosario, Argentina; and †Department of Maternal and Child
Health, School of Hygiene and Public Health, The Johns Hopkins University, Baltimore,
Maryland 21218

Intrauterine growth retardation (IUGR) represents one of the most important perinatal syndromes. Growth-retarded infants have increased perinatal and infant mortality and morbidity and their long-term developmental and physical growth handicaps are well recognized. We shall discuss here some clinical and epidemiological factors that relate to characteristics of IUGR infants and to the long-term prognosis for this group of newborns.

EPIDEMIOLOGICAL CONSIDERATIONS

We shall discuss here only those epidemiological issues that are relevant to the IUGR infant's postnatal experiences. The epidemiology of IUGR is discussed extensively elsewhere in this volume.

Unfortunately, there are not enough reports in the literature to estimate the incidence and distribution of IUGR in different countries. In an effort to explore this distribution, we have analyzed available statistics of low birthweight (LBW) ($\leq 2,500$ g) from different areas in the world (1). The incidence of LBW infants at term underestimates the problem of IUGR, since an important number of IUGR deliveries weigh more than 2,500 g (i.e., between 2,500 g and about 2,900 g, which is the tenth percentile of weight for gestational age).

A distinction can be made between developed and developing countries in relation to the distribution of LBW babies and the different types of IUGR. In an analysis of 25 developing areas where gestational age and birthweight had been recorded (1), we observed a linear correlation between total LBW incidence and the incidence of IUGR–LBW ($r = 0.95$; $b = 0.98$; $p < 0.001$), where IUGR–LBW was defined as birthweight below 2,500 g and gestation ≥ 37 weeks. In contrast, the LBW incidence was not significantly associated with preterm delivery ($r = 0.007$;

$b = 0.024$). Data from developed countries showed the opposite; a significant correlation between LBW and preterm delivery ($r = 0.87$; $b = 0.73$; $p < 0.01$) and a nonsignificant correlation between LBW and IUGR–LBW ($r = 0.054$; $b = 0.26$). From this study we can conclude that in developing countries, the increase in the incidence of LBW is due to an increase in the incidence of IUGR–LBW. The proportion of preterm delivery remains almost unchanged. Therefore, no more than 5% to 7% of all LBW infants can be expected to be premature and any excess of this figure will be IUGR–LBW.

The epidemiological characteristics of prematurity and intrauterine growth retardation are also different. Table 1 shows data from the Guatemalan Nutritional Study, comparing adjusted odds ratios and 95% confidence limits for preterm and IUGR infants calculated using the log-linear model (2). Each odds ratio represents the independent effect of that variable, after controlling for all remaining variables. As Table 1 illustrates, low energy supplementation during pregnancy (<33.2 kcal/day), no protein supplementation, and a small maternal arm circumference (<21.4 cm), independently, and after controlling for the other variables, increased the risk of delivering a preterm newborn approximately two-fold but did not influence the risk of having an IUGR infant. On the other hand, maternal small head circumference, an indicator of early persistent undernutrition, increased the risk of an IUGR infant, but not of a preterm delivery.

Interestingly, socio-economic status lost its significant association with both IUGR and preterm delivery after controlling for variables reflecting maternal nutritional status. Therefore, these indicators of nutritional status are an important pathway between socio-economic status and fetal growth. These data are in agreement with a study from a population in England (3), although here the mediating factors

TABLE 1. *Adjusted odds ratios and 95% confidence intervals (CI) for selected maternal variables for the intrauterine growth retardation (IUGR) and preterm groups*

	Preterm (n = 61)		IUGR (n = 173)	
Variable	Adjusted[a] odds ratios	95% CI	Adjusted[a] odds ratios	95% CI
Energy supplementation (< 33.2 kcal/day)[b]	1.89	1.33–2.46	1.09	0.67–1.51
Protein supplementation (No supplementation)	2.26	1.70–2.83	1.28	0.92–1.64
Maternal arm circumference (< 21.4 cm)	2.27	1.62–2.93	1.08	0.61–1.55
Maternal head circumference (< 50.1 cm)	0.76	0.05–1.47	1.42	1.02–1.82
Sex (male vs. female)	2.04	1.48–2.60	1.61	1.25–1.97

[a]Log linear model: reference group NBW (n = 389).
[b]Cutoff points correspond to the 25th percentile of the total population.
From ref. 2.

were maternal height, preeclampsia-hypertension, history of IUGR, and smoking. Therefore socio-economic status appears to affect fetal growth through different mechanisms in different populations.

Finally, we found in our study (2) that prematurity was associated exclusively with indicators of current nutritional status (supplementation and arm circumference). Data from a well-nourished population (4) also showed that two indicators of current nutritional status were significantly associated with preterm delivery. Thus, published evidence supports the concept of different epidemiological factors associated with prematurity and IUGR.

MATERNAL NUTRITION AND IUGR

There is a general consensus in the literature that maternal nutritional status, expressed as pre-pregnancy weight or height, is significantly associated with birthweight. The magnitude of the relationship is approximately 9 g of birthweight for each additional kg above mother's pre-pregnant weight, and around 10 g of birthweight for each additional centimeter of maternal height (5,6). Weight gain during pregnancy is also independently associated with birthweight but there is no evidence that it correlates with gestational age (2).

Several nutritional interventions during pregnancy have recently been reviewed by us and the following conclusions were drawn (7):

a. Maternal supplementation during pregnancy has, in general, a positive effect on birthweight. This effect is more dramatic the more malnourished the mother was before pregnancy. Malnourished mothers in a hospital in India had an increase in birthweight of up to 458 g when given food supplementation and bed rest (8).
b. The effect on birthweight of nutritional supplementation during pregnancy has been found consistently to be rather modest in well nourished or moderately malnourished women, with an average increase of less than 100 g (7).
c. Data from Guatemala suggest that in chronic moderately malnourished women the main nutritional factor limiting fetal growth is energy (9).
d. The New York study showed that among women with adequate protein intake, high protein supplementation is associated with a small increase in preterm births and neonatal mortality (10). Caution should be exercised in interpreting these results.
e. Nutritional supplementation during pregnancy is also associated with a reduction of the incidence of LBW in developing countries, e.g., Guatemala, Mexico (9,11), and in developed populations, e.g., the Special Supplemental Food Program for Women, Infants, and Children in the United States (12).

In a recent analysis of the Guatemalan study, Villar et al. (2) have shown that the effect on birthweight produced by caloric and/or protein supplementation is predominantly explained by an increase in gestational age rather than an effect on fetal growth. The effect was significant after controlling for interfering variables such as other nutritional factors, morbidity processes, and socio-demographic characteristics. These observations are in agreement with a previous report by Delgado et al. (13), who showed an increase of 4.2 days per 10,000 kcal of supplementation.

Villar and Rivera (14) analyzed the impact of nutritional supplementation on chronically yet moderately malnourished women in two consecutive pregnancies and in the lactation period in between. Birthweight of the second offspring was the outcome variable. Groups were divided according to the levels of caloric supplementation into three periods: the first pregnancy, the present pregnancy, and the period between them. The adjusted mean birthweight of the second offspring of women with high supplementation during the entire period (about 110 extra kcal/day) was up to 301 g greater than that of the low supplementation group. Women with high supplementation while lactating their first offspring and during the second pregnancy had babies up to 150 g heavier than the reference group; those mothers with high supplementation only during the second pregnancy had infants about 124 g heavier than those of the low supplementation group (Table 2). This study showed that nutritional supplementation during two consecutive pregnancies and the intermediate lactation period among women with chronic moderate malnutrition increased the mean birthweight by a value three times higher than the effect shown in many of the previous reports on this topic.

On the interpretation of supplementation studies, we therefore concluded that for women with acute malnutrition, food supplementation during pregnancy does produce a biologically significant increase in birthweight of over 200 g, as has been shown in the Gambia study during the wet season (15). On the other hand, chronically but moderately malnourished mothers would benefit significantly from extra

TABLE 2. *Crude and adjusted birthweight of the second offspring for the four supplementation groups. Level of supplementation as total caloric intake*

Supplementation group			Unadjusted			Adjusted analysis: mean differences from LLL group					
						Parity, maternal height		Parity, maternal height and length of gest., second infant		Parity, maternal height and birthweight, first infant	
1st preg.	Lactation	2nd preg.	n	Mean (g)	SD	Mean (g)	SE	Mean (g)	SE	Mean (g)	SE
H	H	H	21	3,290^c	(514)	301^b	(123)	267^b	(123)	246^a	(157)
L	H	H	55	3,105	(474)	150^a	(91)	113^a	94	193^a	(123)
L	L	H	27	3,056	(378)	124	(112)	100	(112)	202	(163)
L	L	L	50	2,944	(501)	—	—	—	—	—	—

H, high supplementation: > 20,000 kcal pregnancy and > 40,000 kcal lactation; L, low supplementation: ≤ 20,000 kcal pregnancy and ≤ 40,000 kcal lactation.
^{a}p < 0.05.
^{b}p < 0.025 one-tailed t-test compared with the LLL group.
^{c}p < 0.05 (F-test for trend).
From ref. 14.

food if the period of treatment is long enough to supply their long-lasting nutritional deficits, though a poor result (around 100 g) is to be expected if supplementation is given only during the present pregnancy.

DIFFERENT PATTERNS OF INTRAUTERINE GROWTH RETARDATION

As will be described below, fetal growth is a heterogeneous process. The identification of two different types of IUGR derived from this heterogeneous pattern of growth is of great relevance. The implications of this identification are that there will be differences in clinical diagnosis and management of pregnant women and newborns, different postnatal growth patterns and developmental performance of affected children, and therefore different priorities for health interventions in populations, depending on the predominant type of IUGR.

In a previous article we described the different types of IUGR (16). Those fetuses who experience insults early in pregnancy will show alterations in both length and weight growth. If the insult begins around the 27th to 30th week of gestation, it will produce weight retardation but will have less effect on length growth. This different pattern is explained by the fact that the greatest velocity of length growth is reached around the 20th week, and weight increase is at a maximum by the middle of the third trimester (16).

These different types of IUGR can be identified at birth by weight and height measurements and by the calculation of the ponderal index (PI):

$$PI = \text{weight g/(length cm)}^3 \times 100$$

Using the ponderal index, the two different types of IUGR can be described as:

a. "Proportionate" (also called "symmetric" or "chronic") IUGR, with a normal ponderal index, includes newborns who are both short in length and low in weight so that there is, consequently, a linear relationship between these two measurements.

b. "Disproportionate" (also "asymmetric" or "subacute") IUGR, with a low ponderal index, consists of newborns whose length is almost normal but who have a reduced weight so that, consequently, a disproportion between these two measurements is present (16). The deficit in weight is principally due to a reduction in fat deposition, particularly during the third trimester of pregnancy.

Clinical evidence supporting this assumption has been described in two previous articles (16,17). Factors that are present from the inception of pregnancy or earlier can be related to proportionate growth retardation in fetuses. A population in Central America with chronic severe maternal malnutrition (18) has been shown to have an incidence of IUGR of 34%; the mean birthweight for the IUGR infants was $2,366 \pm 150$ g and the mean length was 43.5 ± 0.1 cm. Both values are below a standard population, but the mean ponderal index was 2.24, a value that is close to

TABLE 3. *Maternal factors associated with the two types of intrauterine growth retardation (IUGR) in comparison with a control group*

	Proportionate IUGR (n = 31)	Disproportionate IUGR (n = 38)	Normal birthweight (n = 69)
Age (years)	27.2[a]	28.9	29.2
	(3.8)	(6.3)	(4.9)
Parity	1.7[a]	2.1	2.4
	(1.1)	(1.1)	(1.3)
Maternal preconceptional	54.0[a]	58.0	60.0
weight (kg)	(8.9)	(8.4)	(7.8)
Maternal weight	11.0	11.2	12.2
increase (kg)	(4.2)	(4.0)	(4.8)
Toxemia	8.7	32.0[b]	7.5

Results are means (SD).
[a]Significant difference with control group.
[b]Significant difference with the other two groups.

the 50th percentile in all the curves available. In a recent case-control study, we compared antenatal factors associated with the two types of IUGR with a control group of newborns of normal birthweight (Table 3). As can be appreciated, proportionate (chronic) fetal growth retardation is associated with preconceptional factors such as maternal age and maternal weight. On the other hand, toxemia of pregnancy is associated with disproportionate growth retardation. A similar pattern of association was observed by us in another series from Argentina (19) as well as in a report from the U.S.A. by Miller (20). It has been suggested that smoking during pregnancy is associated with proportionate IUGR. Data from Miller et al. (21) show that smoking mothers have a five times greater risk of having proportionate IUGR infants than non-smokers, after controlling for weight gain during pregnancy. Moreover, Davies et al. (22) presented findings of overall growth retardation (weight, length, and head circumference) among 1,159 infants whose mothers' smoking habits were ascertained early in pregnancy. Relatively well-nourished women with low weight gain during pregnancy had a significantly higher incidence of disproportionate growth retardation (21).

POSTNATAL GROWTH

Short-Term Outcome of IUGR

Neonatal Morbidity

Overall, IUGR infants have higher incidence of asphyxia, hypoglycemia, hypothermia, and hyperviscosity in the neonatal period than normal birthweights (23–

25). Walther and Ramaekers (26) have demonstrated in a population from the Netherlands that disproportionate IUGR (low ponderal index) had higher incidences of asphyxia, acidosis, hypoglycemia, and hypothermia than proportionate IUGR (normal ponderal index). This higher incidence of hypothermia in disporportionate IUGR (35% compared to 8% in proportionate IUGR) (26) can be related to their low subcutaneous fat that should have been deposited during the third trimester of pregnancy. It is this ''fatness'' of newborns that is responsible for reducing heat loss after birth.

Furthermore, a recent large prospective follow-up study of a population from a developing country showed similar morbidity patterns (27). As can be seen in Table 4, the disproportionate (low ponderal index) group has, in this population as well, a higher risk for all morbidity indicators than the normal ponderal index group, with the exception of hyperbilirubinemia and infections.

TABLE 4. *Adjusted neonatal morbidity of intrauterine growth retardation (IUGR) subgroups*

	IUGR subgroups[a] PI Level		
Morbidity	Low (n = 393)	Intermediate (n = 871)	Normal (n = 1,860)
Apgar score			
1 min ≤ 6	2.0[b] (1.4–2.8)	1.4 (1.1–1.9)	1.0
5 min ≤ 6	1.7 (0.7–3.7)	1.2 (0.6–2.4)	1.0
Aspiration syndrome	11.3 (3.4–37.2)	3.6 (1.0–12.2)	1.0
Metabolic alterations	2.9 (0.8–10.2)	1.9 (0.6–6.6)	1.0
Perinatal asphyxia	3.1 (1.3–7.2)	1.6 (0.7–3.7)	1.0
Hyperbilirubinemia	1.1 (0.5–2.6)	1.1 (0.5–2.3)	1.0
Infections	1.1 (0.3–4.8)	2.0 (0.7–5.7)	1.0
Morbidity index[c]	1.9 (1.1–3.1)	1.3 (0.8–2.1)	1.0
Age at discharge (> 7 days)	1.8 (0.9–3.9)	1.6 (0.8–3.2)	1.0

PI, ponderal index.
[a]Low PI: ≤ 10th percentile; intermediate PI: > 10th − ≤ 25th percentile; normal PI: > 25th − ≤ 90th percentile of a PI − gestational age distribution.
[b]Odds ratios (95% confidence interval) adjusted (logistic regression) by birthweight and duration of labor. The normal PI group is used as reference group: odds ratios = 1.0.
[c]Morbidity index: the presence of at least: Apgar score ≤ 3 at 1 min, aspiration syndrome, metabolic alterations, perinatal asphyxia, and infections.
From ref. 27.

Physical Growth

Several reports suggest that IUGR infants do not reach the weight or length of normal birthweight newborns during the first year of life (28,29). However, the heterogeneity of the IUGR group has not always been recognized. In a population of well-nourished mothers in England, disproportionate IUGR (low ponderal index) infants had a weight gain of 228 g per week, significantly higher than the 160 g/week gained by the proportionate (normal ponderal index) infants ($p<0.01$) (30). A similar pattern was observed for length and head circumference growth (30). A different ethnic group of exclusively breast-fed infants of chronically malnourished mothers in Guatemala showed similar growth patterns. The infants with disproportionate IUGR had, in the early neonatal period (first 2 weeks), a weekly weight gain of 298 g, significantly higher than the 126 g per week gained by the proportionate IUGR infants ($p<0.001$) (31). By the third month, infants with disproportionate IUGR continued to have a greater weight gain (219 g per week) than proportionate IUGR infants (199 g a week), although these differences were not statistically significant.

This phenomenon can be explained by differences in postnatal fat deposition patterns between the IUGR subgroups. Triceps skinfold growth velocity in the first three months was 0.23 mm per week for disproportionate IUGR infants and 0.17 mm per week for proportionate IUGR infants (31). Subscapular skinfold growth velocity during the same period was 0.21 and 0.14 mm per week for the same groups, and a similar pattern was found for calf skinfold thickness (0.47 versus 0.40 mm per week) (31). These results suggest that the extra postnatal weight gain and fat deposition is reserved for those newborns who are underweight for length at birth (i.e., who have had disproportionate fetal growth retardation). Independent of their ethnic background, these infants, while remaining lighter and shorter at 1 year of life than normal weight infants, do become better proportioned than at birth through a greater relative increase in weight (31,32). When the ponderal index was used to monitor postnatal growth in these infants, the values became near normal as early as the third month of extrauterine life (31).

This early catch-up growth in IUGR infants with low ponderal index may be possible because they did not experience any deficit in growth during the most critical periods of development, in contrast with symmetric IUGR infants, who suffered a chronic fetal insult.

Long-Term Outcome

Physical Growth

Holmes et al. (33) studied IUGR infants up to 9 months of age in a population from the U.S.A. They showed that the disproportionate IUGR (low ponderal index) infants reached the weight of a control group (normal birthweight) by the 6th month of postnatal life. The proportionate IUGR infants had significantly lower weight, length, and head circumference that persisted up to 9 months of age. In a study in which we followed up Guatemalan children from rural areas we have shown that infants with proportionate IUGR remained significantly lighter and shorter, with smaller head circumference, up to 3 years of age (34). In comparison with a normal birthweight group, the disproportionate IUGR group experienced marked catch-up growth in weight, more evident during the first 2 weeks of postnatal life but continuing from the 6th through the 9th month of age. Length and head circumference of this group were similar to those of the control normal birthweight group from birth to the end of the period under study.

We can therefore conclude that IUGR infants tend to follow postnatal growth patterns that are conditioned by their physical characteristics at birth. Those proportionate IUGR infants who were chronically retarded *in utero* (e.g., maternal undernutrition, smoking) will remain shorter and lighter, and with smaller head circumferences, up to 3 years of age. In contrast, disproportionate IUGR infants, who suffered an intrauterine insult late in pregnancy (e.g., toxemia, low maternal weight gain) but were able to achieve relatively adequate lengths and head circumferences, will recuperate from their growth impairment early in the first month of life, reaching values close to those of their normal counterparts by 12 months of age. Furthermore, weight gain of infants with disproportionate IUGR is inversely related to the degree of undernutrition at birth: The lower the weight for length (i.e., the lower the ponderal index), the higher the weight gain during the neonatal period. There is also a suggestion that the late intrauterine damage of disproportionate IUGR infants remains latent and becomes a handicap when they are exposed to adverse nutritional and sanitary conditions during childhood (34). Whether or not this late effect is present in disproportionate IUGR infants suffering from acute diseases and adverse conditions related to poverty in developed societies remains to be demonstrated.

MENTAL DEVELOPMENT

Due to the fact that there are still controversial findings on the mental development of children who suffered from IUGR, we are going to enlarge on this subject with an update of findings and opinions.

Follow-up studies focused on the development of full-term IUGR infants have been more numerous than those focused on preterm IUGR infants. In addition, for full-term IUGR infants follow-up periods have been longer and the range of developmental outcomes has been greater. As in other areas of IUGR research, studies of developmental sequelae vary in their definition of IUGR (e.g., 10th and 3rd percentile birthweight for gestational age) and in the birthweight standards used.

The developmental outcomes reported most frequently are the results of infant development tests, performance on childhood intelligence tests, and the presence of physical and mental disabilities. Various specific tests of development and intelligence have been used, and the definition of disability has differed across investigations. The issue of the limited predictability of infant test performance (35) must be taken into account when the follow-up period does not exceed 2 years. This consideration may be somewhat less serious for those infants with very low level performance (35), and for very low birthweight preterm infants (36), especially if tested after 14 months of age (37).

General Findings

Although developmental follow-up findings have sometimes been conflicting, some general conclusions are possible. Based on a comprehensive review of IUGR developmental follow-up studies, Allen (38) was able to draw several conclusions about the development of full-term IUGR infants. The vast majority of these infants, when examined in the preschool and school years, demonstrate normal intelligence test performance. The mean IQ of the IUGR group has often been somewhat lower than that of comparison groups, but the difference has not usually been statistically significant. In addition, the vast majority of full-term IUGR infants do not show evidence of major handicap at follow-up, but there is a suggestion of a slightly increased risk of cerebral palsy and mental retardation. Furthermore, evidence exists for increased risk of minimal cerebral dysfunction, including greater occurrence of speech and language problems, minor neurologic findings, attention deficits, and school failures, despite normal intelligence.

Conclusions regarding developmental sequelae of IUGR preterm infants are of necessity more limited and tentative. As noted by previous authors, sample sizes have been small (38,39), comparison groups have varied across studies (38), and almost no information has been reported about development at school age (38). Also the changing nature of the preterm, very low birthweight population must be considered, given that most available information on the developmental sequelae of preterm IUGR infants is based on births occurring between 1974 and 1976 (39–45). Allen's conclusions (38) reflect the caution necessary at this time: Preterm IUGR infants appear to have a higher incidence of major handicap than the general population, probably have a higher incidence of major handicap than term IUGR infants, and perhaps have a higher incidence of major handicap than preterm appropriate-for-gestational age infants.

The number (and particular combinations) of possible influences on the development of IUGR infants is large. The occurrence of intrauterine growth retardation and the subsequent development of the IUGR infant take place in the context of maternal health conditions, family conditions, medical conditions of the fetus, infant, and child, and the postnatal experiences of the child. Many of these factors are themselves related to a child's development. Several authors (34,38,46) have emphasized the need to subdivide the heterogeneous IUGR population into more homogeneous groupings. Investigations of subgroups of the IUGR population offer the possibility of gaining a better understanding of the development of these infants and consequently of establishing more accurate prognoses and more appropriate plans for postnatal services.

Developmental Sequelae of IUGR Subgroups

Studies that have examined developmental sequelae of IUGR subgroups can be classified in three categories: those that have subdivided the population based (a) on the timing of the intrauterine insult, (b) on maternal complications during pregnancy, and (c) on neonatal medical conditions. Available information is greatest for the timing of insult grouping.

Maternal Conditions during Pregnancy

Developmental sequelae of IUGR infants have been studied in relation to maternal hypertension, estimates of placental function, antepartum hemorrhage, and composite indices of maternal conditions (e.g., indices of maternal delivery complications and medical conditions of pregnancy). Conclusions are very limited. Findings are sometimes conflicting, as in the case of hypertensive disorders (46,47). Some developmental differences were found in one study (46) but not in another (47). In the case of placental function estimates, only short follow-up periods have been reported, namely 12 months (48) and 18 months (49). Antepartum hemorrhage (50) and composite maternal indices (51) have been found to have relatively little association with performance on developmental testing in childhood (i.e., in the 5- to 10-year-old period). In general, comparisons of findings across these studies are complicated by variation in definitions of maternal conditions, definitions of IUGR, other population characteristics, developmental outcomes, postnatal environments, approaches to statistical analysis, and the (sometimes unspecified) proportion of preterm and full-term infants in the samples.

Neonatal Medical Conditions

Studies of developmental sequelae have differentiated IUGR infants on the basis of several neonatal medical conditions and complications, including asphyxia (39,47,52), neonatal hypoglycemia and neonatal polycythemia (52), perinatal cerebral distress (53), and a neonatal problems index (51). Methodological variations noted for the maternal conditions studies apply to these investigations as well (e.g., differences in definitions of IUGR and medical conditions). For neonatal conditions, comparisons and conclusions are particularly limited by restricted sample sizes and frequent absence of statistical testing. For example, 33 full-term IUGR children who were not asphyxiated as newborns were tested at a mean age of 16.5 years and had a higher mean IQ than 11 IUGR children who had experienced asphyxia in the newborn period, but no statistical comparison was reported (52). In another study (39), several neonatal complications in addition to asphyxia were examined relative to developmental outcomes of preterm IUGR infants during the first 2 years of life. The only statistically significant association found was between developmental handicap and cerebral depression on admission to the neonatal intensive care unit, but the authors noted that birth asphyxia was an earlier complication in 21 of the 24 surviving infants admitted with cerebral depression.

As the discussion in this and the immediately preceding section indicates, relatively little is known about the developmental course of IUGR infants in relation to neonatal and maternal medical conditions. Somewhat more information about maternal/infant conditions and later development is available for other population groups (38,54–56). Consideration of this type of information is of obvious importance when dealing with issues of developmental prognosis and follow-up care. Detailed recommendations are available regarding procedures for generating developmental prognoses for IUGR infants, and for planning clinical follow-up of their developmental progress (38).

Timing of the Intrauterine Insult

Serial ultrasonic cephalometry during pregnancy (57–60) and ponderal index values in the neonatal period (34,61) have been used to estimate the timing of the intrauterine insult in IUGR sequelae studies. In the ultrasound studies, onset of slow head growth has been the timing indicator, and was defined as the time when the weekly increment in biparietal diameter fell below the 5th percentile over two or more weeks.

Work on subgroups timed in this way has been done with full-term IUGR infants in England (57–60), Guatemala (34), and the Netherlands (61). Mean ages at follow-up assessment have ranged from 6 months to 7.2 years. Developmental functioning has been measured in a number of areas, including general cognition, performance on motor, perceptual, verbal, and memory tasks, behavioral indicators, and school achievement. Findings have been similar across the studies. Those IUGR groups estimated to have experienced insults beginning early in pregnancy (i.e., those with slowed head growth before the 26th week of gestation and those with ponderal index values indicating proportionate effects on weight and length) consistently demonstrated the lowest developmental performance (Table5). Those infants presumed to have experienced late gestation insult (i.e., those with slowed head growth after 26 weeks of gestation and those with ponderal index values suggesting a disproportionate effect on weight) usually performed at developmental levels between those of the early insult group and the appropriate-for-gestational age comparison groups (Table 5).

Clearly there is need for continuing efforts to delineate the developmental sequelae of subgroups of the IUGR population. As part of this type of investigation, it would be valuable to attempt to differentiate those infants whose IUGR status reflects normal adaptation to pregnancy conditions from those whose IUGR reflects a pathologic insult (62,63). Similarly, there is need for greater attention to possible explanatory mechanisms underlying relationships between IUGR and later development.

TABLE 5. *Developmental characteristics of term intrauterine growth retardation (IUGR) infants classified by the time of onset of fetal growth retardation*

Mean postnatal age; Scale used (Ref.)	Time of onset of IUGR		Reference population
	Early onset[a]	Late onset[b]	
3 years; Cognitive composite percentile score (34)	38 (n = 25)	48 (n = 20)	63 (n = 110)
4 years; Griffiths scale development quotient (57)	93.3 ± 8.05[c] (n = 13)	102.0 ± 10.86[c] (n = 47)	—
5.1 years; McCarthy scales	102.9 ± 11.7[c,d] (n = 10)		118.0 ± 12.9[d] (n = 10)
General cognitive index (60)		113.2 ± 16.4[c] (n = 41)	115.0 ± 15.2 (n = 41)
7.2 years; Overall school achievement (59)	40.7 ± 15.4[c] (n = 9)	49.3 ± 23.1[e] (n = 14) 56.4 ± 16.3[f] (n = 22)	38.0 ± 13.0[c] (n = 19)

Results are means ± SD.
[a]IUGR-normal ponderal index (3 years); ultrasonic cephalometry growth retardation < 26 weeks of gestation (4–7.2 years).
[b]IUGR-low ponderal index (3 years); ultrasonic cephalometry growth retardation > 26 weeks or IUGR without evidence of biparietal diameter (BPD) growth retardation.
[c,d]($p < 0.05$) Significantly different from results with same superscript letter.
[e]Slow head growth between 27 and 34 weeks of gestation.
[f]Slow head growth after 35 weeks of gestation (n = 4) or no evidence of slow head growth (n = 18).

FINAL COMMENTS

We have presented evidence from several sources that IUGR infants are a hetero-geneous group. It can be concluded also that these infants tend to follow growth patterns that were conditioned during their fetal life. The timing and duration of the intrauterine insult together determine the physical condition of the infant at birth. Those infants with proportionate IUGR, whose growth has been chronically retarded *in utero*, will remain shorter and lighter and have a smaller head circumference. In contrast, infants with disproportionate IUGR, with a low ponderal index, who suffered growth retardation late in pregnancy can recuperate early in the first months of life, reaching values similar to those of their normal counterparts by 1 year of age. However, some evidence indicates that the intrauterine damage of disproportionate IUGR can remain latent and become a handicap during the second year of life. Developmental performance of IUGR infants is also associated with their physical characteristics at birth. A "time effect" relationship appears to emerge in the data, between the timing of the intrauterine damage and the later developmental performance.

Risk factors associated with IUGR must be detected, if possible, before pregnancy, so that they can be modified. Diagnosis of IUGR should be made as early as possible and corrective measures of associated maternal characteristics or diseases implemented. At birth, in addition to the usual classification, an IUGR newborn should be evaluated according to its ponderal index in order to prevent medical complications that are more prevalent in those infants with low ponderal indices. Follow-up of infants with IUGR should involve a multidisciplinary approach including both physical and mental development.

From a public health viewpoint, IUGR is most frequent in less-developed societies. Using standards from well-nourished populations, it can be estimated that the incidence of IUGR in developing countries is about 20% in urban areas, reaching figures as high as 50% in some rural populations. Furthermore, different distributions can be observed in different populations in relation to the two types of IUGR infants. Table 6 presents available information on this topic (64). Countries are listed in order of the incidence of proportionate (chronic) growth retardation. In developing populations between 67.5% and 79.1% of infants with IUGR have proportionate growth impairment. On the other hand, reports from developed countries show that proportionate IUGR accounts for only 20% to 40% of cases, with the exception of the Dutch population. Occupying an intermediate position (55.6%) is an Argentine population of middle socio-economic status.

In developing countries, factors associated with proportionate IUGR, such as chronic poor nutritional status in the mother, low socio-economic status, extremes

TABLE 6. *Pecentage of chronic proportionate growth retardation among intrauterine growth retardation (IUGR) newborns in developed and developing populations*

Population	No. IUGR in sample	Chronic or proportionate IUGR (%)
Urban Guatemala	848	79.1
Rural Guatemala	143	68.5
Rural South Africa	188	67.5
The Netherlands	119	61.3
Urban Argentina	54	55.6
United States	33	39.4
England	47	34.0
Canada	83	22.9
Yugoslavia	118	20.3
United States	165	20.0
England	51	19.6

From ref. 64.

in maternal age, and infections, are more prevalent. This explains, in part, the higher incidence of proportionate IUGR in these populations. As we have shown above, such children have poorer physical and mental development. This situation imposes a vicious cycle of underdevelopment, poor employment, poor nutrition, and chronic malnutrition continuing when those girls arrive at their reproductive age, a cycle which it is imperative to break in order to assure better growth and development for future generations.

REFERENCES

1. Villar J, Belizan JM. The relative contribution of prematurity and fetal growth retardation to low birth weight in developing and developed societies. *Am J Obstet Gynecol* 1982;143:793–8.
2. Villar J, Khoury MJ, Finucane FF, Delgado H. Differences in the epidemiology of prematurity and intrauterine growth retardation. *Early Hum Dev* 1986;14:307–20.
3. Scott A, Moar V, Ounsted M, et al. The relative contribution of different maternal factors in small-for-date pregnancies. *Eur J Obstet Gynecol Reprod Biol* 1981;12:157–65.
4. Berkowitz G. An epidemiologic study of preterm delivery. *Am J Epidemiol* 1981;113:81–92.
5. Anderson JD, Blinder IN, McClemont S, Sinclair JC. Determinants of size at birth in a Canadian population. *Am J Obstet Gynecol* 1984;150:236–44.
6. Dougherty CRS, Jones AD. The determinants of birth weight. *Am J Obstet Gynecol* 1982;144:190–200.
7. Villar J, Gonzalez-Cossio T. Nutritional factors associated with low birthweight and short gestational age. *Clin Nutr* 1986;5:78–85.
8. Iyengar L. Urinary estrogen excretion in undernourished pregnant Indian women. Effect of dietary supplement on urinary estrogens and birthweight of infants. *Am J Obstet Gynecol* 1968;102:834–8.
9. Lechtig A, Habicht JP, Delgado H, Klein RE, Yarbrough C, Martorell R. Effect of food supplementation during pregnancy on birthweight. *Pediatrics* 1975;56:508–20.
10. Rush D, Stein B, Susser M. A randomized controlled trial of prenatal nutritional supplementation in New York City. *Pediatrics* 1980;65:683–97.
11. Chaves A, Martinez C. The effect of maternal supplementation on infant development. *Arch Latinoam Nutr* 1979;29(Suppl 1):143–53.
12. Kennedy ET, Kotelchick M. The effect of WIC supplemental feeding on birthweight: a case control analysis. *Am J Clin Nutr* 1984;40:579–85.
13. Delgado H, Martorell R, Brineman E, Klein RE. Nutrition and length of gestation. *Nutr Res* 1982;2:117–26.
14. Villar J, Rivera J. Nutritional supplementation during two consecutive pregnancies and the interim lactation period: its effect on birth weight. *Pediatrics* 1988;81:51–7.
15. Prentice AM, Whitehead RG, Watkinson M, Lamb WH. Prenatal dietary supplementation of African women and birthweight. *Lancet* 1983;1:489–91.
16. Villar J, Belizan JM. The timing factor in the pathophysiology of the intrauterine growth retardation syndrome. *Obstet Gynecol Surv* 1982;37:499–506.
17. Villar J, Belizan JM. Growth and development of intrauterine growth retarded infants. *Clin Nutr* 1984;3:198–206.
18. Mata L. The children of Santa Maria Cauque. A prospective field study of health and growth. Cambridge, MA: MIT Press, 1978.
19. Belizan JM. Patterns of fetal growth in pregnancy induced hypertension. Centro Rosarino de Estudios Perinatales (CREP), internal publication, July 1986.
20. Miller HC, Hassanein K. Diagnosis of impaired fetal growth in newborn infants. *Pediatrics* 1971;48:511–22.
21. Miller H, Hassanein K, Hensleiger P. Fetal growth retardation in relation to maternal smoking and weight gain in pregnancy. *Am J Obstet Gynecol* 1976;125:55–60.
22. Davies DP, Abernethy M. Cigarette smoking in pregnancy. Associations with maternal weight gain and fetal growth. *Lancet* 1976;1:385–7.

23. Lubchenco LO, Bard H. Incidence of hypoglycemia in newborn infants classified by birthweight and gestational age. *Pediatrics* 1971;47:831–8.
24. Sinclair JC. Heat production and thermoregulation in the small-for-date infant. *Pediatric Clin North Am* 1970;17:147–58.
25. Wirth FH, Goldberg KE, Lubchenco LO. Neonatal hyperviscosity, I. Incidence. *Pediatrics* 1979; 63:833–36.
26. Walther FJ, Ramaekers LHJ. The ponderal index as a measure of the nutritional status at birth and its relation to some aspects of neonatal morbidity. *J Perinat Med* 1982;10:42–7.
27. deOnis M, Villar J, Kestler E, Berendes H. Differential neonatal morbidity of term intrauterine growth retarded infants. *Pediatr Res* 1989 (in press).
28. Brand I. Growth dynamics of low birthweight infants with emphasis on the perinatal period. In: Falkner F, Tanner JM, eds. *Human growth.* New York: Plenum Publishing Corp., 1978;557–617.
29. Cruise MO. A longitudinal study of the growth of low birthweight infants. I. Velocity and distance growth, birth to 3 years. *Pediatrics* 1973;51:620–8.
30. Davies DP, Platts P, Pritchard JM, Wilkinson PW. Nutritional status of light-for-date infants at birth and its influence on early postnatal growth. *Arch Dis Child* 1979;54:703–6.
31. Villar J, Belizan JM, Spalding J, Klein R. Postnatal growth of intrauterine growth retarded infants. *Early Hum Dev* 1982;6:265–71.
32. Davies DP, Beverly D. Changes in body proportions over first year of life: Comparison between "light-for-dates" and "appropriate-for-dates" term infants. *Early Hum Dev* 1979;3:263–5.
33. Holmes GE, Miller HC, Hassanein K, Goggin JE. Postnatal somatic growth in infants with atypical fetal growth pattern. *Am J Dis Child* 1977;131:1078–83.
34. Villar J, Smeriglio V, Martorell R, Klein RE. Heterogeneous growth and mental development of intrauterine growth retarded infants during the first three years of life. *Pediatrics* 1984;74:783–91.
35. Kopp CB, McCall RB. Predicting later mental performance for normal, at-risk, and handicapped infants. In: Baltes PB, Brim OG Jr, eds. *Life-span development and behavior.* Vol 4. New York: Academic Press, 1982;33–61.
36. Ross G, Lipper EG, Auld AM. Consistency and change in the development of premature infants weighing less than 1,501 grams at birth. *Pediatrics* 1985;76:885–91.
37. Fitzsimons RB, Ashby SA, Fitzhardinge PM. The prediction of school age I.Q. during infancy in the premature child. *Pediatr Res* 1978;12:370.
38. Allen MC. Developmental outcome and follow-up of the small for gestational age infant. *Semin Perinatol* 1984;8:123–56.
39. Commey JOO, Fitzhardinge PM. Handicap in the preterm small-for-gestational age infant. *J Pediatr* 1979;94:779–86.
40. Koops BL. Neurologic sequelae in infants with intrauterine growth retardation. *J Reprod Med* 1978;21:343–51.
41. Fitzhardinge PM, Kalman E, Ashby S, et al. Present status of the infant of very low birth weight treated in a referral neonatal intensive care unit in 1974. In: Ciba Foundation Symposium 59 (New Series): *Major mental handicap: methods and costs of prevention.* New York: Elsevier, 1978; 139–50.
42. Vohr BR, Oh W, Rosenfield AG, et al. The preterm small-for-gestational age infant: a two-year follow-up study. *Am J Obstet Gynecol* 1979;133:425–31.
43. Vohr BR, Oh W. Growth and development in preterm infants small for gestational age. *J Pediatr* 1983;103:941–5.
44. Lipper E, Lee K, Gartner LM, et al. Determinants of neurobehavioral outcome in low-birthweight infants. *Pediatrics* 1981;67:502–5.
45. Hack M, Fanaroff AA, Merkatz IR. The low-birthweight infant—evolution of a changing outlook. *N Engl J Med* 1979;301:1162–5.
46. Winer EK, Tejani NA, Alturu VL, et al. Four-to-seven-year evaluation in two groups of small-for-gestational age infants. *Am J Obstet Gynecol* 1982;143:425–9.
47. Ounsted MK, Moar VA, Scott A. Small-for-dates babies at the age of four years: health, handicap, and developmental status. *Early Hum Dev* 1983;8:243–58.
48. Low JA, Galbraith RS, Muir D, et al. Intrauterine growth retardation: a preliminary report of long-term morbidity. *Am J Obstet Gynecol* 1979;130:534–45.
49. Leijon I, Billstrom G, Lind I. An 18-month follow-up study of growth-retarded neonates. Relation to neurobehavioural condition in the newborn period. *Early Hum Dev* 1980;4:271–85.
50. Neligan GA, Kolvin I, Scott DMcL. Born too soon or born too small: A follow-up study to seven years of age. In: *Clinics in developmental medicine,* No. 61. Philadelphia: Lippincott, 1976.

51. Illsley R, Mitchell RG. *Low birth weight: a medical, psychological, and social study.* New York: Wiley, 1984.
52. Westwood M, Kramer MS, Munz D, et al. Growth and development of full-term nonasphyxiated small-for-gestational age newborns: follow-up through adolescence. *Pediatrics* 1983;71:376–82.
53. Stave U, Ruvalo C. Neurological development in very-low-birth weight infants. Application of a standardized examination and Prechtl's optimality concept in routine evaluations. *Early Hum Dev* 1980;4:229–41.
54. Wade RW, Searby J, Pepperell RJ, et al. Paediatric follow-up of pregnancies complicated by subnormal oestriol excretion. *Br J Obstet Gynaecol* 1985;92:662–82.
55. Skouteli HN, Dubowitz LMS, Levene MI, et al. Predictors for survival and normal neurodevelopmental outcome of infants weighing less than 1001 grams at birth. *Dev Med Child Neurol* 1985;27:589–95.
56. Low JA, Galbraith RS, Muir DW, et al. The contribution of fetal-newborn complications to motor and cognitive deficits. *Dev Med Child Neurol* 1985;27:578–87.
57. Fancourt R, Campbell S, Harvey DR, et al. Follow-up study of small-for-dates babies. *Br Med J* 1976;1:1435–7.
58. Harvey DR, Prince J, Bunton J, et al. Abilities of children who were small-for-dates at birth and whose growth *in utero* was measured by ultrasonic cephalometry. *Pediatr Res* 1976;10:891.
59. Parkinson CE, Wallis S, Harvey DR. School achievement and behaviour of children who are small-for-dates at birth. *Dev Med Child Neurol* 1981;23:41–50.
60. Harvey DR, Prince J, Bunton J, et al. Abilities of children who were small-for-gestational-age babies. *Pediatrics* 1982;69:296–300.
61. Walther FJ, Ramaekers LHJ. Developmental aspects of subacute fetal distress: behaviour problems and neurological dysfunction. *Early Hum Dev* 1982;6:1–10.
62. Read MS, Catz C, Grave G, et al. Introduction: intrauterine growth retardation—Identification of research needs and goals. *Semin Perinatol* 1984;8:2–4.
63. Washaw JB. Intrauterine growth retardation: adaptation or pathology? *Pediatrics* 1985;76:998–9.
64. Villar J, Altobelli LC, Kestler E, Belizan JM. A health priority for developing countries. The prevention of chronic fetal malnutrition. *Bull Wld Hlth Org* 1987;64:147–51.

DISCUSSION

Dr. Alves-Filho: We have a major problem of IUGR in Brazil. We have 2,500,000 births per year in this country, 350,000 of which are of small-for-dates (SFD) infants. In this meeting the local neonatologists have not heard enough about what we can do for these SFD babies. In the service where I work we have 25 deliveries per day a quarter of whom may be small-for-dates, and we sometimes have 10 to 15 premature infants to look after as well. The SFD infants on the whole don't die of respiratory problems because we can usually cope with them. Our babies die of infection and nutrition-related problems. How can we treat these babies? We need practical ideas from investigators in developed countries to help us. We have had detailed discussions about local growth curves, without recognizing that the only way we can show our governments that there is a big problem with nutrition in our population is by showing them how small our babies are compared with babies from developed countries. We can't really be interested in intrauterine nutritional support, parenteral nutrition in the mother, and so on. We need to know what kind of milk to give our babies after they have been born. Personally, I think the best kind of milk for small-for-dates babies is their own mother's milk. I think it is better for a baby of 1,100 g to be at home having his mother's milk than to stay in hospital, with the kinds of problems I have in my hospital. We have tried milk banks but we get milk infected with cytomegalovirus, infectious mononucleosis, and now, AIDS. And also, how can we feed a baby with formula when the mother cannot afford to buy it?

Dr. Villar: I can only answer with a parable. A drunk man came home at 3 o'clock in the morning and couldn't find the key to his house. He went to a street lamp and started searching under the light. Eventually the police came by and asked him what he was doing. "Looking for the keys to my house," he said. "Are you sure you lost your keys here?" the policeman asked. "No, but there is a good light here!" he replied. You will not find the problem of your malnourished SFD babies in this room just because the light is here! The solution lies where you lost your keys.

Dr. Alves-Filho: I agree with that, but it is still very important that investigators from developed countries participate in our problems, our practical problems, that is.

Dr. Chessex: I was certainly very concerned when I came here that I would not be able to provide the message that you wanted. The research we do in my country has to be done with the means available. Just because we have investigated formula-fed small-for-gestational-age (SGA) infants does not mean that such babies should necessarily be fed on formulas. The data I presented were intended to show basic nutritional phenomena, rather than to provide a model for management.

Dr. Senterre: I agree with Dr. Alves-Filho that the best milk for SFD babies is their own mother's milk but I think that if they are growing poorly, supplementation with a standard infant formula will be beneficial. When the mother cannot afford to buy it, I would advise to supplement breast-feeding with 30 ml/kg/day of ordinary cow's milk which will provide a supplement of about 1 g protein, 36 mg calcium, and 27 mg phosphorus as well as 20 kcal per kg body weight per day, facilitating the catch-up growth.

Dr. Rosso: I have a comment for Dr. Alves-Filho. I think our main aim in developing countries must be to try to *prevent* SFD infants. This is where we should put the emphasis. One particular element, which is to some extent in our hands and which we know how to handle, is maternal nutrition. In Chile, although officially 60% of cases of IUGR are of unknown cause, when you look at them carefully you see that in reality only 20% are really unknown—where you don't have an inkling of what went wrong. The remainder occur in women who are either of low weight for height or who gain little weight in pregnancy. Therefore I think we can say that, in this population, over 50% of cases of IUGR are likely to be connected with preventable nutritional problems.

Dr. Bossart: May I return to one thing I said yesterday in relation to the antenatal management of IUGR that has practical implications for developing countries. If we allow babies with IUGR to go to term they will be damaged by the time they are born. I strongly feel that no growth-retarded baby should go to term, since he will either die of asphyxia or be handicapped. So I suggest that if everyone could ensure that such babies are delivered at 37 to 38 weeks, we would see an improvement.

Dr. Belizan: If you follow that policy you will undoubtedly increase the rate of premature deliveries and all the problems they bring for countries without good neonatal intensive care units.

Dr. Villar: I don't think there are any good data to show that you will have a better outcome if you deliver babies with proportional IUGR early. It may be a clinical impression that they do better but there are no data to support this view. It is quite a different matter if you have a baby who stops growing altogether at 34 weeks; you are not going to let that baby go to term. But I think the proportional small baby who is growing along, say, the 5th percentile should be allowed to go to term, because the epidemiologic data tell you that 80% of all babies in developing countries are below the 10th percentile, in other words, may be regarded as normal small infants. If you deliver all these babies early you will have a major epidemic of preterm infants. In developed countries the situation is totally different because the majority of babies below the 10th percentile are not normal small babies but are growth-retarded.

Dr. Bossart: I wanted to be provocative. It is of course clear that it is most important to deliver early those infants who are not growing, rather than those small babies who are continuing to grow. But what about the question of minimal brain damage? Must we simply accept this as a fact of life and not do anything about it?

Dr. Villar: The problem of IUGR prevention is more political and related to the socioeconomical situation than a medical one in countries like ours.

Dr. Marini: A comment about neurological follow-up: We started a long-term follow-up of low birthweight babies 15 years ago and we found initially that SFD babies had more problems than appropriate-for-gestation (AGA) babies. But as time went on we found that the situation gradually reversed until now we see more problems in premature AGA infants, probably because of the increased numbers of very small babies who are surviving problems such as bronchopulmonary dysplasia and intraventricular hemorrhage, with resulting handicap. On the other hand, as Dr. Bossart has said, our obstetricians have also improved a great deal in their handling of IUGR and their selection of the best time for delivery. It is now very unusual for such babies to be born with asphyxia. With good neonatal care these babies do quite well, even if they had severe IUGR. I think good antenatal monitoring is very important, with elective cesarean section as soon as there are biochemical and other indications that the baby has stopped growing. This is a policy that works very well in developed countries.

Dr. Villar: Unfortunately, what we have heard in the last couple of days about early identification of IUGR is not optimistic. For example, it appears that the measurement of urinary estriol does not predict fetal growth retardation.

Dr. Marini: I was referring to fetal sampling, cardiotocography, etc.

Dr. Seeds: It seems clear to me that everyone is right. We need to improve nutrition in the first half of pregnancy, or even before conception, so that we can prevent chronic malnutrition producing proportionate small babies with long-term neurological deficits, albeit subtle ones; we need to avoid perinatal asphyxia to achieve the best outcome in disproportionate IUGR infants with low ponderal index (and this may be the most important aim in such babies); and we need to prevent prematurity while at the same time delivering babies who have stopped growing before it's too late—that is a matter of careful assessment and good timing as we have heard today. In my institution, our approach to the latter problem is to do what we can to detect impaired growth; to determine whether growth is proportionate or disproportionate; to identify babies who, in addition to impaired growth, are facing respiratory failure from inadequate placental gas transfer; and to deliver the baby before he is asphyxiated but hopefully when he is reasonably mature. The only think I disagree with that has been said here is that there could be an absolute gestational age beyond which such infants should not be delivered. I think each case should be taken on its merits in this regard.

Dr. Canosa: I should like to comment on catch-up growth. If we look at the literature on this phenomenon it is clear that not everyone is talking about the same thing. One publication will show good catch-up growth by a year, another not until 6 or 7 years, and still another, never. I think we must come to some kind of agreement about what kind of population we are talking about when presenting results of catch-up growth so that we can be sure we are all using the same terminology.

Dr. Villar: I think this all depends on what measures are being used. Disproportionate SFD babies with severe weight deficit, mainly of fat, will catch up in weight growth in 15 to 30 days if you provide enough nutrients. But if you consider head growth, these infants may not recuperate before a year or 18 months, or perhaps never. After all, almost 80% of adult head circumference is achieved by 2 years of age so there is not much scope for catch-up. With height it is different because it takes 7 years to achieve 80% of adult height so you have a longer period for catch-up. But if by 7 years you are still short, you will remain so because the adolescent growth spurt is relatively small to help much. Thus we are talking about catch-up in head growth by the end of the first year, and in linear growth by school entry.

Dr. Chessex: I should like to ask Dr. Belizan a question about breast milk. I was interested in what you said about prolonged breast-feeding. Do you have any experience of mothers breast-feeding right through into the next pregnancy and then continuing to breast-feed both the toddler and the new baby? I think if this occurs it could be nutritionally very important. We had one such case in a mother who delivered a preterm baby while she was still breast-feeding the previous one. When we analyzed her milk we found it was very low in substrate.

Dr. Belizan: There was one unpublished study of Delgado at the Institute of Nutrition of Central America and Panamá (INCAP) of Guatemalan women who breast-fed during pregnancy. Fetal growth was found to be impaired in comparison with mothers who were not breast-feeding. We must try to persuade mothers to stop breast-feeding when they become pregnant again.

Dr. Villar: The cost of one pregnancy and the lactation period, total time about 17 months in a Guatemalan rural population, is about 7 kg of net weight loss for the mother. So this certainly can't be good for fetal development.

Dr. Martins-Filho: Dr. Fabio and myself have carried out some studies in Brazil in which we showed that the postnatal growth curves of babies did not differ between mothers who were well-nourished and mothers who were poorly nourished. However, what can we do about the undernourished lactating mother anyway? If we give her food supplements she gives them all to her family. The problem of nutrition of SFD babies may well be a problem of the mothers' nutrition, but at least we can say that breast-feeding small babies who are growing below the 25th percentile results in improved mortality figures compared with formula-feeding.

Dr. Villar: Breast-feeding has often been shown to reduce infant mortality. There is a problem with these studies, however, in that most of them did not adjust for birthweight. When you do control for birthweight the preventive effects on mortality become lower. There is a paper showing exactly this effect. So, we have to be careful what kind of babies we are considering since it is apparently not too difficult to "save" normal birthweight infants.

REFERENCE

1. Barros FC, Victoria CG, Vaughan JP, et al. Birthweight and the duration of breast-feeding: are the beneficial effects of breast-feeding being overestimated? *Pediatr* 1986;78:656–61.

Intrauterine Growth Retardation, edited by
Jacques Senterre. Nestlé Nutrition Workshop
Series, Vol. 18. Nestec Ltd., Vevey/Raven Press,
Ltd., New York © 1989.

Nutritional Problems and Catch-Up Growth in Infants with Intrauterine Growth Retardation

Philippe Chessex

*Centre de recherche et service de néonatologie, Hôpital Sainte-Justine,
Montreal, H3T 1C5 PQ, Canada*

In the past, it was common practice to relate low birthweight to prematurity. However, a number of environmental, maternal, placental, and fetal factors have been recognized as causing intrauterine growth retardation (IUGR) in babies who are small-for-gestational-age (SGA). In the more affluent societies, one-third of the low birthweight babies are SGA. Yet in communities where protein-energy malnutrition and common infections are predominant environmental factors, the incidence of growth retardation due to intrauterine malnutrition can increase to 80% in low birthweight infants (1). The infant who has suffered from intrauterine malnutrition early in the third trimester of pregnancy is potentially at risk of continued growth retardation (2–4) as well as of learning and behavioral problems (5–7). Therefore, perinatal problems must be focused on the prevention of intrauterine growth retardation (1).

In the presence of a newborn baby with intrauterine growth retardation, one of the challenging therapeutic problems is to decide when, what, and how to feed this low birthweight infant. In this chapter we shall be concerned with some physiological adaptations and metabolic consequences which modulate such decisions.

INTRAUTERINE MALNUTRITION

Several different etiological factors are associated with IUGR (8–11), explaining the considerable heterogeneity of physical appearance at birth. At least 60% of the variation of birthweight could be attributed to "environmental" factors and only a small proportion to genetic or chromosomal factors (12). Indeed, many small-for-date newborn infants show clinical and biochemical features indicating intrauterine malnutrition. Clinical observations, supported by measurements of subcutaneous fat thickness (13), ponderal or anthropometric indices (14–16), and body composition (17,18), point to a majority of SGA babies being malnourished *in utero* (19). At birth they also present biochemical abnormalities which are characteristic of protein malnutrition, such as changes in serum and urine amino acid patterns (20), de-

281

creased levels of total serum protein (20), and retinol-binding protein (21) concentrations. If those infants with congenital malformations are excluded, birth can be seen to release many SGA babies from a nutritionally inadequate ''environment'' caused either by maternal malnutrition or impaired utero-placental blood flow. We shall discuss how the postnatal period should provide the necessary opportunity to recover the growth deficit attributed to those ''environmental'' factors. We will consider the nutritional problems encountered during three separate periods: the perinatal period with the adaptations to the extrauterine environment; the neonatal period, characterized by its increased nutrient requirements; and finally, the period of catch-up growth.

EXTRAUTERINE ADAPTATION

The major perinatal sequelae of intrauterine growth retardation resulting from impairment of nutrient flow from mother to fetus include low birthweight, hypoglycemia, polycythemia, and birth asphyxia. Therefore, during the period of adaptation to extrauterine life, nutritional policies should be guided by the following aims:

1. to restore normal glucose homeostasis;
2. to control hyperviscosity resulting from polycythemia;
3. to avoid aggravating complications induced by birth asphyxia; and
4. to favor early feeding.

The appropriate-for-gestational age term neonate can remain euglycemic despite a prolonged initial fast, thanks to hepatic gluconeogenesis. The high incidence of hypoglycemia reported in the IUGR infant (22) is probably related to the combined influence of depleted liver glycogen content, increased substrate utilization, and depressed enzymatic activity necessary for gluconeogenesis (23). As these infants are also hypoketonemic (24), it is thought that the low rate of gluconeogenesis could be secondary to reduced lipolysis (25) of small endogenous fat depots and a low rate of fatty acid oxidation (25). Indeed, oral or intravenous administration of triglycerides has been shown to cause a hyperglycemic response in hypoglycemic SGA infants (26,27) by increasing the production of glucose (27). The combination of low glucose with low levels of ketones is potentially deleterious for the brain, which has elevated energy requirements during the neonatal period (28,29). These metabolic consequences of IUGR stress the importance of early feeding.

More recently, research efforts have been directed towards the effect of medium-chain triglyceride (MCT:C6:0-C12:0) feeding on glucose homeostasis. The MCT are more efficient than long-chain triglycerides in correcting fasting-induced hypoglycemia (30). The MCT yield more ketone bodies than long-chain fatty acids (31) and can sustain an active gluconeogenesis (30). Feeding an MCT formula produces a blood ketone body concentration comparable to that of term infants who have been breast-fed (32). Ketone bodies may be particularly important in the developing infant and it has been shown in the newborn that acetoacetate and β-hydroxybutyrate are readily oxidized (33) and serve as key substrates for lipogenesis in the brain (34). This situation is quite relevant in the IUGR newborn, since high concentrations of ketone bodies could decrease the oxidation of glucose in the peripheral tissues, and thus contribute to glucose sparing (30). Therefore, during the first hours of extrauterine adaptation, when maternal milk production is not yet initiated, the early feeding of an MCT-rich solution to the hypoglycemic growth-retarded newborn can be an effective adjunct to the rapid intravenous correction of the glucose homeostasis.

Because of their rapid portal absorption and hepatic oxidation, MCT have been added to several infant formulas. Although oxidation of lipids and synthesis of ketone bodies may be enhanced, the appropriate quantity of MCT in infant formulas has not been clearly established. Storage of medium-chain triglycerides in adipose tissue of orally fed infants has been recently demonstrated (35). Figure 1 shows that in infants fed *ad libitum*, dietary fat is a major determinant of adipose tissue composition, confirming the saying: "You are what you eat." Furthermore, under normal nutritional conditions, MCT are not used solely as a source of energy but can also be re-esterified or serve for chain elongation before being deposited in fat stores. Those infants receiving formulas with higher MCT content had up to 10% of medium-chain fatty acids in their adipose tissue (35). The long-term physiological effects of MCT-rich diets should be carefully evaluated, as dietary lipids are known to influence both cellular properties (36) and membrane structure (37).

IUGR neonates have a high incidence of chronic fetal distress and birth asphyxia (38). Therefore, the early feeding of these infants should be initiated with caution. Erythropoiesis is stimulated by chronic fetal distress with hypoxia. This results in an

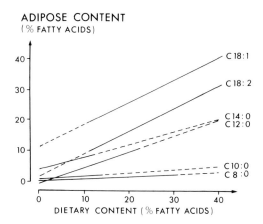

FIG. 1. Significant linear regressions are plotted for individual fatty acids, between the content of medium chain fatty acids (C8:0, C10:0, C12:0) and long-chain fatty acids (C14:0, C18:1, C18:2) in commonly used sources of diet (mother's milk, formulas) on adipose tissue content of these fatty acids. For C18:2, $Y = 0.75X + 1.8$, $n = 29$, $r = 0.87$; for C18:1, $Y = 0.74X + 10.9$, $n = 29$, $r = 0.93$; for C14:0, $Y = 0.41X + 3.6$, $n = 29$, $r = 0.71$; for C12:0, $Y = 0.53X - 3.5$, $n = 29$, $r = 0.95$; for C10:0, $Y = 0.1X + 0.5$, $n = 29$, $r = 0.8$; for C8:0, $Y = 0.08X + 0.2$, $n = 29$, $r = 0.9$. (From ref. 35.)

increase in fetal hemoglobin synthesis (39). Many SGA infants are polycythemic (38,40), and polycythemia is generally associated with hyperviscosity (41), resulting in a sluggish gastrointestinal blood flow. Gastrointestinal disturbances may be apparent in the form of feeding intolerance and in the more severe cases of necrotizing enterocolitis (NEC) (42). Necrotizing enterocolitis is characterized by signs of sepsis in addition to bile-stained vomiting, bloody stools, intestinal perforation, peritonitis, and shock (43). Fetal hypoxia will also result in decreased gastrointestinal perfusion, and again cause increased vulnerability to NEC (44). It was thought that delaying oral-feeding might reduce the incidence of NEC (45,46). Although enteral substrates may be important in the development of NEC, studies conducted in a prospective fashion have demonstrated that delaying feeding failed to prevent necrotizing enterocolitis (47,48). Moreover, functional gut maturation is dependent on enteral substrates (49). In the animal model of NEC (50,51), fresh breast milk protected newborn rats from a similar disease (50,51). However, NEC can occur in neonates fed exclusively on human milk (52,53).

Therefore, during this period of extrauterine adaptation a slowly progressive feeding schedule should be advocated (49,54). When breast milk is not available, early enteral feeding should be initiated with a low volume of low osmolar, medium-chain triglyceride containing formula (48). During this early stage of feeding it is not so much the global energy intake which is to be emphasized, but the quality of available substrate.

INCREASED NUTRIENT REQUIREMENTS

The effects of intrauterine malnutrition on gastrointestinal development in humans have not been investigated. Before increasing the nutrient intake in growth-retarded infants up to full feedings, one should be aware that neonatal animal data suggest subnormal gastrointestinal function as the result of intrauterine malnutrition. A decrease in both intestinal and pancreatic weight secondary to a reduction in the number of cells has been documented in rats undernourished during fetal life (55,56), along with a reduction in total pancreatic enzymes (55). In humans, malnutrition in early infancy has been associated with atrophy of the pancreas and intestinal mucosa in fatal cases of kwashiorkor (57). On the other hand, it has also been shown (58) that there was comparable pancreatic endocrine activity in 48-hr-old SGA and appropriate-for-gestational-age (AGA) infants after an oral glucose load and protein stimulation.

A quantitative evaluation of the energy metabolism of IUGR low birthweight infants has been carried out (29). By combining energy and macronutrient balances with open-circuit indirect calorimetry, the absorption, utilization, and storage of energy and macronutrients were compared between SGA and AGA low birthweight infants. Fourteen studies were performed in six SGA infants (mean ± SEM birthweight: 1.12 ± 0.03 kg; gestational age: 33.1 ± 0.3 weeks; postnatal age: 26 ± 3 days). Twenty-two studies were undertaken in 13 AGA infants (birthweight: 1.15 ± 0.04 kg; gestational age: 29.3 ± 0.4 weeks; postnatal age: 21 ± 2 days). The

TABLE 1. *Macronutrient intake and partition of losses in excretion*

	IUGR	AGA
Intake		
Macronutrients (g/kg-day)		
Fat	8.0 ± 0.1	7.5 ± 0.2
Carbohydrate	16.0 ± 0.2	15.2 ± 0.4
Protein	3.3 ± 0.1	3.2 ± 0.1
Energy		
(kcal/kg-day)	156 ± 2	149 ± 4
(kJ/kg-day)	651 ± 9	621 ± 16
Losses		
Macronutrients (g/kg-day)		
Stool		
Fat	2.5 ± 0.3	1.5 ± 0.1*
Carbohydrate	0.05 ± 0.01	0.05 ± 0.02
Protein	1.1 ± 0.1	0.55 ± 0.05*
Urine		
Carbohydrate	0.10 ± 0.01	0.10 ± 0.01
Protein	0.73 ± 0.04	0.73 ± 0.03
Energy		
(kcal/kg-day)	30 ± 3	18 ± 2*
(kJ/kg-day)	125 ± 11	76 ± 6*

Results are expressed as mean ± SEM.
IUGR, intrauterine growth retardation; AGA, appropriate-for-gestational-age
*$p < 0.05$.
Adapted from ref. 29.

routine feeding schedule provided SGA and AGA infants with similar volumes of long-chain triglycerides (84%) containing formula (185 ± 2 versus 180 ± 3 ml/kg-day). The comparison between macronutrient and energy intakes and the partition of losses in excretion are presented in Table 1. Macronutrient and energy utilization was determined by respiratory gas exchange measurements using the principles of indirect calorimetry. The results of macronutrient and energy utilization and deposition are presented in Table 2. The IUGR infants demonstrated different metabolic responses to the diet in nutrient absorption, energy metabolism, and newly deposited tissues.

Protein absorption was significantly lower in the IUGR infants (69 ± 3 versus 83 ± 2%). Figure 2 shows that there were increased protein losses in these infants. A lower protein digestibility has also been documented in a smaller number of comparative studies on protein turnover in IUGR and AGA low birthweight infants (59). The whole body protein turnover was 26% higher in SGA infants. In older infants treated for malnutrition, the protein turnover rate almost doubled during recovery from undernutrition (60). SGA infants show the same adaptation of their protein metabolism as they recover from intrauterine growth retardation (59). Furthermore, protein synthesis and breakdown were both significantly increased in the growth-

TABLE 2. *Macronutrient utilization and deposition*

	Metabolizable intake		Utilization		Deposition	
	IUGR	AGA	IUGR	AGA	IUGR	AGA
Fat (g/kg-day)	5.5 ± 0.2	6.0 ± 0.2	1.2 ± 0.3	0.6 ± 0.3	4.3 ± 0.4	5.4 ± 0.3*
Carbohydrate (g/kg-day)	15.85 ± 0.2	15.05 ± 0.4	13.2 ± 0.6	13.3 ± 0.5	2.6 ± 0.4	1.8 ± 0.4
Protein (g/kg-day)	2.2 ± 0.1	2.65 ± 0.1*	0.73 ± 0.04	0.73 ± 0.03	1.57 ± 0.12	1.92 ± 0.08*
Energy						
(kcal/kg-day)	126 ± 3	130 ± 4	67 ± 1	63 ± 1*	59 ± 4	68 ± 3
(kJ/kg-day)	526 ± 10	545 ± 14	282 ± 5	261 ± 5*	244 ± 15	283 ± 12

Results are expressed as mean ± SEM.
IUGR, intrauterine growth retardation; AGA, appropriate-for-gestational-age.
Metabolizable intake: intake − losses; Deposition: metabolizable intake − utilization.
*$p < 0.05$.
Adapted from ref. 29.

retarded newborn infants (59), explaining the lack of difference in urinary nitrogen excretion between SGA and AGA infants (29,59). For a similar protein intake received by the SGA and AGA preterm infants (Table 1), the protein retention (as calculated from the nitrogen retention) was significantly lower in the SGA infants (Table 2). Although these protein intakes fell within requirements for IUGR infants (61) the retention (1.6 g/kg-day) fell short of intrauterine accretion rates (Fig. 3). Therefore, the published values of protein requirements (Table 3) for IUGR infants (61) might be somewhat underestimated, because of a lower than anticipated protein digestibility. However, the protein turnover data (59) show that these infants can

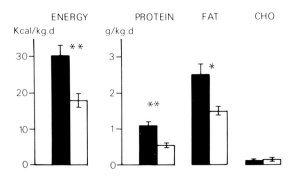

FIG. 2. Energy and macronutrient losses (mean ± SEM) measured during 14 balance studies in 6 IUGR preterm infants (black columns) and 22 balance studies in 13 AGA preterm infants (white columns) receiving similar intakes. The energy losses in excreta were significantly greater in the IUGR infants, due to the combined effect of greater losses in protein (**$p<0.001$) and fat (*$p<0.005$). (From ref. 29.)

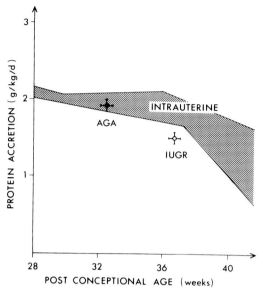

FIG. 3. Protein accretion (mean ± SEM) measured during 14 balance studies in 6 IUGR preterm infants at a postconceptional age of 36 ± 1 week (open circle) and 22 balance studies in 13 AGA preterm infants at a postconceptional age of 32 ± 1 week (closed circle). Results are compared with the range of third trimester fetal accretion rates. (From refs. 19 and 62.)

adapt to a subnormal intake by more intense reutilization of endogenous amino acids.

Fat absorption was significantly worse (69 ± 3 versus 83 ± 2%) in the SGA preterm infants (29); Fig. 2 shows the greater fat loss in these infants. Severe malabsorption of nitrogen and fat is also present in malnourished infants (63). The diminished enzymatic activities of lipase and trypsin documented in animal studies on malnutrition (64) offer a pathophysiological basis for the finding of relative fat and protein malabsorption in IUGR preterm infants. Fat oxidation was 50% higher

TABLE 3. *Protein requirements for IUGR infants in the first 3 months of life*

Age (month)	Protein requirements (g/kg-day)	Protein requirements (g/100 kcal)
0	3.2	2.5
1	2.5	2.0
2	2.2	1.7
3	1.9	1.5

IUGR, intrauterine growth retardation.
Adapted from ref. 61.

in the growth-retarded infants compared to the AGAs; however, this difference did not reach statistical significance (Table 2). Others (65,66) have documented a lower respiratory quotient in SGA infants, pre- as well as postprandially. Such a difference in metabolic response reflects a greater dependence on fat metabolism by the IUGR infant. This is confirmed by a study showing that after the oral administration of lipids, the blood concentration of ketone bodies increased by 120% in SGA infants, compared to only 40% in AGA infants (27). On the other hand, after an intravenous lipid test, significantly higher concentrations of triglycerides and free fatty acids were found in IUGR infants (67). These data have been interpreted as showing a limited capacity of the IUGR infant to hydrolyze triglycerides and utilize the fatty acids. However, the poor utilization of intravenously administered lipids is contrary to the indirect evidence of greater oxidation documented in the orally fed IUGR infants. Therefore, the prolonged elevation of free fatty acid levels (67) may rather be evidence of a low free fatty acid uptake by the reduced mass of adipose tissue in the growth-retarded infant. The higher fatty acid oxidation of the orally fed IUGR infant suggests a higher substrate demand in order to cover the increased energy expenditure found in these babies.

The fecal losses of carbohydrate were similar in IUGR and AGA infants (Table 1). However, a significant impairment of D-xylose absorption is present in growth-retarded infants over the first few weeks of postnatal life (68). Moreover, the small intestine of rats with experimentally induced intrauterine growth retardation has a reduced lactase content compared with appropriately grown controls (69). With the hydrogen breath test (70) it has been shown that a substantial proportion of lactose escapes absorption in the small intestine before being fermented by colonic bacteria. During fermentation this carbohydrate would be converted into rapidly absorbed volatile fatty acids (71). This process could explain the low fecal recovery of carbohydrate as shown in Table 1. The relative functional importance of this carbohydrate salvaging mechanism remains to be explored for different sources of carbohydrates (lactose, glucose, sucrose, dextrin-maltose) in IUGR as well as AGA newborn infants.

Delayed bone mineralization has been found in SGA infants (72). In one study bone mineral content was found to be significantly reduced at birth in term growth-retarded infants compared with term AGA infants (73). During the 12 weeks of that study, the postnatal increase in bone mineral content of the SGA infants lagged significantly behind that of AGA infants. This delayed skeletal maturation might be responsible for the deficit in height described in IUGR infants at follow-up through adolescence (3). On the other hand, preterm SGA infants do not have a delayed bone mineral content compared to preterm AGA infants (73,74). It has been suggested that neither hepatic hydroxylation of vitamin D nor renal hydroxylation of 25-hydroxyvitamin D is delayed in SGA infants (73). Malabsorption of fat has been shown to impede calcium absorption (75). Several pathophysiological explanations have been suggested for this controversial observation (75). Long-chain saturated fatty acids form insoluble soaps with calcium (Ca) in the intestine, preventing its absorption, an observation supported by the finding that MCT have been shown to improve fat as well as Ca absorption in low birthweight infants (76,77). On the other hand, a decrease in fat absorption with increasing Ca intake could take place because of an inhibition of lipase activity. Thus it seems possible that a poor mineral balance, associated with the fat malabsorption described in the IUGR infants, could play a role in poor bone growth.

The relative hypermetabolism of malnourished newborns has been documented by a number of authors (29,78–80). Oxygen consumption was found to be significantly higher (9.37 ± 0.2 versus 8.66 ± 0.1 ml/kg-day), and the global energy expenditure (Table 2) as well as the resting preprandial metabolic rate (57.6 ± 1.0 versus 54.2 ± 1.3 kcal/kg-day; or 241 ± 4 versus 226 ± 5 kJ/kg-day) were increased in the growth-retarded infants (29). Age, weight, relative organ size, growth rate, energy intake, thermal environment, and activity are the major factors influencing metabolic rate (81). The hypermetabolism of SGA infants is unlikely to be due to an increase in the energy cost of activity since the higher energy expenditure persisted under resting conditions. When attempting to predict the energy expenditure of an individual from clinical variables, metabolic rate is best correlated with the active cell mass (82). Thus the hypermetabolic undergrown baby appears to have a higher ratio of metabolically active cell mass to total body mass which is consistent with his longer gestation (78). New tissue deposition is an energy-consuming process (Fig. 4), and with increasing energy intake, the energy cost of tissue synthesis also increases, as does the metabolic rate. Since the energy cost of tissue synthesis is measured as part of the global energy expenditure, the faster growth rate (catch-up growth) exhibited by some IUGR infants could explain part of their relative hypermetabolism. From postmortem analysis of organ size in growth-retarded and normal

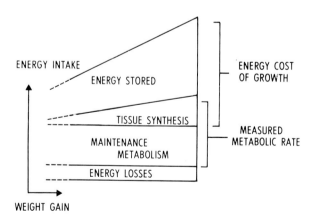

FIG. 4. Diagrammatic representation of the partition of energy metabolism in growing infants cared for under resting conditions in a thermoneutral environment. Energy cost of tissue synthesis is measured as part of the global energy expenditure (metabolic rate). With increasing energy intake the weight gain is greater, but the energy cost of tissue synthesis increases and so does the metabolic rate. Therefore the catch-up growth of IUGR infants could explain part of their relative hypermetabolism. (From ref. 81.)

infants (83) it is apparent that the heavier brain weight of SGA infants is the single major organ size difference. As the brain has the greatest energy requirement of all organs during the neonatal period (28), it has been speculated that the larger brain size to body weight ratio of IUGR infants could account for their hypermetabolism (29,78).

A rise in basal metabolic rate is a well-known phenomenon during recovery from malnutrition (84). Infants with growth failure due to maternal deprivation have an increase in postprandial heat production during the recovery phase (85). This specific dynamic action or thermic effect of food was best correlated with weight gain. Furthermore, the energy cost of growth could explain part of the relative hypermetabolism, as IUGR infants often exhibit a faster growth rate or "catch-up" growth. The increased protein synthesis documented in these infants (59) could account for the higher energy expended for growth (86). Thus, the hypermetabolism of IUGR infants is probably due to two factors: higher rate of growth and larger brain size.

For a comparable volume of milk, IUGR infants have a lower storage of energy than AGA infants (Table 2). Therefore, growth-retarded infants require high-energy feedings in order to satisfy their higher metabolic rate and their increased requirement for catch-up growth.

CATCH-UP GROWTH

A considerable number of follow-up studies point to the fact that IUGR infants show an accelerated growth pattern during the first 6 months of life. From then on, their average weight and height follow a constant course along the same percentile line (2,19,87–89). Therefore, when reaching adolescence the infants born with growth retardation are, as a group, significantly smaller in weight, height, and head circumference than matched controls of normal birthweight (3). This holds true for both term and preterm IUGR infants. The "catch-up" describes the accelerated growth which follows a period of growth retardation and tends to return the infant to a normal growth trajectory. However, the means whereby SGA infants catch up are not fully understood and there seems to be a time-limited potential for catch-up growth.

Because of increased energy requirements (29), high-energy feeding is advocated as nutritional support for the growth-retarded infant. Similarly, high-energy feeding in protein-energy malnutrition produces an accelerated rate of growth (90). However, the long-term effects of such a treatment on spontaneous food intake are poorly understood. The influence of appetite control on energy intake and catch-up growth has been investigated in two groups of SGA infants with distinct etiologies: (a) in those wasted infants born with clinical evidence of intrauterine malnutrition (decreased ponderal index) (91), and (b) in a group of infants who were genetically at the bottom end of the normal range (92) (normal ponderal index). The wasted SGA infants fed *ad libitum* consumed significantly more milk per unit weight than larger babies in the first two months after birth (91). The mean weight gain per kg and per day was significantly higher in these babies. On the other hand, in an elegant study (92), genetically growth-retarded infants fed *ad libitum* were randomly allocated to receive a high-energy (87 kcal/dl; 364 kJ/dl) or a standard energy formula (65 kcal/dl; 270 kJ/dl). Infants on high-energy feeds consumed lower volumes throughout the 3 months of the study. Thanks to the increased energy density of the feeds, the metabolizable energy intake of these infants was significantly greater in the early weeks of the study. After 2 months of age, energy intakes were similar in both groups. The high-energy formula group gained weight at a faster rate than did the other group. These data demonstrate that the hypothalamic center for appetite control is functional in the earliest months of life. The fact that the energy intakes of the two groups were no longer different after three months offers an explanation for the limited time during which catch-up growth is to be found in IUGR infants.

SUMMARY

Intrauterine growth-retarded infants present specific postnatal metabolic and nutritional problems. They have a decreased absorption of fat and protein, hence increased energy loss in excreta. The relative hypermetabolism of these infants is associated with a larger brain size, increased fat oxidation and protein synthesis, as well as accelerated rate of growth. Unless high-energy feeding is offered in the earliest weeks of life, catch-up growth might not occur. Breast milk should specifically be advocated when there is a risk of gastrointestinal disturbances associated with chronic fetal distress and/or asphyxia.

REFERENCES

1. Belizan JM, Lechtig A, Villar J. Distribution of low birthweight babies in developing countries. *Am J Obstet Gynecol* 1978;132:704–5.
2. Fitzhardinge PM, Steven EM. The small-for-date infant. I. Later growth patterns. *Pediatrics* 1972;49:671–81.
3. Westwood M, Kramer MS, Munz D, Lovett JM, Watters GV. Growth and development of full-term nonasphyxiated small-for-gestational-age newborns: follow-up through adolescence. *Pediatrics* 1983;71:376–82.
4. Commey JO, Fitzharding PM. Handicaps in the preterm small-for-gestational age infant. *J Pediatr* 1979;94:779–86.
5. Fitzhardinge PM, Steven EM. The small-for-date infant. II. Neurological and intellectual sequelae. *Pediatrics* 1972;50:50–7.
6. Parkinson CE, Wallis S, Harvey D. School achievement and behaviour of children who were small-for-dates at birth. *Dev Med Child Neurol* 1981;23:41–50.
7. Harvey D, Prince J, Bunton J, Partinson C, Campbell S. Abilities of children who were small-for-gestational-age babies. *Pediatrics* 1982;69:296–300.
8. Federick J, Adelstein P. Factors associated with low birthweight of infants delivered at term. *Br J Obstet Gynaecol* 1978;85:1–7.
9. Cnattingius S, Axelsson O, Eklund G, Lindmark G, Meirik O. Factors influencing birthweight for gestational age, with special respect to risk factors for intrauterine growth retardation. *Early Hum Dev* 1984;10:45–55.
10. Bhargava V, Chatterjee M, Prakash A, Mishara A. Fetal growth variations—I. Influence of maternal size and nutrition on identification of fetal growth. *Indian Pediatr* 1983;20:549–59.

11. Metcoff J, Cole TJ, Luff R. Fetal gowth retardation induced by dietary imbalance of threonine and dispensable amino acids, with adequate energy and protein-equivalent intakes, in pregnant rats. *J Nutr* 1981;111:1411-24.
12. Robinson JS, Falconer J, Owens JA. Intrauterine growth retardation: clinical and experimental. *Acta Paediatr Scand* 1985;Suppl 319:135-42.
13. Hill RM, Verniaud WM, Deter RL, et al. The effect of intrauterine malnutrition on the term infant. *Acta Paediatr Scand* 1984;73:482-7.
14. Walther FJ, Ramaekers LHJ. Neonatal morbidity of SGA infants in relation to their nutritional status at birth. *Acta Paediatr Scand* 1982,71.437-40.
15. Miller HC, Hassanein K. Diagnosis of impaired fetal growth in newborn infants. *Pediatrics* 1971; 48:511-22.
16. Georgieff MK, Sasanow SR, Mammel MC, Pereira GR. Mid-arm circumference/head circumference ratios for identification of symptomatic LGA, AGA, and SGA newborn infants. *J Pediatr* 1986;109:316-21.
17. Gruenwald P. Chronic fetal distress and placental insufficiency. *Biol Neonate* 1963;5:215-65.
18. Mettau JW, Degenhart HJ, Visser HKA, Holland WPS. Measurement of total body fat in newborns and infants by absorption of nonradioactive xenon. *Pediat Res* 1977;11:1097-101.
19. Davies DP. Growth of "small-for-dates" babies. *Early Hum Dev* 1981;5:95-105.
20. Faus MJ, Gil A, Robles R, Sanchez-Pozo A, Pita ML, Sanchez-Medina F. Changes in serum albumin, transferrin and amino acid indices during the first month of life in small-for-date infants. *Ann Nutr Metab* 1984;28:70-6.
21. Howells DW, Levin GE, Brown IRF, Brooke OG. Plasma retinol and retinol-binding protein in pre-term infants born small-for-gestational-age or appropriate-weight-for-age. *Human Nutrition* 1983;38C:107-11.
22. Lubchenko LO, Bard H. Incidence of hypoglycemia in newborn infants classified by birthweight and gestational age. *Pediatrics* 1971;47:831-8.
23. Hay WW. Fetal and neonatal glucose homeostasis and their relation to the small-for-gestational age infant. *Semin Perinatol* 1984;8:101-16.
24. Haymond MW, Karl I, Pagliara AS. Increased gluconeogenesis substrates in the small-for-gestational age infant. *N Engl J Med* 1974;291:322-8.
25. Sabel KG, Olegard R, Hildingsson K, Karlberg P. Effects of injected lipid emulsion on oxygen consumption, RQ, triglyceride, free-fatty-acid and beta hydroxybutyrate levels in small-for-gestational-age (SGA) infants. *Acta Paediatr Scand* 1982;71:63-9.
26. Sabel KG, Olegard R, Mellander M, Hildingsson K. Interrelation between fatty acid oxidation and control of gluconeogenic substrates in small-for-gestational-age (SGA) infants with hypoglycemia and with normoglycemia. *Acta Paediatr Scand* 1982;71:53-61.
27. Sann L, Divry P, Lasne Y, Ruitton A. Effect of oral lipid administration on glucose homeostasis in small-for-gestational-age infants. *Acta Paediatr Scand* 1982;71:923-7.
28. Holliday MA. Metabolic rate and organ size during growth from infancy to maturity and during late gestation and early infancy. *Pediatrics* 1971;47:169-79.
29. Chessex P, Reichman B, Verellen G, Putet G, Smith JM, Heim T, Swyer PR. Metabolic consequences of intrauterine growth retardation in very low birthweight infants. *Pediat Res* 1984;18: 709-13.
30. Pegorier JP, Leturque A, Ferre P, Turlan P, Girard J. Effects of medium-chain triglyceride-feeding on glucose homeostasis in the newborn rat. *Am J Physiol* 1983;244:E329-34.
31. Wu PK, Edmond J, Auestad N, Rambathla S, Benson J, Picone T. Medium-chain triglycerides in infant formulas and their relation to plasma ketone body concentrations. *Pediat Res* 1985;20: 338-41.
32. Lucas A, Boyes S, Bloom SR, Ansley-Green A. Metabolic and endocrine response to a milk fed in six-day-old term infants: differences between breast- and cow's milk formula-feeding. *Acta Paediatr Scand* 1981;70:195-200.
33. Adam PAJ, Raiha N, Rahiala EL, Kekomaki M. Oxidation of glucose and D-beta-hydroxybutyrate by the early human fetal brain. *Acta Paediatr Scand* 1975;64:17-24.
34. Patel MS, Johnson CA, Rajan R, Owen OE. The metabolism of ketone bodies in developing human brain: development of ketone body utilizing enzymes and ketone bodies as precursors for lipid synthesis. *J Neurochem* 1975;25:905-8.
35. Sarda P, Lepage G, Roy CC, Chessex P. Storage of medium-chain triglycerides in adipose tissue of orally fed infants. *Am J Clin Nutr* 1987;45:399-405.

36. Wheeler TG, Benolken RM, Anderson RE. Visual membranes: specificity of fatty acid precursors for the electrical response to illumination. *Science* 1975;188:1312–4.
37. Putnam JC, Carlson SE, DeVoe PW, Barness LA. The effect of variations in dietary fatty acids on the fatty acid composition of erythrocyte phosphatidylcholine and phosphatidylethanolamine in human infants. *Am J Clin Nutr* 1982;36:106–14.
38. Bard H. Neonatal problems of infants with intrauterine growth retardation. *J Reprod Med* 1978; 21:359–64.
39. Bard H, Makowski EL, Meschia G, Battaglia F. Relative rates of synthesis of hemoglobins A and F in immature red cells of newborn infants. *Pediatrics* 1970;45:766–72.
40. Humbert JR, Abelson H, Hathaway WE, Battaglia F. Polycythemia in small-for-gestational-age infants. *J Pediatr* 1969;75:812–9.
41. Black VD, Lubchenco LO. Neonatal polycythemia and hyperviscosity. *Pediatr Clin North Am* 1982;29:1137–48.
42. Leblanc MH, D'Cruz C, Pate K. Necrotizing enterocolitis can be caused by polycythemic hyperviscosity in the newborn dog. *J Pediatr* 1984;105:804–9.
43. Walsh MC, Kliegman RM. Necrotizing enterocolitis: treatment based on staging. *Pediatr Clin North Am* 1986;33:179–201.
44. Goplerud JM, Delivoria-Papadopoulos M. Principles in cellular oxygenation: fetal and neonatal intestines. *Clin Perinatol* 1986;13:191–6.
45. Yu VYH, James B, Hendry P, MacMahon RA. Total parenteral nutrition in very low birthweight infants: a controlled trial. *Arch Dis Child* 1980;54:653–61.
46. Eyal F, Sagi E, Arad I, Avital A. Necrotizing enterocolitis in the very low birthweight infant: expressed breast milk feeding compared with parenteral feeding. *Arch Dis Child* 1982;57:274–6.
47. LaGamma EF, Ostertag SG, Birenbaum H. Failure of oral feedings to prevent necrotizing enterocolitis. *Am J Dis Child* 1985;139:385–9.
48. Ostertag SG, LaGamma EF, Reisen CE, Ferrentino FL. Early enteral feeding does not affect incidence of necrotizing enterocolitis. *Pediatrics* 1986;77:275–80.
49. Aynsley-Green A. Metabolic and endocrine interrelations in the human fetus and neonate. *Am J Clin Nutr* 1985;41:399–417.
50. Barlow BB, Santulli TV, Heird WC, Pitt J, Blanc WA, Schullinger JN. An experimental study of acute neonatal enterocolitis—the importance of breast milk. *J Pediatr Surg* 1974;9:587–95.
51. Pitt J, Barlow B, Heird WC. Protection against experimental necrotizing enterocolitis by maternal milk. I. Role of milk leukocytes. *Pediat Res* 1977;11:906–9.
52. Kleigman RM, Pittard WB, Fanaroff AA. Necrotizing enterocolitis in neonates fed human milk. *J Pediatr* 1979;95:450–3.
53. Moriartey RR, Finer NN, Cox SF, et al. Necrotizing enterocolitis and human milk. *J Pediatr* 1979;94:295–6.
54. Brown EG, Sweet AY. Preventing necrotizing enterocolitis in neonates. *JAMA* 1978;240:2452–4.
55. Lebenthal E, Nitzan M, Chrzanowski BL, Krantz B. The effect of reduced materno-fetal blood flow on the development of fetal pancreatic acinar cells and zymogens. *Pediat Res* 1980;14:1356–9.
56. Lebenthal E, Nitzan M, Lee PC, Chrzanowski BL, Krasner J. Small intestinal enzymes during normal development and the effect of intrauterine growth retardation in fetal rats. *Biol Neonate* 1981;39:14–21.
57. Stransky E, David-Laws DF. On kwashiorkor (infantile pellagra, malignant malnutrition). *Ann Pediat* 1950;174:226–46.
58. Salle BL, Ruiton-Ugliengo A. Effects of oral glucose and protein load on plasma glucagon and insulin concentrations in small for gestational age infants. *Pediat Res* 1977;11:108–12.
59. Pencharz PB, Masson M, Desgranges F, Papageorgiou A. Total-body protein turnover in human premature neonates: effects of birthweight, intrauterine nutritional status, and diet. *Clin Sci* 1981;61:207–15.
60. Picou D, Taylor-Roberts T. The measurements of total protein synthesis and catabolism and nitrogen turnover in infants in different nutritional status and receiving different amounts of dietary protein. *Clin Sci* 1969;36:283–96.
61. Villar J, Belizan JM. Protein requirement for intrauterine growth-retarded infants. *Am J Clin Nutr* 1980;33:536–41.
62. Reichman B, Chessex P, Putet G, et al. Diet, fat accretion and growth in premature infants. *N Engl J Med* 1981;305:1495–500.
63. Viteri FE, Flores JM, Alvarado J, Behar M. Intestinal malabsorption in malnourished children be-

fore, and during recovery. Relation between severity of protein deficiency and the malabsorption process. *Am J Dig Dis* 1973;18:201–11.

64. Hatch TF, Lebenthal E, Krasher J, Branski D. Effect of postnatal malnutrition on pancreatic zymogen enzymes in the rat. *Am J Clin Nutr* 1979;32:1224–30.

65. Senterre J, Karlberg P. Respiratory quotient and metabolic rate in normal full-term and small-for-date newborn infants. *Acta Paediatr Scand* 1970;59:653–8.

66. Brooke OG, Alvear J. Postprandial metabolism in infants of low birthweight. *Hum Nutr* 1982; 36C:167–75.

67. Andrew G, Chan G, Schiff D. Lipid metabolism in the neonate. I. The effects of Intralipid infusion on plasma triglyceride and free fatty acid concentrations in the neonate. *J Pediatr* 1976;88:273–8.

68. Ducker DA, Hughes CA, Warren I, McNeish S. Neonatal gut function, measured by the one hour blood D(+)xylose test: influence of gestational age and size. *Gut* 1980;21:133–6.

69. Lebenthal E, Nitzan M, Lee PC, Chrzanowski BL, Krasner J. Effect of intrauterine growth retardation on the activities of fetal intestinal enzymes in rats. *Biol Neonate* 1981;39:14–21.

70. MacLean WC, Fink BB. Lactose malabsorption by premature infants: magnitude and clinical significance. *J Pediatr* 1980;97:383–8.

71. Bond JH, Levitt MD. Fate of soluble carbohydrate in the colon of rats and man. *J Clin Invest* 1976;57:1158–64.

72. Scott KE, Usher R. Epiphyseal development in fetal malnutrition syndrome. *N Engl J Med* 1964; 270:822–4.

73. Minton SD, Steichen JJ, Tsang RC. Decreased bone mineral content in small-for-gestational-age infants compared with appropriate-for-gestational-age infants: normal serum 25-hydroxyvitamin D and decreasing parathyroid hormone. *Pediatrics* 1983;71:383–8.

74. Helin I, Landin LA, Nilson BE. Bone mineral content in preterm infants at age 4 to 16. *Acta Paediatr Scand* 1985;74:264–7.

75. Senterre J. Calcium and phosphorus retention in preterm infants. In: Stern L, Oh W, Friis-Hansen B, eds. *Intensive care in the newborn, II*. New York: Masson, 1978;205–15.

76. Tantibhedhyangkul P, Hashim SA. Medium-chain triglyceride feeding in premature infants: effects on fat and nitrogen absorption. *Pediatrics* 1975;55:359–70.

77. Tantibhedhyangkul P, Hashim SA. Medium-chain triglyceride feeding in premature infants: effects on calcium and magnesium absorption. *Pediatrics* 1978;61:537–45.

78. Sinclair JC, Silverman WA. Intrauterine growth in active tissue mass of the human fetus, with particular reference to the undergrown baby. *Pediatrics* 1966;38:48–62.

79. Scopes JW, Ahmed I. Minimal rates of oxygen consumption in sick and premature newborn infants. *Arch Dis Child* 1966;41:407–16.

80. Hill JR, Robinson DC. Oxygen consumption in normally grown, small-for-dates and large-for-dates newborn infants. *J Physiol (Lond)* 1968;199:685–703.

81. Chessex P, Reichman BL, Verellen G, et al. Influence of postnatal age, energy intake and weight gain on energy metabolism in the very low birthweight infant. *J Pediatr* 1981;99:761–6.

82. Rosa AM, Shizgal HM. The Harris-Benedict equation reevaluated: resting energy requirements and the body cell mass. *Am J Clin Nutr* 1984;40:168–82.

83. Gruenwald P. Chronic fetal distress and placental insufficiency. *Biol Neonate* 1963;5:215–65.

84. Spady DW, Picou D, Waterlow JC. Energy balance during recovery from malnutrition. *Am J Clin Nutr* 1976;29:1073–89.

85. Krieger I, Whitten CF. Energy metabolism in infants with growth failure due to maternal deprivation, undernutrition, or causes unknown. *Pediatrics* 1969;75:374–79.

86. Catzeflis C, Schutz Y, Micheli JL, Welsch C, Arnaud MJ, Jéquier E. Whole body protein synthesis and energy expenditure in very low birthweight infants. *Pediat Res* 1985;19:6779–87.

87. Walther FJ, Ramaekers LHJ. Growth in early childhood of newborns affected by disproportionate intrauterine growth retardation. *Acta Paediat Scand* 1982;71:651–6.

88. Ounsted M, Moar V, Scott A. Growth in the first four years: II. Diversity within groups of small-for-dates and large-for-dates babies. *Early Hum Dev* 1982;7:29–39.

89. Davies DP, Platts P, Pritchard M, Wilkinson PW. Nutritional status of light-for-date infants at birth and its influence on early postnatal growth. *Arch Dis Child* 1979;54:703–6.

90. Brooke OG, Wheeler EF. High energy feeding in protein-energy malnutrition. *Arch Dis Child* 1976;51:968–71.

91. Ounsted M, Sleigh G. The infant's self-regulation of food intake and weight gain. *Lancet* 1975; 1:1393–7.

92. Brooke OG, Kinsey JM. High energy feeding in small-for-gestation infants. *Arch Dis Child* 1985;60:42–6.

DISCUSSION

Dr. Guesry: I enjoyed your talk very much and would like to come back to a few of the things you said. In the first place, you rightly said that we need to give more energy to the baby, but on the other hand, the feed osmolality must be low and we must avoid high-protein intakes. If you want to do all these things, you must give fat. We all know that fat is not well absorbed unless you give medium-chain triglycerides (MCT), but, and this is my second point, you raised doubts by speaking of the potential danger of deposition of MCT in adipose tissue. You also said that this deposition was mainly of C12 fatty acids and a little of C10. The MCT which are used in formulas designed for low birthweight infants are made almost exclusively from C6 to C10 fatty acids, with very little C12, unless coconut oil is used. So I am sorry that you should raise doubt about this particular aspect of formulas for premature babies, which in my view is all to the good.

Dr. Chessex: About your first comment: I think you may have misinterpreted what I said. I was specifically referring to the early period immediately after birth, at which time I think that it is very important to have low-volume feeding with a low osmolar load. Later on we must accept some compromises if we want to increase the energy intake. I specifically avoided laying down any ground rules about how much energy should be provided. Your comments about MCT are interesting. In North America MCT-containing formulas have a lot of C8 and very little C6, and some of them contain up to 20% C12, in other words, quite large amounts. I agree that it has been clearly shown that the shorter the chain-length the greater the oxidation and the less the storage, but if there are significant amounts of C12 in the formula they will appear in the tissues. My concerns are not limited to MCT. I am also concerned about excess linoleic acid or any blend of fatty acids which might change the properties of cells and cell membranes, particularly in the brain at this period of life when a lot of fat deposition is going on. It has been suggested (1) that altering the linoleic acid content of a formula produces significant changes in the erythrocyte deformability, documenting a direct effect of dietary lipid composition on cellular properties. I don't have anything specifically against MCT, but I think their use should be limited to the early feeding period; later on, I am not sure they have much of a place. I don't think it is important to have very sophisticated formulas after the first few weeks. Perhaps they are financially acceptable in industrialized societies, but I think they might be unnecessarily sophisticated for developing countries.

Dr. Guesry: I should like to answer your last point. We recently conducted a study with Alan Rothberg in a large maternity hospital in South Africa (2). The infants were fed with their own mother's milk or with ordinary formula or with a special formula for low birthweight infants. The use of the low birthweight formula resulted in a reduction by 20 days (from 65 to 45 days) in the average length of stay in the nursery. This is very important in such hospitals because they often do not have enough cots for small infants.

Dr. Chessex: But afterwards, when they leave hospital, should they have to pay more for special formulas? Will the special formula influence their long-term outcome?

Dr. Senterre: I should like to return to the question of the use of MCT in SFD infants, since I am not convinced by your arguments for excluding them. From what I understood you to say, you feel that they should be excluded because you have shown that they are incorporated in the fat deposited by infants fed with MCT-containing formulas. But the absolute level of incorporation is bound to be low. A proportion of ingested MCT are indeed elongated and incorporated in depot fat; the remainder, say, 60%, are readily oxidized, as has been shown with stable isotope work (3). There will be much greater incorporation of C18:2, for example, so why not exclude that? On the other hand, there are a lot of advantages in giving a formula containing about 40% MCT. It improves fat and calcium absorption and leads to better nitrogen retention for the same energy intake. So there are a lot of advantages in using such formulas and I am personally in favor of them. For obtaining a good fat absorption, the alternative is to use formulas with fat containing high levels of polyunsaturated fatty acids and/or high lauric and myristic acid levels. This would be worse than MCT in my opinion.

Dr. Chessex: My response is that you have seen only the mean values for the data; it is important to note that MCT deposition is much greater in infants who are growing faster, as it is related to weight gain. Also, with reference to your remarks about MCT oxidation, I should say that most of the work on this has been in rats. Guy Putet did a study a few years ago (4) which showed a much lower rate of oxidation. I am concerned that oxidation is not as great as we have thought, particularly in rapidly growing infants, and this obviously applies to SGA infants. In relation to your comments about formulas with high linoleic acid content, I agree entirely. It is just a question of balance. I believe that the use of formulas with modest amounts of MCT has a place in the early management but I don't think they should be used later on.

Dr. Marini: I think the situation with regard to MCT is still controversial. For example, there are two papers showing no improvement in growth in preterm infants fed MCT formulas (5). In the second place, Tibor Heim has shown differences in plasma concentrations of cholesterol and triglyceride in infants fed with MCT formulas (6). I should say, however, that we have been unable to confirm this finding. Finally, a more general point: When you change dietary fat composition, tissue fat changes rapidly. Thus I am not too concerned about the possible long-term effects of MCT incorporation.

Dr. Chessex: In the adult it takes about 3 years to change the fat composition in adipose tissue (7). But in the infant it takes about 6 weeks. We have confirmed this in biopsies taken at fortuitous surgery. However, 6 weeks is quite a long time when the brain is growing rapidly and accumulating lipids.

Dr. Guesry: One short point about your last statement concerning the composition of the brain: It has been shown (8) that the main fat which is incorporated in the brain is docosahexaenoic acid, and only about one-third of this is derived from diet. The rest of the fatty acids deposited in the brain are synthesized.

Dr. Bracci: There is another point we haven't considered in relation to early diet in SFD infants. These infants must be considered to have some degree of immunologic depression; for example, there are data which show depression of T-cell function and phagocytosis. Thus they are at risk of infection and we may lose some of them for this reason in the early weeks. I think therefore that the value of the protective properties of human milk should not entirely give way to nutritional considerations. I would be in favor of human milk with nutritional supplementation.

Dr. Priolisi: To follow that, I should like your comment on studies by Räihä's group on very low birthweight infants fed at three different levels of protein intakes: 2.92 g/kg/day from human milk, 3.22 and 4.06 g/kg/day from formula. The increase in protein intake was accompanied by an increased level of serum total α-amino-nitrogen concentration, a concomitant decrease in the intraluminal bile acid concentration. This is an indirect evidence of decreased bile flow in VLBW on excessive oral protein intake (9).

Dr. Senterre: It is well-known that there is a positive relationship between plasma amino acid concentration and protein intake, but this results in an increase in the amino acid supply to the cells and increased protein anabolism, which is just what we want. As to the effect on bile acid production, I accept that there is indeed a correlation between the serum alpha amino nitrogen and serum bile acid concentration; however, the correlation is not linear. Thus, if you increase protein intake by 50% from 2 to 3 g/kg daily, which is a big increase, serum bile acid concentration remains low. Although we know that infants fed on TPN with high methionine intakes may get cholestasis, there is no justification for extrapolating from Räihä's data that if we give a 3 g/kg protein intake enterally in these babies we shall then get biliary stasis. I should also like to comment on Dr. Chessex's protein turnover data. You told us that protein turnover, both synthesis and breakdown, was increased in SFD babies. But you also said that you saw no increase in urinary nitrogen excretion. Since recycling of amino acids is never 100%, a higher protein turnover is bound to be associated with increased urinary nitrogen excretion.

Dr. Chessex: How then would you explain the fact that we had exactly the same nitrogen excretion in our two groups? Do you think it was because we had a sufficient protein intake in both groups, so that they did not have to increase their protein turnover?

Dr. Senterre: No. I think urinary nitrogen excretion in those babies was chiefly related to nitrogen utilization in new tissue synthesis rather than to protein turnover. You showed that your SFD babies were growing faster than preterm infants, especially in the first 3 weeks of life, so nitrogen retention and new tissue synthesis were important. Thus they used their amino acid pool for synthesis, so blood urea nitrogen and excretion decreased. On the other hand, I did not understand why, when you gave too much energy, the energy cost of growth increased so much when energy stores were only increasing slowly.

Dr. Chessex: Brooke found the same thing (10). There must be a point at which you are relatively efficient in relation to the amount of the energy intake and the cost of depositing that energy. Above that point there will be an increase in the energy cost of growth.

Dr. Senterre: I agree that if you push in too much energy you don't see a proportionate increase in energy deposition because the metabolic rate is increased. But to my mind this does not mean that the energy cost of growth is increased; it means that you are wasting energy in other metabolic pathways.

Dr. Chessex: However, the way those tissue synthesis data were derived was by measuring the difference between pre- and postprandial energy expenditures. The postprandial energy expenditure increases with energy intake and with weight as shown previously in numerous studies by Krieger (11), Brooke (12), and Ashworth (13). I accept that this is partly due to energy wasting in other pathways, as in brown fat, for instance. However, during those studies we found no change in deep colonic temperature and mean skin temperature as could be expected if brown fat was active in eliminating excess energy as heat. We have recently repeated some of the experiments during TPN and showed clearly that just by changing substrates—without changing overall energy intake—there was an increase in deep body and subscapular temperature, which is an indirect sign of brown fat activity.

Dr. Pearse: When we tried to determine the energy cost of growth using simultaneous direct and indirect calorimetry, we found that increased postprandial metabolism (specific dynamic action) in SFD infants but not in well-fed appropriate-for-gestation infants. I don't know what this means, but we know that SFD babies tend to appear hungry and much of the original work on specific dynamic action was in malnourished children.

Dr. Chessex: We did find specific dynamic action in appropriate-for-gestation infants, both in the study I have described here and also in numerous other studies, so I cannot explain your findings.

Dr. Toubas: What about heat loss in these babies? An SFD infant must have a larger body surface area than an appropriate-for-gestation infant of similar weight. The infant will lose more heat through the skin. Should we thus be giving more fat to increase subcutaneous fat and thermal insulation?

Dr. Chessex: The babies in our study had a minimal heat loss via this route since they were in a neutral thermal environment. Indeed, the adequate provision of substrate ensures that thermoregulation is more readily achieved. This is why at the beginning I stated that we should try when possible to achieve nutritional accretion before birth.

Dr. Villar: I should like to make a comment on another matter. I do not think one should regard the SGA population as homogeneous. If you look at SFD infants of the same birthweight but different fat and body length, you find that they have quite different *ad libitum* intakes; some for example will eat more than others, some will have a preference for a higher glucose intake. We should be looking at subgroups of SFD infants and not lumping them all together. I also have a question. We have been looking at tryptophan concentration in human milk in a population with a low tryptophan intake, and it occurs to me that this could reduce appetite and change sleeping patterns by increasing the synthesis of serotonin in the brain. There are data from adults which suggest that alterations in appetite and sleep can occur when the ratio of tryptophan to the other large neutral amino acids (LNAA) is changed. Do you have any experience or views on the effect of tryptophan ratios on appetite in SGA infants?

Dr. Chessex: No, I don't, but it is an interesting question.

Dr. Guesry: We have been working on this subject for 5 years. It originates from studies by Wurtman (14) at M.I.T. who showed competition between tryptophan and the other LNAA in crossing the blood-brain barrier. If you give tryptophan together with a protein meal you don't get any effect, but if you give it alone with carbohydrates (which increase the uptake of LNAA into muscle) you find a doubling of the tryptophan:LNAA ratio entering the brain. This increases serotonin synthesis and reduces appetite.

Dr. Senterre: Some SFD infants do not show adequate catch-up growth, and I think in these cases the problem must lie in regulation by the various growth factors. It was shown about 10 years ago (15) that SFD babies who were growing fast had much higher insulin levels than ones who were not growing, or were growing slowly. I think it is important during the first weeks of life to try to promote growth by increasing insulin secretion, which can be done by giving a relatively high protein intake, especially if the protein contains appreciable amounts of the branched chain amino acids (and also by giving carbohydrates, of course). Thus I feel that it is important to supplement the diets of SFD babies with more protein, or with sucrose, but not with additional fat.

Dr. Chessex: There have been other data documenting a linear correlation between growth rate and plasma insulin, metabolic rate and weight gain, as well as metabolic rate and insulin (16). It seems possible that it could answer the question about what determines the plateauing of catch-up growth which is seen after a while. Could this phenomenon be due to a tailing-off of insulin response? However, there is the usual question of which is the cart and which is the horse.

Dr. Villar: If you give *ad libitum* feeds to infants of diabetic mothers, who have high plasma insulin concentrations, these infants will have *lower* glucose intake. We offered, in a preliminary study, feeds of 5%, 10%, and 20% glucose *ad libitum* to such infants and there was a tendency among those with high insulin levels to prefer the 5% feed. This could be related to what I was saying about serotonin. If you have high insulin concentrations in plasma you will increase transport of large neutral amino acids and, more proportionally, tryptophan, into the brain. You thus increase serotonin production, which will reduce appetite. I accept that insulin is a growth hormone, but in my opinion it is not the increase in insulin which makes you grow more, but the increase of substrate which stimulates the increase in insulin release.

Dr. Senterre: I don't think it is as straightforward as that. Infants of diabetic mothers will probably not have had IUGR; in fact they are likely to have macrosomia, so they are not comparable. We are dealing with babies in whom we wish to promote growth, and in such infants an infusion of insulin could be a way to achieve this. Also, you spoke about *ad libitum* feeding, but very small-for-dates infants cannot be fed *ad libitum*—they must be tube-fed, so we have to choose their energy intakes for them, and under these conditions it is likely that we shall get it wrong in some of them.

Dr. Girard: The correlation between plasma insulin and growth cannot take into account variations in tissue sensitivity to insulin. Take an obese adult, for example: He will have very high plasma insulin but his tissues will be quite insensitive. There is very little information about change in insulin-sensitivity in relation to growth or increase in body weight, so I think it is too naive to claim that a correlation between plasma insulin and growth means that the growth is due to the increased insulin.

Dr. Chessex: It is of interest that some SGA babies could have increased insulin receptors (17).

Dr. Girard: In obese diabetic adults there are sometimes a normal number of insulin receptors per cell but the tissues are insensitive to insulin. Although the binding to its receptor is the first step in insulin action, there are intracellular steps which could also be affected and responsible for insulin resistance. The exploration of insulin sensitivity in newborn babies with IUGR and during catch-up growth could be a fruitful field of study.

REFERENCES

1. Carlson SE. Impact of infant feeding on blood and membrane lipids. In: Levy RI, ed: *Primary prevention of atherosclerosis in childhood: the role of lipids. Proceedings of a video conference.* New York: Biomedical Information Corp., 1985;19–24.
2. Cooper PA, Rothberg AD, Davies VA, Argent AC. Comparative growth and biochemical response of very low birthweight infant fed own mother's milk, a premature infant formula or one of two standard formulas. *J Pediatr Gastroenterol Nutr* 1985;4:786–94.
3. Putet G, Thélin A, Philippossian G, et al. Medium-chain triglycerides as a source of energy in premature infants. In: Horisberger M, Bracco V, eds. *Lipids in modern nutrition.* New York: Nestlé Nutrition, Raven Press, 1987;43–9.
4. Putet G, Thélin A, Arnaud MJ, Philippossian G, Senterre J, Fahmy N, Salle BL. Oxidative metabolism of 13C medium-chain triglycerides (MCT) fed to preterm infants (PT) [Abstr.]. *Pediatr Res* 1984;18:344A.
5. Spencer SA, Stammers JP, Hull D. Evaluation of a special low birthweight formula, with and without the use of medium-chain triacylglycerols. *Early Hum Dev* 1986;13:87–95.
6. Carnielli V, Dunn M, Shennan AT, et al. Lipid lowering effect of medium chain triglyceride (MCT) diet in the premature infant. *Ped Res* 1986;20:236A.
7. Hirsch J. Fatty acid pattern in human adipose tissue. In: Renold AE, Ciahill GF, eds. *Handbook of physiology. Adipose tissue, Section 5.* Washington DC: American Physiological Society, 1965;181–90.
8. Bourre JM. Acides gras cérébraux. Synthèse in situ et apports alimentaires. *Diabète Metab* 1984;10:324–31.
9. Senger H, Boehm G, Beyreiss K, Braun W, Räihä N. Evidence for amino acid induced cholestasis

in very low birthweight infants with increasing enteral protein intake. *Acta Paediatr Scand* 1986;75:724–8.
10. Brooke OG. Nutritional requirements of low and very low birthweight infants. *Ann Rev Nutr* 1987;7:91–116.
11. Krieger I, Whitten CF. Energy metabolism in infants with growth failure due to maternal deprivation, undernutrition, or causes unknown. II. Relationship between nitrogen balance, weight gain, and post-prandial excess heat production. *J Pediatr* 1969;75:374–9.
12. Brooke OG, Ashworth A. The influence of malnutrition on the postprandial metabolic rate and respiratory quotient. *Br J Nutr* 1972;27:407–15.
13. Ashworth A. Metabolic rates during recovery from protein-calorie malnutrition: the need for a new concept of specific dynamic action. *Nature* 1969;223:407–9.
14. Wurtman RS. Nutrients that modify brain function. *Sci Am* 1982;246:42–51.
15. Colle E, Schiff D, Andrew G, Bauer CB, Fitzhardinge R. Insulin responses during catch-up growth of infants who were small-for-gestational age. *Pediatrics* 1976;57:363–71.
16. Payne Robinson HM, Cocks T, Kerr D, Picon D. Hormonal control of weight gain in infants recovering from protein energy malnutrition. I. The effect of insulin and metabolic rate. *Pediatr Res* 1980;14:28–33.
17. Hill DE. Effect of insulin on fetal growth. *German Perinatol* 1978;2:319–28.

SUBJECT INDEX